Crosstalk between Depression, Anxiety, and Dementia: Comorbidity in Behavioral Neurology and Neuropsychiatry

Crosstalk between Depression, Anxiety, and Dementia: Comorbidity in Behavioral Neurology and Neuropsychiatry

Editor

Masaru Tanaka

MDPI • Basel • Beijing • Wuhan • Barcelona • Belgrade • Manchester • Tokyo • Cluj • Tianjin

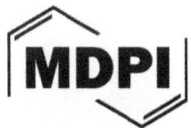

Editor
Masaru Tanaka
University of Szeged
Hungary

Editorial Office
MDPI
St. Alban-Anlage 66
4052 Basel, Switzerland

This is a reprint of articles from the Special Issue published online in the open access journal *Biomedicines* (ISSN 2227-9059) (available at: https://www.mdpi.com/journal/biomedicines/special_issues/neuropsychiatry).

For citation purposes, cite each article independently as indicated on the article page online and as indicated below:

LastName, A.A.; LastName, B.B.; LastName, C.C. Article Title. *Journal Name* **Year**, *Volume Number*, Page Range.

ISBN 978-3-0365-4001-6 (Hbk)
ISBN 978-3-0365-4002-3 (PDF)

© 2022 by the authors. Articles in this book are Open Access and distributed under the Creative Commons Attribution (CC BY) license, which allows users to download, copy and build upon published articles, as long as the author and publisher are properly credited, which ensures maximum dissemination and a wider impact of our publications.
The book as a whole is distributed by MDPI under the terms and conditions of the Creative Commons license CC BY-NC-ND.

Contents

About the Editor ix

Masaru Tanaka and László Vécsei
Editorial of Special Issue "Crosstalk between Depression, Anxiety, and Dementia: Comorbidity in Behavioral Neurology and Neuropsychiatry"
Reprinted from: *Biomedicines* **2021**, 9, 517, doi:10.3390/biomedicines9050517 1

Sangki Park, Ahream Bak, Sujin Kim, Yunkwon Nam, Hyeon soo Kim, Doo-Han Yoo and Minho Moon
Animal-Assisted and Pet-Robot Interventions for Ameliorating Behavioral and Psychological Symptoms of Dementia: A Systematic Review and Meta-Analysis
Reprinted from: *Biomedicines* **2020**, 8, 150, doi:10.3390/biomedicines8060150 5

Joanna Rog, Anna Błażewicz, Dariusz Juchnowicz, Agnieszka Ludwiczuk, Ewa Stelmach, Małgorzata Kozioł, Michal Karakula, Przemysław Niziński and Hanna Karakula-Juchnowicz
The Role of GPR120 Receptor in Essential Fatty Acids Metabolism in Schizophrenia
Reprinted from: *Biomedicines* **2020**, 8, 243, doi:10.3390/biomedicines8080243 21

Antonio J. López-Gambero, Carlos Sanjuan, Pedro Jesús Serrano-Castro, Juan Suárez and Fernando Rodríguez de Fonseca
The Biomedical Uses of Inositols: A Nutraceutical Approach to Metabolic Dysfunction in Aging and Neurodegenerative Diseases
Reprinted from: *Biomedicines* **2020**, 8, 295, doi:10.3390/biomedicines8090295 35

Ana Sofia Vargas, Ângelo Luís, Mário Barroso, Eugenia Gallardo and Luísa Pereira
Psilocybin as a New Approach to Treat Depression and Anxiety in the Context of Life-Threatening Diseases—A Systematic Review and Meta-Analysis of Clinical Trials
Reprinted from: *Biomedicines* **2020**, 8, 331, doi:10.3390/biomedicines8090331 75

Masaru Tanaka and László Vécsei
Monitoring the Redox Status in Multiple Sclerosis
Reprinted from: *Biomedicines* **2020**, 8, 406, doi:10.3390/biomedicines8100406 91

Eun Young Kim, Hee-Sung Ahn, Min Young Lee, Jiyoung Yu, Jeonghun Yeom, Hwangkyo Jeong, Hophil Min, Hyun Jeong Lee, Kyunggon Kim and Yong Min Ahn
An Exploratory Pilot Study with Plasma Protein Signatures Associated with Response of Patients with Depression to Antidepressant Treatment for 10 Weeks
Reprinted from: *Biomedicines* **2020**, 8, 455, doi:10.3390/biomedicines8110455 127

Vanesa Cantón-Habas, Manuel Rich-Ruiz, Manuel Romero-Saldaña and Maria del Pilar Carrera-González
Depression as a Risk Factor for Dementia and Alzheimer's Disease
Reprinted from: *Biomedicines* **2020**, 8, 457, doi:10.3390/biomedicines8110457 149

Katarzyna Kowalska, Łukasz Krzywoszański, Jakub Droś, Paulina Pasińska, Aleksander Wilk and Aleksandra Klimkowicz-Mrowiec
Early Depression Independently of Other Neuropsychiatric Conditions, Influences Disability and Mortality after Stroke (Research Study—Part of PROPOLIS Study)
Reprinted from: *Biomedicines* **2020**, 8, 509, doi:10.3390/biomedicines8110509 165

Junhyung Kim and Yong-Ku Kim
Crosstalk between Depression and Dementia with Resting-State fMRI Studies and Its Relationship with Cognitive Functioning
Reprinted from: *Biomedicines* **2021**, *9*, 82, doi:10.3390/biomedicines9010082 . . . . **183**

Aida Muntsant, Francesc Jiménez-Altayó, Lidia Puertas-Umbert, Elena Jiménez-Xarrie, Elisabet Vila and Lydia Giménez-Llort
Sex-Dependent End-of-Life Mental and Vascular Scenarios for Compensatory Mechanisms in Mice with Normal and AD-Neurodegenerative Aging
Reprinted from: *Biomedicines* **2021**, *9*, 111, doi:10.3390/biomedicines9020111 . . . . **203**

Katalin Eszter Ibos, Éva Bodnár, Zsolt Bagosi, Zsolt Bozsó, Gábor Tóth, Gyula Szabó and Krisztina Csabafi
Kisspeptin-8 Induces Anxiety-Like Behavior and Hypolocomotion by Activating the HPA Axis and Increasing GABA Release in the Nucleus Accumbens in Rats
Reprinted from: *Biomedicines* **2021**, *9*, 112, doi:10.3390/biomedicines9020112 . . . . **233**

About the Editor

Masaru Tanaka, M.D., Ph.D., has been a Research Fellow in the MTA-SZTE Neuroscience Research Group of the Hungarian Academy of Sciences at the University of Szeged (MTA-SZTE) since 2005. His scientific interests include depression, anxiety, dementia and pain, and their comorbid nature in neurological diseases and psychiatric disorders. His current research focuses on the antidepressant, anxiolytic and nootropic effects of neuropeptides, neurohormones and tryptophan metabolites, and their analogues in animal models of behavior and psychiatric disease. He is an editorial board member of the Journal of Integrative Neuroscience and Advances in Clinical and Experimental Medicine, an advisory board member of Biology and Life Sciences, and a section board member of Biomedicines. He obtained a PhD in Medicine (1998) and an MD in General Medicine from the University of Szeged, and bachelor's degrees in Biophysics (1987) from the University of Illinois, Urbana-Champaign.

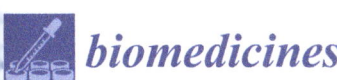

Editorial

Editorial of Special Issue "Crosstalk between Depression, Anxiety, and Dementia: Comorbidity in Behavioral Neurology and Neuropsychiatry"

Masaru Tanaka [1,2,]* and László Vécsei [1,2]

1. MTA-SZTE, Neuroscience Research Group, Semmelweis u. 6, H-6725 Szeged, Hungary; vecsei.laszlo@med.u-szeged.hu
2. Department of Neurology, Interdisciplinary Excellence Centre, Faculty of Medicine, University of Szeged, Semmelweis u. 6, H-6725 Szeged, Hungary
* Correspondence: tanaka.masaru.1@med.u-szeged.hu; Tel.: +36-62-545-597

Keywords: depression; anxiety; dementia; Alzheimer's disease; multiple sclerosis; schizophrenia; stroke; lipid; nutraceutical; diabetes

"Where there is light, there must be shadow, ..."

—Carl Jung
—Haruki Murakami

"Somethings can only be seen in the shadows."

—Carlos Ruiz Zafon

"The world outside you is only a reflection of the world inside you."

—unknown

Depression, anxiety, and dementia are spectra of the most common symptoms experienced by patients with a wide range of diseases. The symptoms often concur and frequently wax and wane in the course of the diseases. However, they may serve as prodromal indicators for and may inflict in sequelae to a certain condition. Indeed, depression and anxiety are risk factors for dementia, but they are not just comorbidities or sequelae of dementia. This Special Issue highlights laboratory, clinical, and statistical studies on the crosstalk between depression, anxiety, dementia, Alzheimer's disease (AD), multiple sclerosis (MS), schizophrenia (SCZ), diabetes mellitus (DM), Down's syndrome, and/or compulsive disorders, presented by 71 authors and edited by 25 referees, three academic editors, and one editor.

Animal research is one of the essential arenas for laboratory sciences in neuropsychiatry. Kisspeptins (KP) are endogenous neuropeptides with L-arginine and L-phenylalanine motif at the C-terminal (RF-amide peptides), which regulate the reproductive system. The N-terminally truncated octapeptide KP-8 induced anxiety-like behavior, reduced ambulatory activity, and suppressed exploratory locomotion by activating the hypothalamic–pituitary–adrenal (HPA) axis and increasing gamma-aminobutyric acid (GABA) release in the nucleus accumbens in rats [1]. The studies on the triple transgenic mouse model of AD model (3xTg-AD) showed higher mortality rates and HPA axis activation in female mice of 3xTg-AD and the wild type, but worse behavioral and cognitive functions, higher cerebral blood flow, and improved cardiovascular phenotypes only in 3xTg-AD female mice. The authors suggested the presence of a sex-dependent compensatory hemodynamic mechanism, proposing a possible target for interventions of dementia in aging [2].

The linkage between late-life depression (LLD) and AD was explored by resting-state functional magnetic resonance imaging (fMRI) studies analyzing the default mode network (DMN), executive control network, and salience network (SN). The dissociated

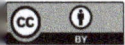

functional connectivity pattern with increased anterior DMN and decreased posterior DMN was commonly observed in LLD and AD. The DMN connectivity increased in LLD and decreased in AD, but the SN connectivity decreased in LLD and increased in AD. The authors proposed that the similarity of dissociation may be a possible mechanism of association between LLD and AD [3]. Depression is a common sequela to stroke attack. Poststroke depression increased the level of disability and mortality rates regardless of stroke severity and other neuropsychiatric symptoms during the first year of stroke or transient ischemic attack. The authors suggested depression as a prognostic biomarker for cerebrovascular accidents [4].

Plasma protein signatures were explored in patients suffering from major depressive disorder (MDD). Longitudinal liquid chromatography tandem mass spectrometry (LC-MS/MS) analysis showed 63 proteins significantly associated with drug response-time interactions, 21 proteins significantly associated with response term, and 15 proteins significantly correlated with psychiatric measurement indices. The authors proposed the LC-MS/MS analysis of the serum proteins for a predictive and prognostic biomarker for MDD [5].

Animal-assisted intervention (AAI) and prerobot intervention (PRI) are interventional strategies for the elderly with cognitive impairment or dementia. Pooled analysis of AAI and PRI on the behavioral and psychological symptoms of dementia (BPSD) revealed that the interventions induced a beneficial impact on the depression component of BPSD, but not on the component of anxiety or quality of life. Thus, the authors revealed that depression is an interventional target for cognitive impairment and dementia [6]. Mushroom-produced psychedelic prodrug psylocibin was shown to be significantly effective in the treatment of depression and anxiety in patients suffering from life-threatening diseases by meta-analysis. The authors emphasized the importance of psilocybin translational research for the treatment of emotional symptoms, especially for the patients resistant to conventional pharmacotherapy [7].

Depression, anxiety, and dementia are common psychobehavioral symptoms in autoimmune demyelinating MS. The disturbance of reduction-oxidation homeostasis was commonly observed in MS. Monitoring various components of reactive chemical species, oxidative enzymes, antioxidative enzymes, and degradation products, including kynurenines was proposed to build personalized treatment plans for a better quality of life in MS [8].

The disturbance of lipid metabolism is gaining increasing attention in neuropsychiatric diseases and their comorbidities. A case-control study revealed that depression, diabetes mellitus, and older age were associated with an increased likelihood of developing AD, and dyslipidemia treatment reduced the likelihood of developing AD. The authors declared that depression and diabetics are risk factors of dementia, treatment of dyslipidemia reduces the risk of dementia, and ageing is a decisive risk factor of dementia [9]. The status of polyunsaturated G-protein coupled receptor (GPR) 120 and its ligands, polyunsaturated fatty acid (PUFA) concentrations was studied in patients suffering from SCZ. Correlations were observed between the serum fatty acids (FAs) and GPR120 concentration in healthy controls (HCs), but no correlation was found in SCZ. Furthermore, alpha-linolenic acid and docosahexaenoic acid were independently associated with GPR120 concentration in the model adjusted for eicosapentaenoic acid in HCs. The authors concluded that a disturbance of PUFA concentrations may play a role in SCZ pathogenesis [10].

The use of nutraceutical compounds was proposed for the prevention of neurodegenerative diseases. A sugar-like compound inositol plays an important role in insulin signaling, oxidative stress, and neuronal activities. Prophylactic and supplemental use of nutraceutical inositol was suggested to prevent development and progression of cognitive impairments in AD, Down's syndrome, anxiety, compulsive disorder, and depressive disorder [11].

Depression, anxiety, and dementia are insufferable burdens experienced by patients and conspicuous findings exhibited to physicians. However, light is versatile and sometimes mischievous. The symptoms may not be the parts of the spectrum emitting or reflecting from the underlying conditions. Maybe the manifestations are footprints left by or shadows embodied through a certain pathogenesis. However, shadow is miscellaneous and multifarious. The clinical, laboratory, and statistical studies in this Special Issue successfully cast some gleams of light on the silhouette of depression, anxiety, and dementia in comorbidities. In order to capture the sharper image, our mission continues (https://www.mdpi.com/journal/biomedicines/special_issues/neuropsychiatry_2).

Author Contributions: Conceptualization, M.T. and L.V.; writing—original draft preparation, writing—review and editing, M.T. and L.V.; supervision, L.V.; project administration, M.T. and L.V.; funding acquisition, L.V. All authors have read and agreed to the published version of the manuscript.

Funding: The current work was supported by the Economic Development and Innovation Operational Programme (GINOP) GINOP 2.3.2-15-2016-00034, GINOP 2.3.2-15-2016-00048, TUDFO/47138-1/2019-ITM, and TKP2020 Thematic Excellence Programme 2020.

Institutional Review Board Statement: Not applicable.

Informed Consent Statement: Not applicable.

Conflicts of Interest: The authors declare no conflict of interest.

References

1. Ibos, K.E.; Bodnár, É.; Bagosi, Z.; Bozsó, Z.; Tóth, G.; Szabó, G.; Csabafi, K. Kisspeptin-8 Induces Anxiety-Like Behavior and Hypolocomotion by Activating the HPA Axis and Increasing GABA Release in the Nucleus Accumbens in Rats. *Biomedicines* **2021**, *9*, 112. [CrossRef] [PubMed]
2. Muntsant, A.; Jiménez-Altayó, F.; Puertas-Umbert, L.; Jiménez-Xarrie, E.; Vila, E.; Giménez-Llort, L. Sex-Dependent End-of-Life Mental and Vascular Scenarios for Compensatory Mechanisms in Mice with Normal and AD-Neurodegenerative Aging. *Biomedicines* **2021**, *9*, 111. [CrossRef] [PubMed]
3. Kim, J.; Kim, Y.-K. Crosstalk between Depression and Dementia with Resting-State fMRI Studies and Its Relationship with Cognitive Functioning. *Biomedicines* **2021**, *9*, 82. [CrossRef] [PubMed]
4. Kowalska, K.; Krzywoszański, Ł.; Droś, J.; Pasińska, P.; Wilk, A.; Klimkowicz-Mrowiec, A. Early Depression Independently of Other Neuropsychiatric Conditions, Influences Disability and Mortality after Stroke (Research Study—Part of PROPOLIS Study). *Biomedicines* **2020**, *8*, 509. [CrossRef] [PubMed]
5. Kim, E.Y.; Ahn, H.-S.; Lee, M.Y.; Yu, J.; Yeom, J.; Jeong, H.; Min, H.; Lee, H.J.; Kim, K.; Ahn, Y.M. An Exploratory Pilot Study with Plasma Protein Signatures Associated with Response of Patients with Depression to Antidepressant Treatment for 10 Weeks. *Biomedicines* **2020**, *8*, 455. [CrossRef] [PubMed]
6. Park, S.; Bak, A.; Kim, S.; Nam, Y.; Kim, H.s.; Yoo, D.-H.; Moon, M. Animal-Assisted and Pet-Robot Interventions for Ameliorating Behavioral and Psychological Symptoms of Dementia: A Systematic Review and Meta-Analysis. *Biomedicines* **2020**, *8*, 150. [CrossRef] [PubMed]
7. Vargas, A.S.; Luís, Â.; Barroso, M.; Gallardo, E.; Pereira, L. Psilocybin as a New Approach to Treat Depression and Anxiety in the Context of Life-Threatening Diseases—A Systematic Review and Meta-Analysis of Clinical Trials. *Biomedicines* **2020**, *8*, 331. [CrossRef] [PubMed]
8. Tanaka, M.; Vécsei, L. Monitoring the Redox Status in Multiple Sclerosis. *Biomedicines* **2020**, *8*, 406. [CrossRef] [PubMed]
9. Cantón-Habas, V.; Rich-Ruiz, M.; Romero-Saldaña, M.; Carrera-González, M.d.P. Depression as a Risk Factor for Dementia and Alzheimer's Disease. *Biomedicines* **2020**, *8*, 457. [CrossRef] [PubMed]
10. Rog, J.; Błażewicz, A.; Juchnowicz, D.; Ludwiczuk, A.; Stelmach, E.; Kozioł, M.; Karakula, M.; Niziński, P.; Karakula-Juchnowicz, H. The Role of GPR120 Receptor in Essential Fatty Acids Metabolism in Schizophrenia. *Biomedicines* **2020**, *8*, 243. [CrossRef] [PubMed]
11. López-Gambero, A.J.; Sanjuan, C.; Serrano-Castro, P.J.; Suárez, J.; Rodríguez de Fonseca, F. The Biomedical Uses of Inositols: A Nutraceutical Approach to Metabolic Dysfunction in Aging and Neurodegenerative Diseases. *Biomedicines* **2020**, *8*, 295. [CrossRef] [PubMed]

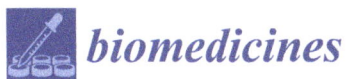

Review

Animal-Assisted and Pet-Robot Interventions for Ameliorating Behavioral and Psychological Symptoms of Dementia: A Systematic Review and Meta-Analysis

Sangki Park [1,†], Ahream Bak [2,†], Sujin Kim [3,†], Yunkwon Nam [3], Hyeon soo Kim [3], Doo-Han Yoo [1,*] and Minho Moon [3,*]

1. Department of Occupational Therapy, Konyang University, 158, Gwanjeodong-ro, Seo-gu, Daejeon 35365, Korea; sangki0222@gmail.com
2. Department of Occupational Therapy, Jeonju Kijeon College, 267, Jeonjucheonseo-ro, Wansan-gu, Junju 54989, Korea; orang43@naver.com
3. Department of Biochemistry, College of Medicine, Konyang University, 158, Gwanjeodong-ro, Seo-gu, Daejeon 35365, Korea; aktnfl3371@naver.com (S.K.); yunkwonnam@gmail.com (Y.N.); sooya1105@naver.com (H.s.K)
* Correspondence: glovia@konyang.ac.kr (D.-H.Y.); hominmoon@konyang.ac.kr (M.M.); Tel.: +82-42-600-8414 (D.-H.Y.); +82-42-600-8691 (M.M.)
† These authors contributed equally to this work.

Received: 11 May 2020; Accepted: 1 June 2020; Published: 2 June 2020

Abstract: Patients with dementia suffer from psychological symptoms such as depression, agitation, and aggression. One purpose of dementia intervention is to manage patients' inappropriate behaviors and psychological symptoms while taking into consideration their quality of life (QOL). Animal-assisted intervention (AAI) and pet-robot intervention (PRI) are effective intervention strategies for older people with cognitive impairment and dementia. In addition, AAI and PRI have been shown to have positive effects on behavioral and psychological symptoms of dementia (BPSD). However, studies into the association between AAI/PRI and BPSD have elicited inconsistent results. Thus, we performed a meta-analysis to investigate this association. We analyzed nine randomized controlled trials on AAI and PRI for dementia patients published between January 2000 and August 2019 and evaluated the impact of AAI/PRI on agitation, depression, and QOL. We found that AAI and PRI significantly reduce depression in patients with dementia. Subsequent studies should investigate the impact of AAI and PRI on the physical ability and cognitive function of dementia patients and conduct a follow-up to investigate their effects on the rate of progression and reduction of symptoms of dementia. Our research will help with neuropsychological and environmental intervention to delay or improve the development and progression of BPSD.

Keywords: dementia; behavioral and psychological symptoms of dementia; systematic review; meta-analysis; animal-assisted intervention; pet-robot intervention

1. Introduction

In 2016, it was estimated that 47 million individuals are living with dementia worldwide, and this figure is projected to increase to 113 million in 30 years. As a result, the public health burden of dementia is anticipated to significantly increase in the coming years [1]. Currently, the World Health Organization is striving to promote dementia prevention and increase dementia awareness by significantly investing in health and welfare and active research into dementia [2]. Furthermore, many countries have implemented national strategies aimed at optimizing dementia management in preparation for the anticipated burden of dementia and its effects on their healthcare system [3]. Dementia patients commonly suffer from behavioral and psychological symptoms of dementia (BPSD) [4]. BPSD include socially inappropriate neurobehavioral symptoms such as mental and emotional symptoms, hyperactivity, and sleep disorders [5]. Depression and agitation are the most common emotional problems that affect dementia patients [4]. The goal of dementia treatment is to manage patients' inappropriate behaviors and psychological symptoms while considering their quality of life (QOL), and active research into cognitive stimulation therapy, a nonpharmacological intervention for dementia, is ongoing [6]. However, previous studies into therapies for dementia have generally focused on their effect on cognitive abilities such as memory, problem-solving ability, and communication skills, and the impact of these therapies on the psychological and social aspects of dementia has been neglected [7]. Recently, many interventions for the treatment of BPSD have received attention [8–10], including animal-assisted interventions [11,12].

Animal-assisted interventions (AAI) are interventions that involve animals. There are various subgroups of AAI, namely animal-assisted activities (AAA), animal-assisted therapies (AAT), and service animal programs (SAP) [13]. These are known to be effective interventions for older people with cognitive impairment, and recent studies have reported that AAI have positive effects on dementia patients [14]. AAA refer to unofficial activities involving animals that meet certain requirements and are characterized by a certain level of flexibility and spontaneity. AAT refer to interventions involving animals that are aimed at improving certain patient outcomes and are incorporated into rehabilitation programs [15]. SAP refers to programs that utilize trained animals to help clients with physical disabilities to overcome functional difficulties in their activities of daily living [16]. These interventions provide joy to patients, increase their motivation, and allow them to rest [17], and patients are able to resolve their unmet physical and emotional needs by being involved in activities related to patients therapeutic goals [18]. In particular, walking a living animal is not only beneficial to dementia patients but also facilitates the rehabilitation of adults who have undergone surgery or have an illness by reacquainting them with ambulation and recovering ambulation speed [19–21]. The first AAI to be developed were found to reduce depression [22], and the ability of AAI to reduce depression and improve QOL in older people with dementia is currently being investigated [11,23–25]. Despite the known benefits of AAI, their use is restricted in some medical environments due to concerns about patients having a fear of animals, possible infection risk, and fright [26].

Recently, pet-robot intervention (PRI) has been proposed as an alternative to AAI. PARO, the most widely studied PRI, is a seal-shaped robot which responds to light, temperature, touch, and posture and monitors the client's emotional changes and health status using sensors [27]. PARO is reported to have various beneficial psychological and social effects such as promoting interaction, reducing stress, and alleviating depression. Furthermore, PRI has similar effects to AAI involving living animals; overcomes the limitations associated with living animals; and has cost, hygiene, and safety benefits [28]. Notably, one study reported that PARO has a positive impact on depression and psychological agitation in older people with dementia and concluded that PARO is a nonpharmacological intervention effective at alleviating neuropsychiatric symptoms [29]. Furthermore, PARO alleviated stress and agitation and reduced the use of antipsychotics and analgesics in older people with dementia [30].

It is well-known that AAI and PRI have beneficial effects on symptoms of dementia [23,30]. In addition, systematic reviews of the effect of AAI or PRI on symptoms of dementia have been performed [31–33]. However, no studies have been conducted into the effects of both AAI and PRI on BPSD. Therefore, the aim of this systemic review and meta-analysis was to investigate the effects of AAI and PRI on BPSD and to present clinical evidence for the application of these interventions.

2. Results

2.1. Characteristics of the Included Studies

Nine studies met the inclusion criteria for this study, and their general characteristics are presented in Table 1. Only studies with a PEDro score of 4–7 and thus deemed to be of "fair" or "good" quality were included [34]. A total of 507 participants were included in the meta-analysis. In the included studies, dementia patients were subjected to various interventions involving living or robotic animals. Each study was systematically analyzed and compared with the rest of the studies. The control group was typically subjected to the conventional treatment program provided at the hospital or facility at which the study was conducted.

Table 1. Characteristics of the included studies.

	Study	Participants (Experimental/Control)			Intervention			Period/Total Number of Sessions	Outcome Measures	Pedro Score
		Age	Sample Size		Experimental Group	Control Group				
1	Majic (2013) [35]	81.33 ± 10.20 /82.07 ± 8.65	27/27	AAI (Dog)	Dog-assisted intervention	Same care and treatment as before the study		10 weeks /10 sessions	MMSE, CMAI, DMAS *	4
2	Friedmann (2015) [23]	79.59 ± 9.74 /82.11 ± 8.36	22/18	AAI (Dog)	Dog-assisted intervention	Social skills and fine motor skills		12 weeks /24 sessions	AES, CSDD, CMAI	6
3	Olsen (2016a) [11]	65 or older	25/26	AAI (Dog)	Petting the dog, feeding the dog a treat, and throwing a toy for the dog to fetch	Music therapy, sensory garden, singing, exercise, cooking, and handicrafts		12 weeks /24 sessions	BARS, CSDD *, QUALID	6
4	Olsen (2016b) [24]	65 or older	22/26	AAI (Dog)	Petting the dog, feeding the dog a treat, and throwing a toy for the dog to fetch	Usual treatment		12 weeks /24 sessions	BBS, QUALID	5
5	Joranson (2015) [29]	83.9 ± 7.2 /84.1 ± 6.7	27/26	PRI (PARO)	Petting, talking to and about, smiling to, and singing to the robotic animal	Usual treatment		12 weeks /24 sessions	BARS *, CSDD *	6
6	Joranson (2016) [36]	83.9 ± 7.2 /84.1 ± 6.7	27/26	PRI (PARO)	Petting, talking to and about, smiling to, and singing to the robotic animal	Usual treatment		12 weeks /24 sessions	CDR, QUALID	7
7	Petersen (2016) [30]	83.5 ± 5.8 /83.3 ± 6.0	35/26	PRI (PARO)	Interaction activity of 5 people one group to PARO	Music therapy, physical activity, and mental stimulation		12 weeks /36 sessions	RAID **, CSDD **, GDS, pulse oximetry **, pulse rate **, GSR	6
8	Liang (2017) [37]	67–98	13/11	PRI (PARO)	Separate PAROs were provided to each participant's home environment	Standard activities (quizzes, exercise, bingo, music, and word activities)		6 weeks /12–18 sessions	CMAI-SF, cognitive score, NPI-Q, depressive symptoms *	6
9	Moyle (2018) [38]	84 ± 8.8 /86 ± 7.6 /85 ± 6.9	67/55/53	PRI (PARO)	Participants were left alone with PARO for 15 min to interact with it as they liked	PARO with all artificial intelligence disabled	Usual treatment	10 weeks /30 sessions	Sense Wear *	7

AAI, animal-assisted intervention; AES, Apathy Evaluation Scale; BARS, Brief Agitation Rating Scale; BBS, Berg Balance Scale; CDR, Clinical Dementia Rating Scale; CMAI, Cohen-Mansfield Agitation Inventory; CMAI-SF, Cohen-Mansfield Agitation Inventory Short Form; CSDD, Cornell Scale for Depression in Dementia; DMAS, Dementia Mood Assessment Scale; GDS, Global Deterioration Scale; GSR, galvanic skin response; MMSE, mini mental state examination; PRI, pet-robot intervention; RAID, Rating for Anxiety in Dementia; QUALID, Quality of Life in Late-Stage Dementia Scale; NPI-Q, Neuropsychiatric Inventory Brief Questionnaire; * $p < 0.05$, ** $p < 0.01$.

2.2. Meta-Analysis of the Effects of AAI and PRI

2.2.1. Meta-Analysis of the Effects of AAI and PRI on Agitation in Dementia Patients

In the meta-analysis of the effects of AAI and PRI on agitation in dementia patients, the effect size was 0.70 (95% confidence interval: $p = 0.12$, $I^2 = 89\%$), which was considered a large effect size. Overall, AAI and PRI did not significantly affect agitation in dementia patients (Figure 1).

Study or Subgroup	Experimental Mean	SD	Total	Control Mean	SD	Total	Weight	Std. Mean Difference IV, Random, 95% CI
Liang 2017 [37]	-10.4	13	13	-7.16	11	11	19.3%	-0.26 [-1.06, 0.55]
Olsen 2016a [11]	-23.75	7.13	24	-24.65	13.95	26	21.1%	0.08 [-0.48, 0.63]
Majic 2013 [35]	-15.87	27	27	-23.34	27	27	21.2%	0.27 [-0.26, 0.81]
Joranson 2015 [29]	-20.2	10.1	27	-24.7	14	27	21.2%	0.36 [-0.17, 0.90]
Friedmann 2015 [23]	-15.53	0.68	19	-20	1.69	18	17.3%	3.43 [2.38, 4.48]
Total (95% CI)			**110**			**109**	**100.0%**	**0.70 [-0.18, 1.57]**

Heterogeneity: Tau² = 0.87; Chi² = 36.16, df = 4 (P < 0.00001); I² = 89%
Test for overall effect: Z = 1.56 (P = 0.12)

Favours [experimental]   Favours [control]

Figure 1. Forest plot of the effect of animal-assisted intervention and pet-robot intervention on agitation in dementia patients.

2.2.2. Meta-Analysis of the Effects of AAI and PRI on Depression in Dementia Patients

In the meta-analysis of the effects of AAI and PRI on depression in dementia patients, the effect size was −0.47 (95% confidence interval: $p < 0.001$, $I2 = 0\%$). Overall, AAI and PRI significantly reduced depression in dementia patients (Figure 2).

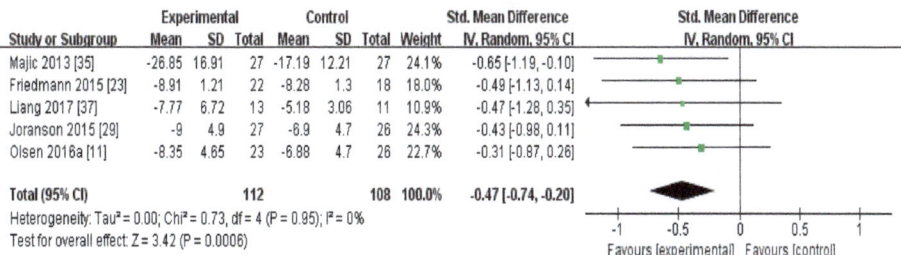

Study or Subgroup	Experimental Mean	SD	Total	Control Mean	SD	Total	Weight	Std. Mean Difference IV, Random, 95% CI
Majic 2013 [35]	-26.85	16.91	27	-17.19	12.21	27	24.1%	-0.65 [-1.19, -0.10]
Friedmann 2015 [23]	-8.91	1.21	22	-8.28	1.3	18	18.0%	-0.49 [-1.13, 0.14]
Liang 2017 [37]	-7.77	6.72	13	-5.18	3.06	11	10.9%	-0.47 [-1.28, 0.35]
Joranson 2015 [29]	-9	4.9	27	-6.9	4.7	26	24.3%	-0.43 [-0.98, 0.11]
Olsen 2016a [11]	-8.35	4.65	23	-6.88	4.7	26	22.7%	-0.31 [-0.87, 0.26]
Total (95% CI)			**112**			**108**	**100.0%**	**-0.47 [-0.74, -0.20]**

Heterogeneity: Tau² = 0.00; Chi² = 0.73, df = 4 (P = 0.95); I² = 0%
Test for overall effect: Z = 3.42 (P = 0.0006)

Favours [experimental]   Favours [control]

Figure 2. Forest plot of the effect of animal-assisted intervention and pet-robot intervention on depression in dementia patient.

2.2.3. Meta-Analysis of the Effects of AAI and PRI on the QOL of Dementia Patients

In the meta-analysis of the effects of AAI and PRI on the QOL of dementia patients, the effect size was 0.13 (95% confidence interval: $p = 0.34$, $I^2 = 0\%$), which was considered a small effect size. Overall, AAI and PRI did not significantly affect the QOL of dementia patients (Figure 3).

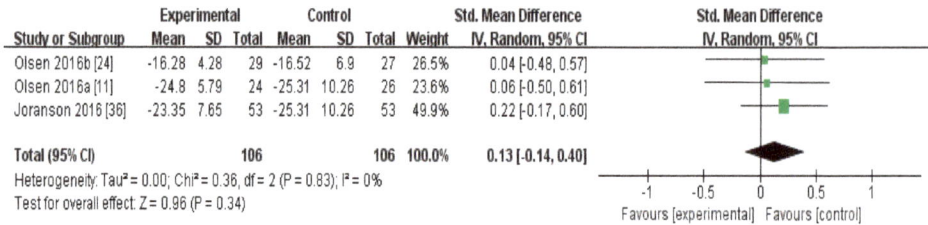

Figure 3. Forest plot of the effect of animal-assisted intervention and pet-robot intervention on the quality of life of dementia patients.

2.2.4. Publication Bias

When publication bias with respect to agitation, four studies were within the 95% confidence interval and were plotted to the left of the overall effect estimate (Figure 4A). When publication bias with respect to depression and QOL with respect to the effect of AAI and PRI was assessed (Figure 4B,C), all plotted dots were within the 95% confidence interval.

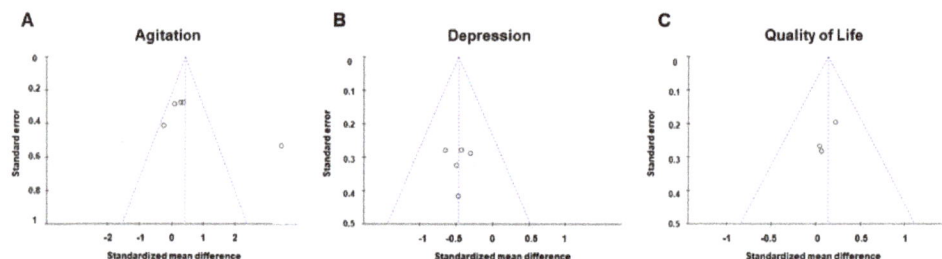

Figure 4. Funnel plots used to assess the existence of publication bias in the included studies. Publication bias of (**A**) agitation, (**B**) depression, and (**C**) quality of life.

3. Discussion

Currently, more than 90% of dementia patients suffer from BPSD [39], which poses major difficulties to both dementia patients and their caregivers. The type of BPSD varies according to dementia type, stage of the illness and various other factors. Particularly, patients of frontotemporal lobar degeneration (FTLD) show more prominent behavioral variants such as disinhibition, impulsivity, aggression, and personality change than those with other types of dementia [40–42]. Another study demonstrated that patients with dementia with Lewy bodies (DLB) present hallucinations and aberrant motor behavior (AMB) more so than Alzheimer's disease (AD) patients [43,44]. An increased rate of anxiety, depression, and psychosis may occur in vascular dementia (VD) [40,43,45]. Depression and agitation are the most common symptoms affecting various dementia patients. Furthermore, it is known that agitation, apathy, disinhibition, irritability, and motor dysfunction become serious as dementia progresses. In particular, depression and anxiety become more severe in the moderate stage of dementia [46–48]. In the early stages of dementia, apathy mainly appears, which is one of the first symptoms of the various forms of dementia. Apathy is a dangerous barrier that affects social interaction and activities of daily living due to lack of interest, enthusiasm, and apathetic response to interpersonal communication [49]. These psychological and behavioral changes from the early stages of dementia can affect aspects of BPSD such as depression and anxiety more seriously as dementia progress. Although BPSD, which varies depending on the type and progression of dementia, contains a range of important symptoms that affect the quality of life, stress, and prognosis of dementia patients and their caregivers, there is little of interest in and study on nonpharmacological interventions to treat BPSD. Thus, we performed a meta-analysis to investigate the effect of AAI and PRI—one of the nonpharmacological interventions using animals— on agitation, depression, and QOL in dementia patients [15,26,27].

The meta-analysis of the effects of AAI and PRI on agitation showed a medium effect size of 0.70 (Figure 1). Three studies that utilized AAI and two studies that utilized PRI were included in the meta-analysis. The studies that used AAI reported larger effect sizes than those that used PRI, but AAI and PRI were not found to significantly affect agitation overall [23,24,35]. Our result contrasts with the results of a previous study which showed an alleviation in the agitation. However, since the level of evidence for the randomized controlled trials (RCTs) in previous studies was very low, we thought that the opposite results were obtained. Accordingly, our results support the suggestion of previous studies that the level of evidence is low [32].

The meta-analysis of the effects of AAI and PRI on depression showed a medium effect size of −0.47 (Figure 2). Three studies that used AAI were included, and two reported that this intervention strategy reduced depression [23,24,35]. Two studies that used PRI were included, and these showed a medium effect size [36,37]. AAI and PRI were found to significantly reduce depression, which serves as evidence that AAI and PRI are effective at reducing depression in dementia patients ($p < 0.001$).

The meta-analysis of the effects of AAI and PRI on QOL showed a small effect size of 0.13, but the results were not statistically significant ($p > 0.05$) (Figure 3). Two studies used AAI, and both reported that these interventions improved QOL [11,24]. One study used PRI, and reported that this intervention did not significantly affect QOL [36]. The meta-analysis results showed that AAI and PRI did not significantly affect QOL, which supports previous findings [32].

The present study analyzed the effects of AAI and PRI on BPSD and found that these interventions did not affect agitation or QOL but significantly reduced depression. It is well known that the brain with depression in dementia has reduced connectivity on amygdala and emotion control regions [50,51]. AAI and PRI provide an emotional effect and a and sense of closeness to dementia patients [52], which may the reduced amygdala connectivity in dementia patients. In addition, AAI and PRI could have a positive effect on hippocampus in the brain with depression through activities that require memory, such as checking the health of animals, walking, and feeding. On the other hand, the agitation-related connectivity is the orbital frontal cortex and anterior cingulate cortex, which is a region that has little association with emotional support obtained through activities with animals. Thus, AAI and PRI did not show a significant effect in agitation. Although AAI and PRI have been effective in improving depression, it is difficult to dramatically relieve all BPSD symptoms. Moreover, it is known that BPSD is specifically related with the patient's low of QOL [53]. Therefore, in this study, it is considered that AAI and PRI were difficult to significantly influence QOL. A previous meta-analysis reported that AAI do not affect activities of daily living, depression, agitation, QOL, or cognitive function. In addition, a number of limitations are associated with interventions involving the use of living animals: patients may be fearful of or allergic to animals, animals may provoke falls in vulnerable patients, and animals may pose an infection risk to patients [32]. Moreover, there are a number of difficulties associated with managing animals—they need to be fed, produce feces, and may smell. However, it is clear that AAI can enhance the emotional wellbeing and QOL of dementia patients. Although robotic animals cannot evoke the same variety of emotions and sensations as living animals, they are easier to manage and could aid patients wherever needed. Subsequent studies should additionally examine the impact of living animals and robotic animals on the emotional wellbeing, cognitive function, and physical ability of dementia patients. Furthermore, patients should be followed-up to investigate the efficacy of these interventions in slowing the progression of dementia.

Several studies have suggested that psychiatric symptoms such as depression and anxiety are associated with dementia and cognitive impairment [54–56]. Indeed, patients with dementia have an increased risk of major depression, and many suffer from anxiety [57,58]. Interestingly, amyloid-beta (Aβ) burden and tau-related pathology are known to worsen in Alzheimer-type dementia with depression [55,59]. In addition, depression and agitation are causative factors of sleep disorders, and they can promote the development of dementia by inhibiting Aβ clearance and inducing systemic inflammation [60–63]. Therefore, it is important to alleviate the psychological symptoms of dementia patients. In this study, we confirmed that AAI and PRI can relieve the psychological symptoms of dementia patients. Several mechanisms by which AAI and PRI may affect BPSD have been proposed. First, AAI and PRI affect hormone levels. Previous studies consistently reported that dog-raising people exhibit higher levels of oxytocin, a hypothalamic neuropeptide [64,65]. Oxytocin is closely related to cognitive function, depression, agitation, and social communication and has been proposed as a pharmacological intervention for neurobehavioral disorders in patients with prefrontal dementia [66,67]. In addition, it has been reported that animal owners exhibit reduced cortisol levels [68]. In AD, cortisol levels substantially increase and this steroid hormone elicits neurotoxic effects in the hippocampus and thus exacerbates Aβ pathology and contributes to cognitive impairment [69]. Therefore, AAI may improve BPSD by increasing oxytocin levels and reducing cortisol levels. Furthermore, the relationship between loneliness and depression is well established, and loneliness has been reported to promote Aβ deposition in the brain of AD patients [70,71]. In addition, loneliness is known to contribute to cognitive decline by lowering cognitive reserve [72]. Surprisingly, AAI is known to reduce the loneliness of residents in long-term care facilities [73]. Therefore, AAI and PRI may effectively reduce loneliness and depression in dementia patients.

Second, it is possible that AAI and PRI modulate brain structure and functional connectivity. Patients with dementia exhibit atrophy of the hippocampus and entorhinal cortex, areas of the brain associated with emotional and spatial memory [74]. In addition, late-stage dementia is associated with dysfunction of the amygdala and cerebral cortex [75,76]. Accordingly, patients with dementia have problems with language, reasoning, emotions, and social behavior. Furthermore, atrophy of the hippocampus and cerebral cortex affects the functional connectivity of frontotemporal and limbic circuits involved in depression and mood regulation [77]. Strikingly, emotion-related brain areas may be affected by dementia patients' relationship and emotional stability. Indeed, improvements in executive function, social skills, mood regulation, learning, memory, and attention were noted in patients receiving cognitive rehabilitation therapy through various AAI [52]. In addition, in children with ADHD, AAI had a calming effect, increased motivation, improved cognitive function, and promoted socialization [78]. It is thought that interaction with a therapy animal enhances functional connectivity between the frontotemporal and limbic systems. Moreover, having to look after an animal and remember to perform tasks such as feeding it is thought to improve memory and learning ability and attenuate hippocampal and cortical atrophy. Social interaction is possible through relationships and walking with animals, and through group meetings, depression will be alleviated. Although the neurological mechanisms underlying the effects of AAI and PRI have not been fully elucidated, accumulating evidence suggests that AAI and PRI can effectively improve BPSD.

Although a number of previous studies have also investigated living- and robotic- animal-assisted interventions for patients with dementia, our study has a number of strengths [31–33]. First, we comprehensively investigated the effects of interventions involving living and robotic animals and, for the first time, compared the effects of AAI and PRI on BPSD. Second, we demonstrated trends in research in this field and confirmed that more research is now being conducted into interventions involving robotic animals for dementia patients. Third, two reviewers independently identified articles that met the inclusion criteria, and a high level of inter-rater agreement was noted. Fourth, we focused on BPSD and dementia. Although AAI and PRI are known to affect various symptoms of dementia patients, we conducted a literature search and meta-analysis focusing on BPSD. Finally, it is difficult to distinguish between mild cognitive impairment (MCI) and dementia patients unless a neurological examination is performed to definitively diagnose dementia. In this study, we aimed to confirm the effect of AAI and PRI in individuals who had been diagnosed with dementia, not MCI.

Nevertheless, our study has a number of limitations. One limitation of the meta-analysis is the small number of included studies, which shows that there is a lack of literature relating to AAI and PRI for dementia patients. In addition, we only selected studies published in peer-reviewed journals and did not include any grey literature, which may have introduced publication bias. Third, we were unable to identify specific subgroups of dementia patients who may benefit most from AAI and PRI. Finally, we searched only a few English language databases, so some relevant studies may have been missed.

4. Methods

4.1. Subsection

A meta-analysis was performed to analyze and validate studies that investigated the effects of AAI and PRI on dementia patients.

4.2. Search Strategy

Studies into the effect of AAI and PRI on dementia patients published between January 2000 and August 2019 were analyzed. Data were collected from three electronic databases—the Cochrane Library, Embase, and PubMed (Figure 5). The search terms used were "Dementia" AND "animal-assisted therapy OR animal-assisted activity OR service animal programs OR animal OR robot". A total of 5364 studies were initially identified, and, after the exclusion of 4858 nonclinical trials, 506 studies underwent further analysis. An additional 506 studies were then excluded: 1 because the original text was unavailable, 9 because they were written in a language other than English, 173 because they were not RCTs, 216 because they were duplicates, 92 because they were inappropriate for the purpose of our study/because they were unsuitable based on a review of their titles and abstracts, and 7 because data were missing or disorganized. Ultimately, nine studies were included in the systematic review and meta-analysis.

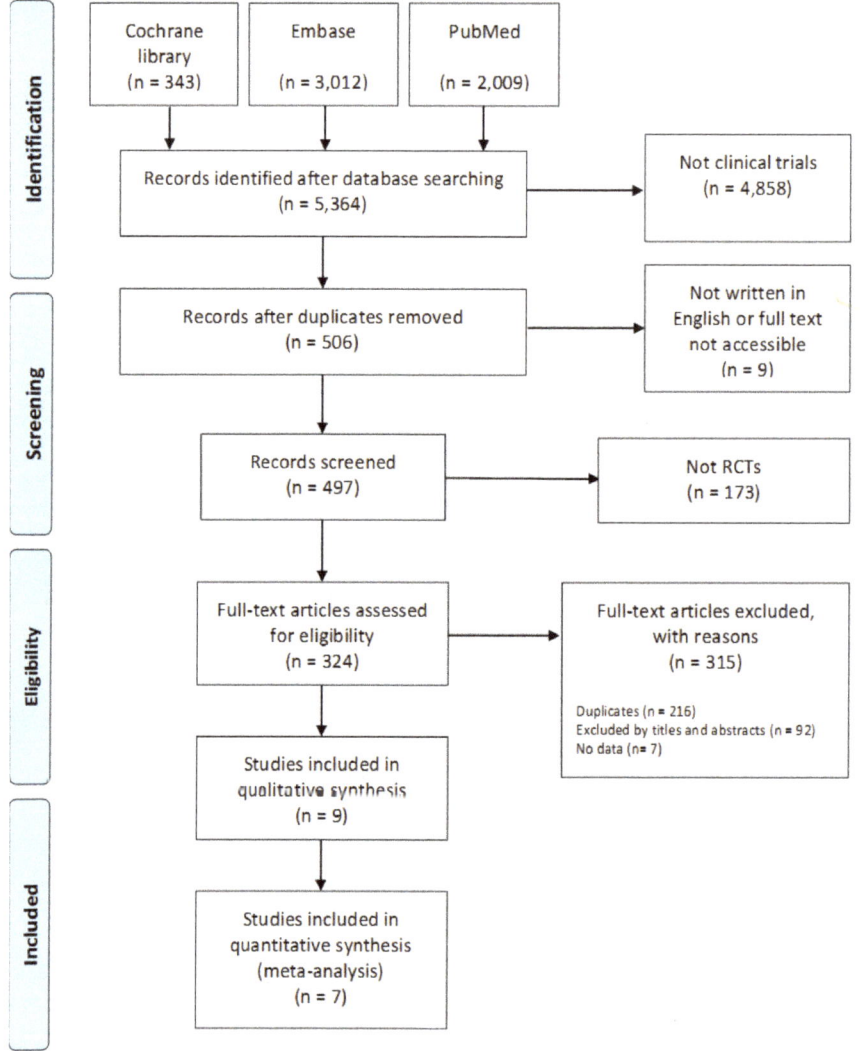

Figure 5. Flow chart of the systematic literature review.

4.3. Selection Criteria

Studies were included if they met all of the following criteria: (i) the study population comprised dementia patients, (ii) the experimental intervention was an AAI or PRI, (iii) the participants were randomized into groups, (iv) standardized evaluations were conducted to compare the effects of the intervention and control treatment, and (v) sufficient data were available to compute the effect size.

4.4. Study Selection and Data Extraction

Two reviewers (S.P. and A.B.) independently identified studies that met the inclusion criteria and performed data extraction. Disagreements between the reviewers were resolved by discussion. From each selected study, the following data were extracted: author, year of publication, mean age of the participants, study design (sample size, intervention type, follow-up duration, and frequency of intervention), and outcome measurement tools.

4.5. Qualitative Assessment of Study Methodology

One reviewer (S.P.) assessed the quality of the nine selected studies by assigning each a PEDro score (OTseeker, 2003), and the results were verified by the other reviewer (A.B.). The PEDro score ranges from 0–10 and the quality of a study is classified as "poor" (≤3), "fair" (4–5), "good" (6–8), or "excellent" (9–10) [34]. Studies deemed to be of "fair" to "good" quality (4–7) were included in this analysis. Any disagreements between the investigators with respect to the qualitative assessment of the studies were resolved by discussion.

4.6. Qualitative Assessment of Study Methodology

For each of the included studies, the following data were presented: name of first author/names of all authors, year of publication, age of participants, sample size, type of intervention/intervention method, duration and frequency of intervention, instruments used to assess primary outcomes, and PEDro score. To analyze the effects of AAI on dementia patients based on these characteristics, the mean, standard deviation, and sample size of the intervention and control groups were computed (Table 1). We examined whether the direction of the effect size was identical across studies and if not, made them equal by multiplying the mean by −1 [79].

4.7. Statistical Analysis

It is inappropriate to determine whether a fixed effect model or random effect model should be employed using the heterogeneity statistic I^2. In order to select an appropriate effect model, the characteristics of the study, the subjects of the study, the method of intervention, and the mean value of the intervention effect were examined. In order to select an appropriate model to determine statistical heterogeneity, the characteristics of individual studies, study design, study subjects, intervention methods, and average values of intervention effects were examined [80].

Effect sizes were calculated to determine and compare the effect of AAI and PRI/different interventions on activities of daily living, stress, depression, and mental health using the sample size, mean, standard deviation, and statistically significant test of the experimental and control groups. According to the analysis criteria suggested by Cohen [81], 0.2 or less was considered a small effect size, 0.5 a medium effect size, and 0.8 or more a large effect size. The quantitative results of the meta-analysis were presented using forest plots. Publication bias was assessed by creating funnel plots. These were assessed by two reviewers and any disagreements were resolved by discussion. The chi-squared test was performed to determine the significance of the Q statistic [82,83]. If the p-value of Q was less than 0.10, there was deemed to be significant statistical heterogeneity between studies. A higher significance level was used since the Q statistic has low statistical power when only a small number of studies are included in a meta-analysis [84]. All statistical analyses were performed using Review Manager 5.3 software (RevMan; the Cochrane Collaboration, Oxford, UK).

5. Conclusions

This study systematically reviewed, compared, and meta-analyzed the impact of AAI and PRI on agitation, depression, and QOL in dementia patients. Interventions involving both living and robotic animals were investigated. The meta-analysis revealed that AAI and PRI interventions significantly reduced depression but did not affect agitation or QOL. Comparison of AAI and PRI showed that each method has its benefits and shortcomings and indicated that the two methods could potentially complement each other. Interventions involving living animals had a more beneficial effect on the emotional wellbeing of dementia patients than PRI. Although robotic animals overcome some limitations of living animals, they were not shown to alleviate BPSD in this study. In the future, more research should be conducted on the impact of living and robotic animals on the emotional wellbeing, cognitive function, and physical ability of dementia patients. Furthermore, we hope that AAI and PRI, which have been found to effectively reduce depression in dementia patients based on follow-ups, are more commonly utilized in clinical practice.

Author Contributions: Conceptualization, M.M. and D.-H.Y.; data curation, S.P. and A.B.; formal analysis, S.K. and Y.N.; funding acquisition, M.M. and D.-H.Y.; investigation, S.P. and A.B.; methodology S.P., A.B. and S.K.; project administration, M.M. and D.-H.Y.; resources, A.B. and S.K.; software, S.P. and D.-H.Y.; supervision, M.M. and D.-H.Y.; validation, S.K. and H.s.K.; visualization, S.K., Y.N. and H.s.K.; roles/writing—original draft, S.P., A.B., and S.K.; writing—review and editing, M.M. and D.-H.Y. All authors have read and agreed to the published version of the manuscript.

Funding: This work was supported by the Basic Science Research Program of the National Research Foundation of Korea (NRF), which is funded by the Ministry of Science, ICT & Future Planning (NRF-2018R1D1A3B07041059 to M.M.; NRF-2019R1G1A1004010 to D.-H.Y.) and by the Cooperative Research Program for Agriculture Science and Technology Development (Project No. PJ01319901 and PJ01428603), Rural Development Administration, Republic of Korea.

Conflicts of Interest: The authors declare no conflicts of interest.

Abbreviations

AMB	aberrant motor behavior
AD	Alzheimer's disease
Aβ	amyloid-β
AAA	animal-assisted activities
AAI	Animal-assisted intervention
AAT	animal-assisted therapies
BPSD	behavioral and psychological symptoms of dementia
DLB	dementia with Lewy bodies
FTLD	frontotemporal lobar degeneration
MCI	mild cognitive impairment
PRI	pet-robot intervention
QOL	quality of life
RCTs	randomized controlled trials
RevMan	Review Manager
SAP	service animal programs
VD	vascular dementia

References

1. Prince, M.; Comas-Herrera, A.; Knapp, M.; Guerchet, M.; Karagiannidou, M. *World Alzheimer Report 2016: Improving Healthcare for People Living with Dementia: Coverage, Quality and Costs Now and in the Future*; Alzheimer's Disease International: London, UK, 2016.
2. World Health Organization. *Global Action Plan on the Public Health Response to Dementia*; World Health Organization: Geneva, Switzerland, 2017.
3. Pimouguet, C.; Bassi, V.; Somme, D.; Lavallart, B.; Helmer, C.; Dartigues, J.F. The 2008–2012 French Alzheimer plan: A unique opportunity for improving integrated care for dementia. *J. Alzheimers Dis.* **2013**, *34*, 307–314. [CrossRef] [PubMed]
4. Kales, H.C.; Gitlin, L.N.; Lyketsos, C.G. Assessment and management of behavioral and psychological symptoms of dementia. *BMJ* **2015**, *350*, h369. [CrossRef] [PubMed]
5. Van der Linde, R.M.; Dening, T.; Matthews, F.E.; Brayne, C. Grouping of behavioural and psychological symptoms of dementia. *Int. J. Geriatr. Psychiatry* **2014**, *29*, 562–568. [CrossRef]
6. Cooper, C.; Mukadam, N.; Katona, C.; Lyketsos, C.G.; Ames, D.; Rabins, P.; Engedal, K.; de Mendonca Lima, C.; Blazer, D.; Teri, L.; et al. Systematic review of the effectiveness of non-pharmacological interventions to improve quality of life of people with dementia. *Int. Psychogeriatr.* **2012**, *24*, 856–870. [CrossRef] [PubMed]
7. Yuill, N.; Hollis, V. A systematic review of cognitive stimulation therapy for older adults with mild to moderate dementia: An occupational therapy perspective. *Occup. Ther. Int.* **2011**, *18*, 163–186. [CrossRef]

8. Gill, S.S.; Bronskill, S.E.; Normand, S.L.; Anderson, G.M.; Sykora, K.; Lam, K.; Bell, C.M.; Lee, P.E.; Fischer, H.D.; Herrmann, N.; et al. Antipsychotic drug use and mortality in older adults with dementia. *Ann. Intern. Med.* **2007**, *146*, 775–786. [CrossRef]
9. Guetin, S.; Portet, F.; Picot, M.C.; Pommie, C.; Messaoudi, M.; Djabelkir, L.; Olsen, A.L.; Cano, M.M.; Lecourt, E.; Touchon, J. Effect of music therapy on anxiety and depression in patients with Alzheimer's type dementia: Randomised, controlled study. *Dement. Geriatr. Cogn. Disord.* **2009**, *28*, 36–46. [CrossRef]
10. Berkheimer, S.D.; Qian, C.; Malmstrom, T.K. Snoezelen Therapy as an Intervention to Reduce Agitation in Nursing Home Patients With Dementia: A Pilot Study. *J. Am. Med. Dir. Assoc.* **2017**, *18*, 1089–1091. [CrossRef]
11. Olsen, C.; Pedersen, I.; Bergland, A.; Enders-Slegers, M.J.; Patil, G.; Ihlebaek, C. Effect of animal-assisted interventions on depression, agitation and quality of life in nursing home residents suffering from cognitive impairment or dementia: A cluster randomized controlled trial. *Int. J. Geriatr. Psychiatry* **2016**, *31*, 1312–1321. [CrossRef]
12. Jones, C.; Moyle, W.; Murfield, J.; Draper, B.; Shum, D.; Beattie, E.; Thalib, L. Does Cognitive Impairment and Agitation in Dementia Influence Intervention Effectiveness? Findings From a Cluster-Randomized-Controlled Trial With the Therapeutic Robot, PARO. *J. Am. Med. Dir. Assoc.* **2018**, *19*, 623–626. [CrossRef]
13. Kruger, K.A.; Serpell, J.A. *Animal-Assisted Interventions in Mental Health*; Academic Press: Cambridge, MA, USA, 2010. [CrossRef]
14. Friedmann, E.; Galik, E.; Thomas, S.A.; Hall, S.; Cheon, J.; Han, N.; Kim, H.J.; McAtee, S.; Gee, N.R. Relationship of Behavioral Interactions during an Animal-assisted Intervention in Assisted Living to Health-related Outcomes. *Anthrozoös* **2019**, *32*, 221–238. [CrossRef]
15. Kamioka, H.; Okada, S.; Tsutani, K.; Park, H.; Okuizumi, H.; Handa, S.; Oshio, T.; Park, S.J.; Kitayuguchi, J.; Abe, T.; et al. Effectiveness of animal-assisted therapy: A systematic review of randomized controlled trials. *Complement. Ther. Med.* **2014**, *22*, 371–390. [CrossRef] [PubMed]
16. American Veterinary Medical Association. *Guidelines for Animal Assisted Activity, Animal-Assisted Therapy and Resident Animal Programs*; Current as of 2007; American Veterinary Medical Association: Schaumburg, IL, USA, 2014.
17. Ohtani, N.; Narita, S.; Yoshihara, E.; Ohta, M.; Iwahashi, K. Psychological Evaluation of Animal-assisted Intervention (AAI) Programs Involving Visiting Dogs and Cats for Alcohol Dependents: A Pilot Study. *Nihon Arukoru Yakubutsu Igakkai Zasshi* **2015**, *50*, 289–295. [PubMed]
18. Ebener, J.; Oh, H. A Review of Animal-Assisted Interventions in Long-Term Care Facilities. *Act. Adapt. Aging* **2017**, *41*, 107–128. [CrossRef]
19. Abate, S.V.; Zucconi, M.; Boxer, B.A. Impact of canine-assisted ambulation on hospitalized chronic heart failure patients' ambulation outcomes and satisfaction: A pilot study. *J. Cardiovasc. Nurs.* **2011**, *26*, 224–230. [CrossRef]
20. Ruzic, A.; Miletic, B.; Ruzic, T.; Persic, V.; Laskarin, G. Regular dog-walking improves physical capacity in elderly patients after myocardial infarction. *Coll. Antropol.* **2011**, *35* (Suppl. 2), 73–75.
21. Rondeau, L.; Corriveau, H.; Bier, N.; Camden, C.; Champagne, N.; Dion, C. Effectiveness of a rehabilitation dog in fostering gait retraining for adults with a recent stroke: A multiple single-case study. *NeuroRehabilitation* **2010**, *27*, 155–163. [CrossRef]
22. Souter, M.A.; Miller, M.D. Do Animal-Assisted Activities Effectively Treat Depression? A Meta-Analysis. *Anthrozoös* **2015**, *20*, 167–180. [CrossRef]
23. Friedmann, E.; Galik, E.; Thomas, S.A.; Hall, P.S.; Chung, S.Y.; McCune, S. Evaluation of a pet-assisted living intervention for improving functional status in assisted living residents with mild to moderate cognitive impairment: A pilot study. *Am. J. Alzheimers Dis. Other Demen.* **2015**, *30*, 276–289. [CrossRef]
24. Olsen, C.; Pedersen, I.; Bergland, A.; Enders-Slegers, M.J.; Ihlebaek, C. Effect of animal-assisted activity on balance and quality of life in home-dwelling persons with dementia. *Geriatr. Nurs.* **2016**, *37*, 284–291. [CrossRef]
25. Travers, C.; Perkins, J.; Rand, J.; Bartlett, H.; Morton, J. An evaluation of dog-assisted therapy for residents of aged care facilities with dementia. *Anthrozoös* **2013**, *26*, 213–225. [CrossRef]
26. Velde, B.; Cipriani, J.; Fisher, G. Resident and therapist views of animal-assisted therapy: Implications for occupational therapy practice. *Aust. Occup. Ther. J.* **2005**, *52*, 43–50. [CrossRef]

27. Bemelmans, R.; Gelderblom, G.J.; Jonker, P.; de Witte, L. Socially assistive robots in elderly care: A systematic review into effects and effectiveness. *J. Am. Med. Dir. Assoc.* **2012**, *13*, 114–120. [CrossRef] [PubMed]
28. Preuss, D.; Legal, F. Living with the animals: Animal or robotic companions for the elderly in smart homes? *J. Med. Ethics* **2017**, *43*, 407–410. [CrossRef]
29. Joranson, N.; Pedersen, I.; Rokstad, A.M.; Ihlebaek, C. Effects on symptoms of agitation and depression in persons with dementia participating in robot-assisted activity: A cluster-randomized controlled trial. *J. Am. Med. Dir. Assoc.* **2015**, *16*, 867–873. [CrossRef]
30. Petersen, S.; Houston, S.; Qin, H.; Tague, C.; Studley, J. The utilization of robotic pets in dementia care. *J. Alzheimers Dis.* **2017**, *55*, 569–574. [CrossRef]
31. Hu, M.; Zhang, P.; Leng, M.; Li, C.; Chen, L. Animal-assisted intervention for individuals with cognitive impairment: A meta-analysis of randomized controlled trials and quasi-randomized controlled trials. *Psychiatry Res.* **2018**, *260*, 418–427. [CrossRef]
32. Zafra-Tanaka, J.H.; Pacheco-Barrios, K.; Tellez, W.A.; Taype-Rondan, A. Effects of dog-assisted therapy in adults with dementia: A systematic review and meta-analysis. *BMC Psychiatry* **2019**, *19*, 41. [CrossRef]
33. Leng, M.; Liu, P.; Zhang, P.; Hu, M.; Zhou, H.; Li, G.; Yin, H.; Chen, L. Pet robot intervention for people with dementia: A systematic review and meta-analysis of randomized controlled trials. *Psychiatry Res.* **2019**, *271*, 516–525. [CrossRef]
34. Moseley, A.M.; Herbert, R.D.; Sherrington, C.; Maher, C.G. Evidence for physiotherapy practice: A survey of the Physiotherapy Evidence Database (PEDro). *Aust. J. Physiother.* **2002**, *48*, 43–49. [CrossRef]
35. Majic, T.; Gutzmann, H.; Heinz, A.; Lang, U.E.; Rapp, M.A. Animal-assisted therapy and agitation and depression in nursing home residents with dementia: A matched case-control trial. *Am. J. Geriatr. Psychiatry* **2013**, *21*, 1052–1059. [CrossRef] [PubMed]
36. Joranson, N.; Pedersen, I.; Rokstad, A.M.; Ihlebaek, C. Change in quality of life in older people with dementia participating in Paro-activity: A cluster-randomized controlled trial. *J. Adv. Nurs.* **2016**, *72*, 3020–3033. [CrossRef] [PubMed]
37. Liang, A.; Piroth, I.; Robinson, H.; MacDonald, B.; Fisher, M.; Nater, U.M.; Skoluda, N.; Broadbent, E. A pilot randomized trial of a companion robot for people with dementia living in the community. *J. Am. Med. Dir. Assoc.* **2017**, *18*, 871–878. [CrossRef] [PubMed]
38. Moyle, W.; Jones, C.; Murfield, J.; Thalib, L.; Beattie, E.; Shum, D.; O'Dwyer, S.; Mervin, M.C.; Draper, B. Effect of a robotic seal on the motor activity and sleep patterns of older people with dementia, as measured by wearable technology: A cluster-randomised controlled trial. *Maturitas* **2018**, *110*, 10–17. [CrossRef]
39. Colombo, M.; Vitali, S.; Cairati, M.; Vaccaro, R.; Andreoni, G.; Guaita, A. Behavioral and psychotic symptoms of dementia (BPSD) improvements in a special care unit: A factor analysis. *Arch. Gerontol. Geriatr.* **2007**, *44* (Suppl. 1), 113–120. [CrossRef]
40. Srikanth, S.; Nagaraja, A.V.; Ratnavalli, E. Neuropsychiatric symptoms in dementia-frequency, relationship to dementia severity and comparison in Alzheimer's disease, vascular dementia and frontotemporal dementia. *J. Neurol. Sci.* **2005**, *236*, 43–48. [CrossRef]
41. Levy, M.L.; Miller, B.L.; Cummings, J.L.; Fairbanks, L.A.; Craig, A. Alzheimer disease and frontotemporal dementias. Behavioral distinctions. *Arch. Neurol.* **1996**, *53*, 687–690. [CrossRef]
42. Warren, J.D.; Rohrer, J.D.; Rossor, M.N. Clinical review. Frontotemporal dementia. *BMJ* **2013**, *347*, f4827. [CrossRef]
43. Kazui, H.; Yoshiyama, K.; Kanemoto, H.; Suzuki, Y.; Sato, S.; Hashimoto, M.; Ikeda, M.; Tanaka, H.; Hatada, Y.; Matsushita, M.; et al. Differences of behavioral and psychological symptoms of dementia in disease severity in four major dementias. *PLoS ONE* **2016**, *11*, e0161092. [CrossRef]
44. McKeith, I.G.; Boeve, B.F.; Dickson, D.W.; Halliday, G.; Taylor, J.P.; Weintraub, D.; Aarsland, D.; Galvin, J.; Attems, J.; Ballard, C.G.; et al. Diagnosis and management of dementia with Lewy bodies: Fourth consensus report of the DLB Consortium. *Neurology* **2017**, *89*, 88–100. [CrossRef]
45. Ballard, C.; Neill, D.; O'Brien, J.; McKeith, I.G.; Ince, P.; Perry, R. Anxiety, depression and psychosis in vascular dementia: Prevalence and associations. *J. Affect. Disord.* **2000**, *59*, 97–106. [CrossRef]
46. Zamboni, G.; Huey, E.D.; Krueger, F.; Nichelli, P.F.; Grafman, J. Apathy and disinhibition in frontotemporal dementia: Insights into their neural correlates. *Neurology* **2008**, *71*, 736–742. [CrossRef] [PubMed]

47. Starkstein, S.E.; Migliorelli, R.; Manes, F.; Teson, A.; Petracca, G.; Chemerinski, E.; Sabe, L.; Leiguarda, R. The prevalence and clinical correlates of apathy and irritability in Alzheimer's disease. *Eur. J. Neurol.* **1995**, *2*, 540–546. [CrossRef] [PubMed]
48. Tanaka, H.; Hashimoto, M.; Fukuhara, R.; Ishikawa, T.; Yatabe, Y.; Kaneda, K.; Yuuki, S.; Honda, K.; Matsuzaki, S.; Tsuyuguchi, A.; et al. Relationship between dementia severity and behavioural and psychological symptoms in early-onset Alzheimer's disease. *Psychogeriatrics* **2015**, *15*, 242–247. [CrossRef]
49. Nobis, L.; Husain, M. Apathy in Alzheimer's disease. *Curr. Opin. Behav. Sci.* **2018**, *22*, 7–13. [CrossRef]
50. Yue, Y.; Yuan, Y.; Hou, Z.; Jiang, W.; Bai, F.; Zhang, Z. Abnormal functional connectivity of amygdala in late-onset depression was associated with cognitive deficits. *PLoS ONE* **2013**, *8*, e75058. [CrossRef]
51. Guo, Z.; Liu, X.; Hou, H.; Wei, F.; Liu, J.; Chen, X. Abnormal degree centrality in Alzheimer's disease patients with depression: A resting-state functional magnetic resonance imaging study. *Exp. Gerontol.* **2016**, *79*, 61–66. [CrossRef]
52. Stapleton, M. Effectiveness of animal assisted therapy after brain injury: A bridge to improved outcomes in CRT. *NeuroRehabilitation* **2016**, *39*, 135–140. [CrossRef]
53. Hurt, C.; Bhattacharyya, S.; Burns, A.; Camus, V.; Liperoti, R.; Marriott, A.; Nobili, F.; Robert, P.; Tsolaki, M.; Vellas, B.; et al. Patient and caregiver perspectives of quality of life in dementia. An investigation of the relationship to behavioural and psychological symptoms in dementia. *Dement. Geriatr. Cogn. Disord.* **2008**, *26*, 138–146. [CrossRef]
54. Ownby, R.L.; Crocco, E.; Acevedo, A.; John, V.; Loewenstein, D. Depression and risk for Alzheimer disease: Systematic review, meta-analysis, and metaregression analysis. *Arch. Gen. Psychiatry* **2006**, *63*, 530–538. [CrossRef]
55. Rapp, M.A.; Schnaider-Beeri, M.; Grossman, H.T.; Sano, M.; Perl, D.P.; Purohit, D.P.; Gorman, J.M.; Haroutunian, V. Increased hippocampal plaques and tangles in patients with Alzheimer disease with a lifetime history of major depression. *Arch. Gen. Psychiatry* **2006**, *63*, 161–167. [CrossRef] [PubMed]
56. Palmer, K.; Berger, A.K.; Monastero, R.; Winblad, B.; Backman, L.; Fratiglioni, L. Predictors of progression from mild cognitive impairment to Alzheimer disease. *Neurology* **2007**, *68*, 1596–1602. [CrossRef] [PubMed]
57. Kitching, D. Depression in dementia. *Aust. Prescr.* **2015**, *38*, 209–211. [CrossRef] [PubMed]
58. Kwak, Y.T.; Yang, Y.; Koo, M.S. Anxiety in dementia. *Dement. Neurocogn. Disord.* **2017**, *16*, 33–39. [CrossRef]
59. Rapp, M.A.; Schnaider-Beeri, M.; Purohit, D.P.; Perl, D.P.; Haroutunian, V.; Sano, M. Increased neurofibrillary tangles in patients with Alzheimer disease with comorbid depression. *Am. J. Geriatr. Psychiatry* **2008**, *16*, 168–174. [CrossRef]
60. Ooms, S.; Ju, Y.E. Treatment of sleep disorders in dementia. *Curr. Treat. Options Neurol.* **2016**, *18*, 40. [CrossRef]
61. Shokri-Kojori, E.; Wang, G.J.; Wiers, C.E.; Demiral, S.B.; Guo, M.; Kim, S.W.; Lindgren, E.; Ramirez, V.; Zehra, A.; Freeman, C.; et al. beta-Amyloid accumulation in the human brain after one night of sleep deprivation. *Proc. Natl. Acad. Sci. USA* **2018**, *115*, 4483–4488. [CrossRef]
62. Cordone, S.; Annarumma, L.; Rossini, P.M.; De Gennaro, L. Sleep and beta-Amyloid deposition in Alzheimer disease: Insights on mechanisms and possible innovative treatments. *Front. Pharmacol.* **2019**, *10*, 695. [CrossRef]
63. Irwin, M.R.; Vitiello, M.V. Implications of sleep disturbance and inflammation for Alzheimer's disease dementia. *Lancet Neurol.* **2019**, *18*, 296–306. [CrossRef]
64. Petersson, M.; Uvnas-Moberg, K.; Nilsson, A.; Gustafson, L.L.; Hydbring-Sandberg, E.; Handlin, L. Oxytocin and cortisol levels in dog owners and their dogs are associated with behavioral patterns: An exploratory study. *Front. Psychol.* **2017**, *8*, 1796. [CrossRef] [PubMed]
65. Nagasawa, M.; Kikusui, T.; Onaka, T.; Ohta, M. Dog's gaze at its owner increases owner's urinary oxytocin during social interaction. *Horm. Behav.* **2009**, *55*, 434–441. [CrossRef] [PubMed]
66. Jesso, S.; Morlog, D.; Ross, S.; Pell, M.D.; Pasternak, S.H.; Mitchell, D.G.; Kertesz, A.; Finger, E.C. The effects of oxytocin on social cognition and behaviour in frontotemporal dementia. *Brain* **2011**, *134*, 2493–2501. [CrossRef]
67. McQuaid, R.J.; McInnis, O.A.; Abizaid, A.; Anisman, H. Making room for oxytocin in understanding depression. *Neurosci. Biobehav. Rev.* **2014**, *45*, 305–322. [CrossRef]

68. Handlin, L.; Hydbring-Sandberg, E.; Nilsson, A.; Ejdebäck, M.; Jansson, A.; Uvnäs-Moberg, K. Short-term interaction between dogs and their owners: effects on oxytocin, cortisol, insulin and heart rate—An exploratory study. *Anthrozoös* **2011**, *24*, 301–315. [CrossRef]
69. Ouanes, S.; Popp, J. High cortisol and the risk of dementia and Alzheimer's Disease: A review of the literature. *Front. Aging Neurosci.* **2019**, *11*, 43. [CrossRef] [PubMed]
70. Cacioppo, J.T.; Hawkley, L.C.; Thisted, R.A. Perceived social isolation makes me sad: 5-year cross-lagged analyses of loneliness and depressive symptomatology in the Chicago Health, Aging, and Social Relations Study. *Psychol. Aging* **2010**, *25*, 453–463. [CrossRef]
71. Donovan, N.J.; Okereke, O.I.; Vannini, P.; Amariglio, R.E.; Rentz, D.M.; Marshall, G.A.; Johnson, K.A.; Sperling, R.A. Association of higher cortical amyloid burden with loneliness in cognitively normal older adults. *JAMA Psychiatry* **2016**, *73*, 1230–1237. [CrossRef]
72. Scarmeas, N.; Stern, Y. Cognitive reserve and lifestyle. *J. Clin. Exp. Neuropsychol.* **2003**, *25*, 625–633. [CrossRef]
73. Banks, M.R.; Banks, W.A. The effects of animal-assisted therapy on loneliness in an elderly population in long-term care facilities. *J. Gerontol. A Biol. Sci. Med. Sci.* **2002**, *57*, M428–M432. [CrossRef]
74. Devanand, D.P.; Pradhaban, G.; Liu, X.; Khandji, A.; De Santi, S.; Segal, S.; Rusinek, H.; Pelton, G.H.; Honig, L.S.; Mayeux, R.; et al. Hippocampal and entorhinal atrophy in mild cognitive impairment: Prediction of Alzheimer disease. *Neurology* **2007**, *68*, 828–836. [CrossRef]
75. Cuenod, C.A.; Denys, A.; Michot, J.L.; Jehenson, P.; Forette, F.; Kaplan, D.; Syrota, A.; Boller, F. Amygdala atrophy in Alzheimer's disease. An in vivo magnetic resonance imaging study. *Arch. Neurol.* **1993**, *50*, 941–945. [CrossRef] [PubMed]
76. De la Monte, S.M. Quantitation of cerebral atrophy in preclinical and end-stage Alzheimer's disease. *Ann. Neurol.* **1989**, *25*, 450–459. [CrossRef] [PubMed]
77. Campbell, S.; Macqueen, G. The role of the hippocampus in the pathophysiology of major depression. *J. Psychiatry Neurosci.* **2004**, *29*, 417–426. [PubMed]
78. Busch, C.; Tucha, L.; Talarovicova, A.; Fuermaier, A.B.M.; Lewis-Evans, B.; Tucha, O. Animal-assisted interventions for children with attention deficit/hyperactivity disorder: A theoretical review and consideration of future research directions. *Psychol. Rep.* **2016**, *118*, 292–331. [CrossRef] [PubMed]
79. Kim, S.Y.; Park, J.E.; Seo, H.J.; Seo, H.S.; Son, H.J.; Sim, C.M.; Lee, Y.J.; Jang, B.H.; Heo, D.S. *NECA's Guidance for Undertaking Systematic Reviews and Meta-Analyses for Intervention*; National Evidence-Based Healthcare Collaborating Agency: Seoul, Korea, 2011; Volume 25.
80. Borenstein, M.; Hedges, L.V.; Higgins, J.P.; Rothstein, H.R. Overview. In *Introduction to Meta-Analysis*; John Wiley & Sons: Hoboken, NJ, USA, 2009; Chapter 15; pp. 103–106. [CrossRef]
81. Cohen, J. *Statistical Power Analysis for the Behavioral Sciences*; L. Erlbaum Associates: Hillsdale, NJ, USA, 1988.
82. Cochran, W.G. Some Methods for Strengthening the Common χ^2 Tests. *Bioethics* **1954**. [CrossRef]
83. Furberg, C.D.; Morgan, T.M. Lessons from overviews of cardiovascular trials. *Stat. Med.* **1987**, *6*, 295–306. [CrossRef]
84. Rosenthal, R.; Rubin, D.B. Comparing effect sizes of independent studies. *Psychol. Bull.* **1982**, *92*, 500–504. [CrossRef]

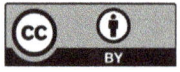

© 2020 by the authors. Licensee MDPI, Basel, Switzerland. This article is an open access article distributed under the terms and conditions of the Creative Commons Attribution (CC BY) license (http://creativecommons.org/licenses/by/4.0/).

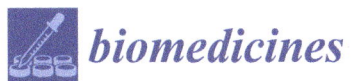

Article

The Role of GPR120 Receptor in Essential Fatty Acids Metabolism in Schizophrenia

Joanna Rog [1,*], Anna Błażewicz [2], Dariusz Juchnowicz [3], Agnieszka Ludwiczuk [4], Ewa Stelmach [5], Małgorzata Kozioł [6], Michal Karakula [7], Przemysław Niziński [2] and Hanna Karakula-Juchnowicz [1,8]

1. 1st Department of Psychiatry, Psychotherapy and Early Intervention, Medical University of Lublin, 20-439 Lublin, Poland; hanna.karakula-juchnowicz@umlub.pl
2. Chair of Chemistry, Department of Analytical Chemistry, Medical University of Lublin, 20-093 Lublin, Poland; anna.blazewicz@umlub.pl (A.B.); pnizinski11@gmail.com (P.N.)
3. Department of Psychiatric Nursing, Medical University of Lublin, 20-093 Lublin, Poland; juchnowiczdariusz@wp.pl
4. Independent Laboratory of Natural Products Chemistry, Department of Pharmacognosy, Medical University of Lublin, 20-093 Lublin, Poland; agnieszka.ludwiczuk@umlub.pl
5. 2nd Department of Psychiatry and Psychiatric Rehabilitation, Medical University of Lublin, 20-439 Lublin, Poland; ewastelmach@umlub.pl
6. Chair and Department of Medical Microbiology, Medical University of Lublin; 20-093 Lublin, Poland; malgorzata.koziol@umlub.pl
7. Student Research Team from Department of Analytical Chemistry, Medical University of Lublin, 20-093 Lublin, Poland; michal.karakula@gmail.com
8. Department of Clinical Neuropsychiatry, Medical University of Lublin, 20-439 Lublin, Poland
* Correspondence: rog.joann@gmail.com

Received: 12 June 2020; Accepted: 21 July 2020; Published: 24 July 2020

Abstract: A growing body of evidence confirms abnormal fatty acid (FAs) metabolism in the pathophysiology of schizophrenia. Omega-3 polyunsaturated fatty acids (PUFAs) are endogenous ligands of the G protein-coupled receptors, which have anti-inflammatory properties and are a therapeutic target in many diseases. No clinical studies are concerned with the role of the GPR120 signaling pathway in schizophrenia. The aim of the study was to determine the differences in PUFA nutritional status and metabolism between patients with schizophrenia (SZ group) and healthy individuals (HC group). The study included 80 participants (40 in the SZ group, 40 in the HC group). There were no differences in serum GPR120 and PUFA concentrations and PUFA intake between the examined groups. In the HC group, there was a relationship between FAs in serum and GPR120 concentration ($p < 0.05$): α-linolenic acid (ALA) ($R = -0.46$), docosahexaenoic acid (DHA) ($R = -0.54$), omega-3 PUFAs ($R = -0.41$), arachidonic acid (AA) ($R = -0.44$). In the SZ group, FA serum concentration was not related to GPR120 ($p > 0.05$). In the HC group, ALA and DHA serum concentrations were independently associated with GPR120 ($p < 0.05$) in the model adjusted for eicosapentaenoic acid (EPA) and accounted for 38.59% of GPR120 variability ($p < 0.05$). Our results indicate different metabolisms of FAs in schizophrenia. It is possible that the diminished anti-inflammatory response could be a component connecting GPR120 insensitivity with schizophrenia.

Keywords: G protein-coupled receptors; GPR120; FFAR4; schizophrenia; polyunsaturated fatty acids; long-chain fatty acids; omega-3; nutritional psychiatry

1. Introduction

Polyunsaturated fatty acid (PUFA) imbalance is linked with various clinical conditions, especially neuropsychiatric diseases, including schizophrenia [1]. Numerous reports confirmed that patients with schizophrenia (SZ) have lower levels of blood omega-3 fatty acids (FAs) compared with healthy individuals [2,3]. The comparison of the erythrocyte FA composition in 429 subjects with schizophrenia and 444 healthy individuals revealed that the patients had lower levels of omega-3 PUFAs fatty acids: docosahexaenoic acid (DHA, 22:6), docosapentaenoic acid (DPA, 22:5), eicosapentaenoic acid (EPA, 20:5), and an omega-6 fatty acid, arachidonic acid (AA, 20:4) [4]. The mechanism of undernutrition of PUFAs in the SZ population is still under examination. Studies indicated that several factors engage in improper FA blood concentrations, including poor nutrition, antipsychotic drug interactions with cell membranes, and disturbances of lipid metabolism, as well as fatty acid-dependent signaling pathways [2,3,5].

The clinical findings support the abnormal metabolism of FAs in SZ, reflected by attenuation of responses to the niacin skin flush test. The dermal application of aqueous methyl nicotinate (AMN) leads to redness, as well as edema of skin as a result of the cascade of inflammatory reactions mediated by phospholipase A2 (PLA2) [6,7]. PLA2 activates the release of omega-6 AA from membrane phospholipids which is related to various physiological processes connected with emotions, motivation, response to stress, and energy homeostasis, including eicosanoid biosynthetic enzymes, as well as promotion of the immune type 2 response and initiation of endocannabinoid signaling in the brain [8,9].

PLA2 activity can be modulated by a G-coupled receptor responsive to fatty acids—GPR120 (also known as an free fatty acid receptor 4: FFAR4). Omega-3 PUFAs are endogenous ligands of the receptor. FA stimulation leads to GPR120–β-arrestin-2 complex formation and contributes to anti-inflammatory signaling pathway activation [10]. GPR120 is a therapeutic target in many diseases, especially diabetes and other inflammatory conditions [11]. Taking into account lipid disturbances in schizophrenia and the mechanistic and genetic connection between schizophrenia and inflammatory disorders, GPR120 could also be a promising target in this condition [12]. An animal study showed that receptor activation in the microglia of the hypothalamus reduces neuroinflammation via a decrease in pro-inflammatory cytokine synthesis [13]. However, little is known about GPR120 in psychiatric disorders. To our best knowledge, no clinical studies are concerned about the role GPR120 signaling together with FA metabolism in schizophrenia.

The aim of the study was to determine the differences in PUFAs nutritional status and metabolism between patients with schizophrenia and healthy individuals. More specifically, we examined and compared serum concentrations of GPR120, polyunsaturated fatty acids (omega-6: AA, omega-3: DHA, EPA, α-linolenic acid (ALA)) and dietary intake of omega-3 and omega-6 FAs (omega-6: LA—linolenic acid (precursor of AA)), omega-3: DHA, EPA, ALA) between patients and healthy individuals. The secondary aim was to find a relationship between PUFA metabolism and clinical/sociodemographic variables in the examined population.

2. Materials and Methods

2.1. Study Participants

The age of eligible participants ranged between 18 and 65. Forty outpatients suffering from schizophrenia (SZ group) according to the Diagnostic and Statistical Manual of Mental Disorders (DSM-5) criteria [14] were recruited in the study. Out of them, 95% were treated with antipsychotic medication. Forty healthy volunteers matched for age and body mass index (BMI) were enrolled in the study, as the control (HC group). Participants from the HC group had no psychiatric, inflammatory-related, metabolic disorders, or other health problems which in the examiner's opinion could have affected FA metabolism, while they were also not taking any medication. Neither group followed any specific diet within the six months prior to the examination. Before entering the study, all subjects gave their informed consent to participate. The study was conducted in accordance with the Declaration of Helsinki [15], and the protocol was approved by the Ethics Committee of Medical University of Lublin, Poland (Project identification code: KE-0254/127/2016, 28 April 2016).

2.2. Blood Collection

Venous blood (10 mL) samples were collected after overnight fasting using S-Monovette® 4.9 mL and a Clotting Activator/Serum blood collection system (Sarstedt, Nümbrecht, Germany). Serum was obtained by centrifugation (at 2000× g, 10 min) and stored at −80 °C for later analyses (but no longer than a six-month period). No hemolysis was observed in any of the samples.

2.3. Fatty Acids Assay

Serum samples were thawed and a mixture of chloroform/methanol (2:1 v/v) was added to a 50-µL aliquot. Samples were flushed with nitrogen gas and stored at 4 °C. The next step was to perform double extraction. After drying, lipids (in lower phase) were saponified (using a mixture of KOH and methanol) and subsequently methylated by boron trifluoride (14%). The analysis was carried out using gas chromatography–mass spectrometry (GC/MS) (Shimadzu GC-2010 PLUS gas chromatograph coupled to a Shimadzu QP2010 Ultra mass spectrometer (Shim-pol, Warsaw, Poland)). Compounds were separated on a fused-silica capillary column SP™-2560 (100 m, 0.25 mm inner diameter (i.d.)) with a film thickness of 0.20 mm (Supelco, Darmstadt, Germany). The injection volume was 1.0 µL, and the temperature of the injection port was 230 °C with a split ratio of 1:20, while helium was used as a carrier gas; the temperature program was 70 °C/2 min, 175 °C/25 min, and 200 °C/17 min. As done by other authors, non-endogenous C17:0 free fatty acid (5 µg of 1 mg/mL stock) was used as an internal standard [16].

2.4. GPR120 Assay

GPR120 serum concentration was assessed using a commercially available kit (O3FAR1 ELISA Kit, EIAab, Gentaur Poland, Sopot, Poland) according to the manufacturer's instruction. The sensitivity of the test was 0.097 ng/mL. The number of studies focusing on membrane proteins in serum is still limited. Nevertheless, this type of analysis has the potential to diagnose and/or treat diseases in further clinical practice [17].

2.5. Dietary Assessment

The intake of FAs was assessed during a face-to-face interview by a registered dietitian (J.R.) using the 24 h recall method referring to the day prior blood collection. The nutritional value of the diet was determined using nutrition analysis software (ESHA Food Processor SQL, version 10.1.1; ESHA, Salem, OR, USA) with additional Polish Food composition tables (the standard reference food composition database of nutrients in foods and dishes commonly consumed in Poland) [18].

2.6. Sociodemographic and Clinical Data

All participants answered questions via a structural interview. The self-created questionnaire was always filled out by the same person. The clinical data of patients were obtained from a supervising physician. The questionnaire was composed of the following parts: sociodemographic/anthropometric information, lifestyle (including dietary habits), medical data (in case of patients, including duration of illness, number of hospitalizations, using medication).

2.7. The Severity of Schizophrenia Symptoms Assessment

The severity of schizophrenia symptoms was assessed using the Polish adaptation of the Positive and Negative Symptom Scale (PANSS) by a well-trained physician [E.S] [19]. The examination was always performed on the same day assessing other variables.

2.8. Statistical Analysis

Statistical analyses were conducted using Statistica software (TIBCO Software Inc., Palo Alto, CA, USA). The Shapiro–Wilk test was performed to explore variable distribution. To determine differences between groups, a chi-square test for categorical variables and a Mann–Whitney U-test for continuous variables were used. To determine the magnitude and direction of the correlation between examined variables, Spearman's rho correlation was used. The multiple-step regression analysis was carried out to explain the variability in GPR120 concentration depending on the nutritional status or sociodemographic data. For all analyses, a value of $p < 0.05$ was considered statistically significant. When multiple statistical tests were performed, Bonferroni correction was applied [20].

3. Results

3.1. Study Participant Characteristics

The sociodemographic and clinical characteristics of the examined group are presented in Table 1. The study included 40 individuals with schizophrenia (SZ group; mean age: 31 years old; 52.5% males) and 40 healthy volunteers as the control (HC group) (mean age: 29 years old; 37.5% males). There were no significant differences between the clinical and control groups in age, gender, and body mass index (BMI) ($p > 0.05$). The median of illness duration was 78 months, and the number of hospitalizations was two. In total, 95% of patients were taking antipsychotic medication. Most of the SZ group was treated with second-generation antipsychotic drugs ($n = 36$; 90%). Other patients ($n = 2$; 5%) received first-generation antipsychotic drugs, one of them together with an anticonvulsant drug. In total, five persons (12.5%) received first-generation treatment, 13 (32.5%) individuals took anticonvulsant medications, and six individuals (15%) received selective serotonin reuptake inhibitors (SSRIs). Two patients (5%) received benzodiazepines. Furthermore, 5% ($n = 2$) of the SZ group was antipsychotic-free due to medication nonadherence. The median modal doses of antipsychotic medication treatment were 15 mg of olanzapine equivalent [21]. The average severity of schizophrenia symptoms measured with the Positive and Negative Symptom Scale (PANSS) scale was 54 points (median) (a maximum score of 210 points).

Table 1. The characteristics of studied population.

Clinical Data	Schizophrenia ($n = 40$)		Healthy Controls ($n = 40$)		SZ vs. HC
	Mean (Median)	SD	Mean (Median)	SD	
Age	31 (30)	7.32	29 (27)	7.93	NS
BMI (kg/m^2)	26.6 (26.6)	5.12	24.6 (24.2)	4.39	NS
Duration of illness (months)	90 (78)	83.43	NA	NA	NA
Number of hospitalization	2.7 (2)	2.25	NA	NA	NA
Olanzapine equivalents	18.12 (15)	13.93	NA	NA	NA
PANSS total	55.35 (54)	26.71	NA	NA	NA

PANSS—Positive and Negative Symptom Scale; SZ—schizophrenia; HC—healthy control; BMI—body mass index; SD—standard deviation; NA—not applicable; NS—not significant. The Mann–Whitney U-test was used.

3.2. Nutritional Status and Metabolism of PUFAs

Table 2 shows the FA and GPR120 concentrations in SZ and HC groups. There were no significant differences in the concentrations of AA, ALA, EPA, DHA, total omega-3, PUFAs, and GPR120 between patients and the control group.

As it was shown in Table 2, the examined groups had a similar intake of total fat, as well as omega-3 and omega-6 PUFAs. The mean intake of EPA + DHA was 88.17 mg and 34.86 mg in the SZ and HC groups, respectively, and the same number of participants from both groups (97.5%) had an intake of omega-3 FAs below the recommended daily intake (RDA; 250 mg) [22].

Table 2. The nutritional fatty acid status and metabolism.

	Schizophrenia (n = 40)		Healthy Controls (n = 40)		SZ vs. HC
	Mean (Median)	SD	Mean (Median)	SD	
Serum Measurement					
ALA (mcg/mL)	1.61 (1.16)	1.74	0.91 (0.67)	0.93	NS
EPA (mcg/mL)	2.03 (1.37)	2.45	1.45 (1.38)	0.89	NS
DHA (mcg/mL)	6.88 (6.81)	2.26	6.80 (6.41)	1.91	NS
AA (mcg/mL)	19.63 (19.48)	4.10	19.92 (19.36)	3.75	NS
PUFAs (mcg/mL)	29.80 (28.61)	7.62	28.57 (27.19)	5.76	NS
Omega-3 (mcg/mL)	10.18 (10.05)	4.50	8.65 (8.34)	3.27	NS
Omega-3/6 ratio [1]	0.52 (0.50)	0.20	0.44 (0.45)	0.18	NS
GPR120 (ng/mL)	2.41 (1.24)	2.72	2.00 (1.02)	2.32	NS
Dietary Assessment					
Fat (g)	81.11 (78.63)	34.65	85.62 (80.26)	39.04	NS
PUFAs (g)	14.01 (10.69)	8.20	12.33 (10.84)	6.22	NS
Omega-3 (g)	2.33 (1.42)	2.78	1.87 (1.66)	1.04	NS
Omega-6 (g)	11.67 (9.35)	7.25	10.45 (9.40)	5.56	NS
18:2 LA (g)	11.55 (9.23)	7.24	10.34 (9.35)	5.51	NS
20:5 EPA (mg)	35.45 (0)	187.63	6.21 (0)	17.54	NS
22:6 DHA (mg)	52.72 (10)	177.18	28.65 (10)	71.07	NS

[1] Expressed as a (DHA + EPA + ALA)/AA concentration; PUFAs—polyunsaturated fatty acids; ALA—α-linolenic acid; EPA—eicosapentaenoic acid; DHA—docosahexaenoic acid; AA—arachidonic acid; GPR120—G protein-coupled receptor 120; LA—linolenic acid; SZ—schizophrenia; HC—healthy control; SD—standard deviation; NS—not significant. The Mann–Whitney U-test was used.

3.3. Effect of Nutritional Status on PUFA Metabolism

In the HC group, there was a relationship between FAs in serum and GPR120 concentration. ALA ($R = -0.46$; $p < 0.05$), AA ($R = -0.44$; $p < 0.05$), DHA ($R = -0.54$, $p < 0.05$), and omega-3 FA ($R = -0.41$; $p < 0.05$) concentrations were inversely associated with GPR120. In the SZ group, FA serum concentration was not related to GPR120 ($p > 0.05$) (see Table 3, and Figure 1). The revealed relationships were not significant after Bonferroni correction for multiple comparisons ($p > 0.0083$).

In the patient group, there were only positive relationships between EPA intake and serum FA concentration: ALA ($R = 0.46$; $p < 0.05$), AA, ($R = 0.44$; $p < 0.05$), DHA ($R = 0.46$; $p < 0.05$), and omega-3/omega-6 PUFA ratio ($R = 0.35$; $p < 0.05$) (see Table 4).

There were various correlations between FA intake and their concentration in serum in the HC group (see Figure 2). The serum concentration of DHA was positively associated with the intake of PUFAs (total amount) ($R = 0.40$; $p < 0.05$), LA ($R = 0.40$; $p < 0.05$), and omega-6 PUFAs ($R = 0.39$; $p < 0.05$) (see Table 4). A higher intake of DHA was associated with a lower serum concentration of ALA ($R = -0.34$; $p < 0.05$).

However, the relationships were not significant after Bonferroni correction for multiple comparisons ($p > 0.0017$).

Table 3. The relationship between GPR120 and PUFA serum concentration.

GPR120	ALA	EPA	DHA	AA	Omega-3	Omega-3/6 Ratio [1]
Healthy controls	−0.46 *	NS	−0.54 *	−0.44 *	−0.41 *	NS
Schizophrenia	NS	NS	NS	NS	NS	NS

[1] Expressed as a (DHA + EPA + ALA)/AA concentration; * $p < 0.05$; NS—not significant. Spearman's rank correlation coefficient was calculated.

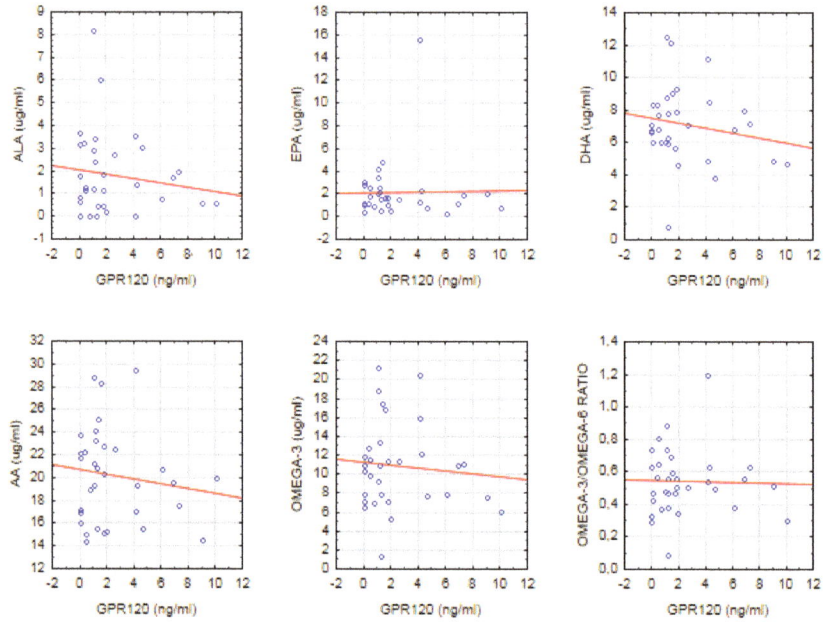

Figure 1. The scatter plot of the relationship between GPR120 and PUFA serum concentration in the SZ group. Spearman's rank correlation coefficient was calculated.

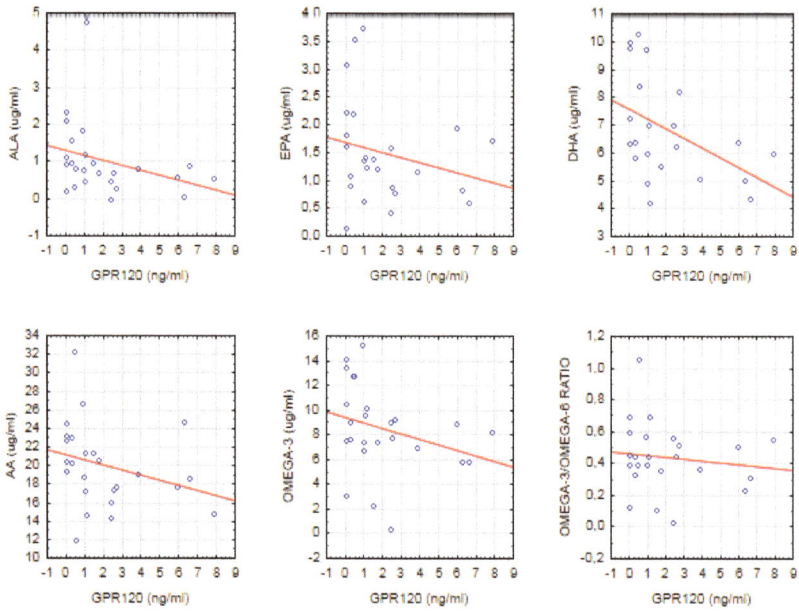

Figure 2. The scatter plot of the relationship between GPR120 and PUFA serum concentration in the HC group. Spearman's rank correlation coefficient was calculated.

Table 4. Relationship between PUFA intake and their metabolism.

Diet \ Blood	ALA	EPA	DHA	AA	Omega-3/6 Ratio [1]	GPR120
SZ group						
20:5 EPA	0.46 *	NS	0.46 *	0.44 *	0.35 *	NS
HC group						
PUFAs	NS	NS	0.40 *	NS	NS	NS
Omega-6	NS	NS	0.39 *	NS	NS	NS
18:2 LA	NS	NS	0.40 *	NS	NS	NS
22:6 DHA	−0.34 *	NS	NS	NS	NS	NS

[1] Expressed as a (DHA + EPA + ALA)/AA concentration; * $p < 0.05$; NS—not significant. Spearman's rank correlation coefficient was calculated.

3.4. Effect of Demographic and Clinical Variables on PUFAs Nutritional Status

In the SZ group, there was a positive correlation between DHA intake and BMI ($R = 0.39$; $p < 0.05$), as well as between duration of illness and BMI ($R = 0.38$; $p < 0.05$). We did not find a relationship between schizophrenia symptoms (measured with PANSS) or clinical data and FA nutritional status or metabolism.

In the HC group, there was a positive relationship between AA serum concentration and age ($R = 0.36$; $p < 0.05$) and BMI ($R = 0.44$; $p < 0.05$), between EPA concentration and BMI ($R = 0.33$; $p < 0.05$), and between DHA concentration and age ($R = 0.41$; $p < 0.05$). There was also an inverse relationship between GPR120 serum concentration and age ($R = −0.50$; $p < 0.05$) and between intake of EPA and age ($R = −0.45$; $p < 0.05$), as well as a positive relationship between intake of LA and BMI ($R = 0.44$; $p < 0.05$) and between intake of total PUFAs and BMI ($R = 0.40$; $p < 0.05$).

3.5. GPR120 Serum Concentration Variability

To further determine the independent predictors of GPR120 serum concentration using a multiple regression model, the following explanatory variables were used: age, BMI, and serum concentration of ALA, AA, EPA, and DHA. In the patient group, there were no relationships between GPR120 concentration and other variables ($p > 0.05$). In the HC group, ALA and DHA serum concentration were independently associated with GPR120 ($p < 0.05$) in a model adjusted for EPA concentration. The model explained 38.59% of GPR120 serum concentration variability. The estimated relationship was not statistically significant after Bonferroni correction ($p > 0.0167$).

4. Discussion

An increasing amount of evidence confirms the role of abnormal lipid metabolism in the pathobiology and clinical course of schizophrenia [2–4]. Despite the fact that research concerning fatty acid metabolism is going on for a long time, there is an insufficient amount of evidence to determine the mechanism and all pathways engaged in lipid disturbances related to schizophrenia [23]. Differences in PUFA levels between patients suffering from schizophrenia and healthy individuals were also reported [4]. Until now there are no guidelines for the routine assessment of serum FA levels or concentrations in patients with psychiatric illness.

In our study, there were no differences in GPR120 levels between patients and healthy individuals. Nevertheless, the negative relationship between GPR120 serum concentration and DHA and ALA concentration was detected only among healthy individuals. We did not find any correlation between GPR120 receptor concentration and FA serum concentration in the SZ group. This phenomenon suggests that patients suffering from schizophrenia may manifest a GPR120 insensitivity with activation becoming impossible (see Figure 3). The revealed relationships were found to be insignificant after Bonferroni correction for multiple comparisons. To some extent, the small sample size could have also affected the lack of relationship after performing multiple comparisons. Further studies with a larger sample size are required.

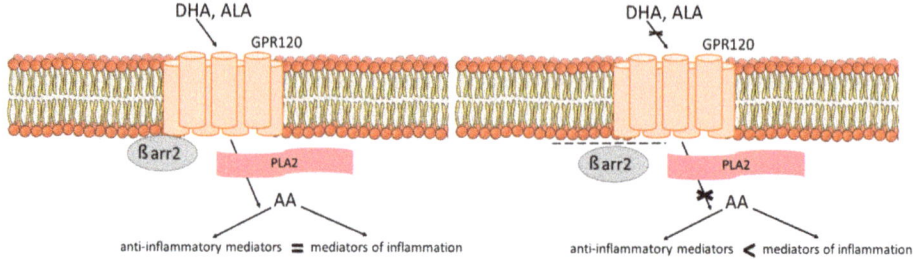

Figure 3. The proposed mechanism of the connection between GPR120 insensitivity and impaired lipid metabolism in schizophrenia. In healthy individuals, GPR120 activation leads to anti-inflammatory effects. Natural ligands (DHA and ALA) stimulate GPR120–β-arrestin complex formation and drive phospholipase A2 (PLA2) activation. Pro-/anti-inflammatory homeostasis is maintained. In schizophrenia patients, GPR120 insensitivity leads to pro/anti-inflammatory imbalance. Natural ligands (DHA and ALA) are unable to stimulate GPR120–β-arrestin complex formation. Overactivity of PLA2 causes a switch to inflammatory pathway stimulation. Pro-/anti-inflammatory homeostasis is disturbed.

It is still unclear whether GPR120 concentration in the serum reflects the expression of the receptor and cell signaling. We decided to examine the serum concentration of GPR120 for some reasons. Firstly, this type of sample is more stable during storage in low temperatures compared to RNA [24]. Gene testing is essential to confirm the results of our study. Introducing serum sample collection in clinical practice from a population health perspective is more convenient and accessible compared to RNA samples. Thus, serum samples may be a more favorable material used as a biomarker of fatty acid metabolism disturbances in further clinical practice [17,25].

In a population of children, lower GPR120 plasma levels were associated with negative outcomes, i.e., insulin resistance and higher BMI [26]. In our study, we did not find any relationship between BMI and GPR120, and lower GPR120 serum concentration was related to the higher concentration of PUFAs in the HC group. It is possible that a higher concentration of PUFAs in serum increases anti-inflammatory status, and GPR120 activation (to restore balance) is not required. On the other hand, an activated GPR120 forms a complex with β-arrestin, which may lead to a reduction in free GPR120 blood concentration [10].

The mechanism linked with GPR120 disruption in schizophrenia may be related to PLA2 activity. According to Horrobin's theory of schizophrenia, PLA2 excess activity is linked with an abnormal skin reaction in the niacin test in schizophrenia patients [27]. PUFAs are able to activate PLA2 via the GPR120 receptor, leading to the production of prostaglandin. This pathway is involved in the anti-inflammatory DHA effects in macrophages [28].

GPR120 activation mediates downstream signaling mechanisms and prevents the expression of proinflammatory cytokines. Thus, GPR120 has the potential to diminish systemic inflammation and manage metabolic functions [10,12]. There is a suggestion that several beneficial effects of omega-3 do not require GPR120. However, GPR120 function is essential to regulate vascular inflammation and neointimal hyperplasia [29]. Disruption of the anti-inflammatory GPR120-related pathway could affect the persistent proinflammatory state in schizophrenia and may be involved in a higher risk of cardiometabolic conditions in the psychiatric population [30]. However, GPR120 participation in dyslipidemia observed in schizophrenia patients remains unclear.

Clinical trials showed the ability of omega-3 PUFAs to reduce clinical symptoms of schizophrenia [31,32]. We did not find any differences in PUFA concentration and intake between schizophrenia patients and healthy individuals. The pharmacological treatment of schizophrenia increases the sterol regulatory element-binding protein type 1 (SREBP1) which regulates the expression of genes related to fatty acid synthesis [33]. This phenomenon to a certain degree may explain the lack of difference in serum FAs between SZ and HC groups. Antipsychotic medication increases the expression and activity of enzymes involved in PUFA metabolism, and changes in the blood plasma lipidome are suggested as a treatment response in psychiatric disorders [5]. On the other hand, in our study, the nutritional assessment concerned short-term omega-3 intake. This short period of dietary habit analysis was performed due to the evaluation of serum as a biomarker of PUFAs. We hypothesize that the severity of symptoms will be more linked to long-term omega-3 intake. However, in patients suffering from schizophrenia, especially those who experienced psychotic symptoms recently, examining long-term intake will be a challenge. People with schizophrenia commonly experience cognitive impairment, lack of motivation, and poor compliance; thus, misreporting could be expected, especially regarding long-term food intake assessment [34,35].

Adequate intake of omega-3 fatty acids plays an important role in maintaining mental health. DHA and EPA are structurally integrated via phospholipid molecules and they ensure the proper structure of neuronal cell membranes [3]. FAs regulate the expression of genes, as well as changes in protein concentration, which could be blocked to some extent in SZ patients [36].

Each omega-3 PUFA has various molecular effects, and EPA levels are several hundred-fold lower than DHA levels [37]. Studies confirmed the anti-inflammatory potential of DHA. However, DHA formulas did not improve schizophrenia symptoms, which suggest an abnormal or lack of response to its supplementation [38]. GPR120 insensitivity and changes in FAs metabolism could, to some extent, explain the better efficacy of EPA in SZ. In our study, we found numerous correlations between the intake of EPA and the concentration of blood PUFAs in patients, which we did not notice in the HC group. These findings may be the result of a different utilization of FAs in metabolic pathways.

Increasing ALA while simultaneously decreasing LA intake is effective in improving omega-3 PUFA status [39]. The scientific community suggests that the dietary ratio of omega-6/omega-3 PUFAs should be from 2:1 to 4:1; however, in the Western diet, the ratio ranges from 15:1 to 17:1 [39]. In our study, 85% of patients and 80% of healthy individuals had a ratio higher than 4:1, and the median ratio was 6.23:1 in the SZ group and 5.23:1 in the HC group. Taking into consideration the variation PUFA metabolism between patients and healthy subjects, it is possible that individuals with psychiatric disorders require a higher intake or different proportions of omega-3/omega-6 FAs for health benefits. The different recommended intake of PUFAs in the psychiatric population should be considered [40]. No differences in the intake of PUFAs between persons with schizophrenia and healthy volunteers was revealed. Nevertheless, we found improper intake of DHA and EPA in 97.5% of the SZ group and 97.5% of the HC group.

5. Conclusions

Our consistent findings report lipid disturbances in schizophrenia patients. Interestingly, no changes in serum FAs or related markers were found. However, our results indicate different transformations and responses to FAs in schizophrenia. Based on our results, it is suggested that a diminished anti-inflammatory response could be a component connecting GPR120 insensitivity with schizophrenia. The interplay involving the inflammatory processes confirmed in psychiatric diseases, the limited ability to extinguish them, and the imbalance in PUFA diet could lead to the worsening course of schizophrenia, with increasing metabolic complication risk.

Further work should concentrate on finding lipid-based biomarkers and lipid-related interventions in patients suffering from schizophrenia. The modulation of lipid homeostasis is a promising target in managing psychiatric disorders.

6. Advantages and Limitations

The study has some potential advantages and limitations. To the best of our knowledge, this is the first work examining GPR120 protein concentration in schizophrenia and the relationship between GPR120 with PUFAs. Fatty acids were determined using a very sensitive and modern analytical technique (GC/MS) that enables accurate and precise measurements even in a very complex sample matrix such as human serum.

The study has some limitations. The sample size was relatively small and we mainly examined patients treated with antipsychotic drugs and in remission. Further studies should concentrate on lipid metabolism at a different stage of illness and include antipsychotic-naïve patients.

Another disadvantage is the dietary assessment using a single 24 h recall. Although it is considered the least biased self-report tool, three or more daily recalls are needed to determine the usual intake [41]. Through contact loss with most of the respondents, we were unable to apply multiple daily recalls.

The obtained data could be considered only as a possible explanation for the lipid disruption in SZ. An examination of gene expression involved in fatty acid metabolism, along with their variants and the main metabolites of PUFAs, is needed to confirm this hypothesis. The quality and the quantity of FAs in the erythrocyte membrane are considered more appropriate markers of the long-term nutritional status of the entire organism. Nevertheless, red blood cell FAs are more inclined to undergo deterioration during storage [42].

We included potential confounding factors related to lifestyle (BMI, age). However, taking into consideration the complexity and interactions of metabolic pathways, the examination of processes affecting the presence of substrates in blood (related to gene expression, enzyme activity) is necessary to determine the exact mechanism and importance of lipid metabolism in schizophrenia [43].

Author Contributions: Conceptualization, J.R. and H.K.-J.; methodology, J.R., A.B., D.J., A.L., and H.K.-J.; formal analysis, J.R., M.K. (Małgorzata Kozioł), M.K. (Michal Karakula) and P.N.; investigation, J.R. and E.S.; writing—original draft preparation, J.R., D.J., and H.K.-J.; writing—review and editing, J.R., A.B., D.J., and H.K.-J.; visualization, J.R. and H.K.-J.; supervision, H.K.-J. All authors have read and agreed to the published version of the manuscript.

Funding: This research was funded by the Medical University of Lublin, Lublin, Poland, grant number DS192.

Conflicts of Interest: The authors declare no conflict of interest. The funders had no role in the design of the study; in the collection, analyses, or interpretation of data; in the writing of the manuscript, or in the decision to publish the results.

Abbreviations

PUFAs	Polyunsaturated fatty acids
FAs	Fatty acids
DHA	Docosahexaenoic acid
DPA	Docosapentaenoic acid
EPA	Eicosapentaenoic acid
AA	Arachidonic acid
SZ	Schizophrenia
AMN	Aqueous methyl nicotinate
PLA2	Phospholipase A2
GPR120	G-coupled receptor responsive to fatty acids
LA	Linolenic acid
ALA	α-Linolenic acid
HC	Healthy control
BMI	Body mass index
PANSS	Positive and Negative Symptom Scale
RDA	Recommended daily intake
SREBP1	Sterol regulatory element-binding protein type 1
DSM-5	The Diagnostic and Statistical Manual of Mental Disorders
GS/MS	Gas chromatography–mass spectrometry

References

1. Clari, R.; McNamara, R.K.; Szeszko, P.R. Omega-3 Polyunsaturated Fatty Acids and Antioxidants for the Treatment of Schizophrenia: A Role for Magnetic Resonance Imaging. In *Neuroimaging in Schizophrenia*; Kubicki, M., Shenton, M.E., Eds.; Springer: Cham, Switzerland, 2020; pp. 367–383.
2. McNamara, R.K.; Almeida, D.M. Omega-3 Polyunsaturated Fatty Acid Deficiency and Progressive Neuropathology in Psychiatric Disorders: A Review of Translational Evidence and Candidate Mechanisms. *Harv. Rev. Psychiatry* **2019**, *27*, 94–107. [CrossRef]
3. Bozzatello, P.; Rocca, P.; Mantelli, E.; Bellino, S. Polyunsaturated Fatty Acids: What is Their Role in Treatment of Psychiatric Disorders? *Int. J. Mol. Sci.* **2019**, *20*, 5257. [CrossRef]
4. Van der Kemp, W.J.M.; Klomp, D.W.J.; Kahn, R.S.; Luijten, P.R.; Hulshoff, H.E.P. A meta-analysis of the polyunsaturated fatty acid composition of erythrocyte membranes in schizophrenia. *Schizophr. Res.* **2012**, *141*, 153–161. [CrossRef]
5. De Almeida, V.; Alexandrino, G.L.; Aquino, A.; Gomes, A.F.; Murgu, M.; Dobrowolny, H.; Guest, P.C.; Steiner, J.; Martins-de-Souza, D. Changes in the blood plasma lipidome associated with effective or poor response to atypical antipsychotic treatments in schizophrenia patients. *Prog. Neuro-Psychopharmacol. Biol. Psychiatry* **2020**, *101*, 109945. [CrossRef]
6. Messamore, E. The niacin response biomarker as a schizophrenia endophenotype: A status update. *Prostaglandins Leukot. Essent. Fatty Acids* **2018**, *136*, 95–97. [CrossRef] [PubMed]
7. Messamore, E.; Yao, J.K. Phospholipid, arachidonate and eicosanoid signaling in schizophrenia. *OCL* **2016**, *23*, D112. [CrossRef]
8. Mouchlis, V.D.; Dennis, E.A. Phospholipase A2 catalysis and lipid mediator lipidomics. *Biochim. Biophys. Acta BBA Mol. Cell Biol. Lipids* **2019**, *1864*, 766–771. [CrossRef]
9. Tallima, H.; El Ridi, R. Arachidonic acid: Physiological roles and potential health benefits—A review. *J. Adv. Res.* **2018**, *11*, 33–41. [CrossRef] [PubMed]
10. Milligan, G.; Alvarez-Curto, E.; Hudson, B.D.; Prihandoko, R.; Tobin, A.B. FFA4/GPR120: Pharmacology and Therapeutic Opportunities. *Trends Pharmacol. Sci.* **2017**, *38*, 809–821. [CrossRef]
11. Im, D.-S. FFA4 (GPR120) as a fatty acid sensor involved in appetite control, insulin sensitivity and inflammation regulation. *Mol. Asp. Med.* **2018**, *64*, 92–108. [CrossRef]
12. Karakuła-Juchnowicz, H.; Róg, J.; Juchnowicz, D.; Morylowska-Topolska, J. GPR120: Mechanism of action, role and potential for medical applications. *Postepy Hig. Med. Dosw.* **2017**, *71*, 942–953. [CrossRef]
13. Dragano, N.R.V.; Solon, C.; Ramalho, A.F.; de Moura, R.F.; Razolli, D.S.; Christiansen, E.; Azevedo, C.; Ulven, T.; Velloso, L.A. Polyunsaturated fatty acid receptors, GPR40 and GPR120, are expressed in the hypothalamus and control energy homeostasis and inflammation. *J. Neuroinflammation* **2017**, *14*, 91. [CrossRef]
14. American Psychiatric Association. *Diagnostic and Statistical Manual of Mental Disorders (DSM-5®)*; American Psychiatric Pub: Washington, DC, USA, 2013.
15. World Medical Association. World Medical Association Declaration of Helsinki: Ethical principles for medical research involving human subjects. *JAMA* **2013**, *310*, 2191. [CrossRef]
16. Dams, S.; Holasek, S.; Tsiountsioura, M.; Edelsbrunner, M.; Dietz, P.; Koefeler, H.; Malliga, D.-E.; Gürbüz, A.; Meier-Allard, N.; Poncza, B.; et al. Effects of a plant-based fatty acid supplement and a powdered fruit, vegetable and berry juice concentrate on omega-3-indices and serum micronutrient concentrations in healthy subjects. *Int. J. Food Sci. Nutr.* **2020**, 1–12. [CrossRef]
17. Dung, N.T.; Van Chi, P. A Survey of Membrane Proteins in Human Serum. *Proteom. Insights* **2012**, *5*, 1–19. [CrossRef]
18. Kunachowicz, H.; Nadolna, I.; Przygoda, B.; Iwanow, K. *Tables of Composition and Nutritional Value*; Food and Nutrition Institute: Warsaw, Poland, 2005; pp. 145–149.
19. Kay, S.R.; Fiszbein, A.; Opler, L.A. The Positive and Negative Syndrome Scale (PANSS) for Schizophrenia. *Schizophr. Bull.* **1987**, *13*, 261–276. [CrossRef]
20. Multiple Significance Tests: The Bonferroni Method|The BMJ. Available online: https://www.bmj.com/content/310/6973/170.short (accessed on 14 July 2020).
21. Leucht, S.; Samara, M.; Heres, S.; Davis, J.M. Dose Equivalents for Antipsychotic Drugs: The DDD Method. *Schizophr. Bull.* **2016**, *42*, S90–S94. [CrossRef]

22. Jarosz, M.; Rychlik, E.; Stoś, K.; Wierzejska, R.; Wojtasik, A.; Charzewska, J.; Mojska, H.; Szponar, L.; Sajór, I.; Kłosiewicz-Latoszek, L.; et al. *Normy żywienia dla populacji Polski*; Instytut Żywności i Żywienia: Warszawa, Poland, 2017.
23. Horrobin, D.F.; Glen, A.I.M.; Vaddadi, K. The membrane hypothesis of schizophrenia. *Schizophr. Res.* **1994**, *13*, 195–207. [CrossRef]
24. The Procurement, Storage, and Quality Assurance of Frozen Blood and Tissue Biospecimens in Pathology, Biorepository, and Biobank Settings. Abstract—Europe PMC. Available online: https://europepmc.org/article/PMC/3982909 (accessed on 17 July 2020).
25. B7-H4 Is a Novel Membrane-Bound Protein and a Candidate Serum and Tissue Biomarker for Ovarian Cancer|Cancer Research. Available online: https://cancerres.aacrjournals.org/content/66/3/1570.short (accessed on 17 July 2020).
26. Gozal, D.; Kheirandish-Gozal, L.; Carreras, A.; Khalyfa, A.; Peris, E. Obstructive sleep apnea and obesity are associated with reduced GPR120 plasma levels in children. *Sleep Med.* **2013**, *14*, e142. [CrossRef]
27. Horrobin, D.F. Fatty Acids, Phospholipids, and Schizophrenia. In *Handbook of Essential Fatty Acid Biology*; Yehuda, S., Mostofsky, D.I., Eds.; Humana Press: Totowa, NJ, USA, 1997; pp. 245–256.
28. The Fish Oil Ingredient, Docosahexaenoic Acid, Activates Cytosolic Phospholipase A2 via GPR120 Receptor to Produce Prostaglandin E2 and Plays an Anti-Inflammatory Role in Macrophages. *Immunology* **2014**, *143*, 81–95. Available online: https://onlinelibrary.wiley.com/doi/full/10.1111/imm.12296 (accessed on 23 April 2020). [CrossRef]
29. Li, X.; Ballantyne, L.L.; Che, X.; Mewburn, J.D.; Kang, J.X.; Barkley, R.M.; Murphy, R.C.; Yu, Y.; Funk, C.D. Endogenously Generated Omega-3 Fatty Acids Attenuate Vascular Inflammation and Neointimal Hyperplasia by Interaction With Free Fatty Acid Receptor 4 in Mice. *J. Am. Heart Assoc.* **2015**, *4*, e001856. [CrossRef] [PubMed]
30. Khandaker, G. Causal Associations between Inflammation, Cardiometabolic Markers and Schizophrenia: The known unknowns. *Int. J. Epidemiol.* **2019**, *48*. [CrossRef] [PubMed]
31. Omega-3 Fatty Acids in Cause, Prevention and Management of Violence in Schizophrenia: Conceptualization and Application|Elsevier Enhanced Reader. Available online: https://reader.elsevier.com/reader/sd/pii/S1359178918302064?token=0848FEFBEFB483C5BCDA97AA2A003B03AA91EE74DFB0C03D62CB53B0889C696177E1BF7FE8CBB5BBE28CC13B39F4C801 (accessed on 23 April 2020).
32. Tang, W.; Wang, Y.; Xu, F.; Fan, W.; Zhang, Y.; Fan, K.; Wang, W.; Zhang, Y.; Zhang, C. Omega-3 fatty acids ameliorate cognitive dysfunction in schizophrenia patients with metabolic syndrome. *Brain Behav. Immun.* **2020**. [CrossRef] [PubMed]
33. Sterol Regulatory Element Binding Protein 1 Couples Mechanical Cues and Lipid Metabolism|Nature Communications. Available online: https://www.nature.com/articles/s41467-019-09152-7 (accessed on 23 April 2020).
34. Dipasquale, S.; Pariante, C.M.; Dazzan, P.; Aguglia, E.; McGuire, P.; Mondelli, V. The dietary pattern of patients with schizophrenia: A systematic review. *J. Psychiatr. Res.* **2013**, *47*, 197–207. [CrossRef]
35. Teasdale, S.B.; Ward, P.B.; Samaras, K.; Firth, J.; Stubbs, B.; Tripodi, E.; Burrows, T.L. Dietary intake of people with severe mental illness: Systematic review and meta-analysis. *Br. J. Psychiatry* **2019**, *214*, 251–259. [CrossRef]
36. Yang, X.; Sun, L.; Zhao, A.; Hu, X.; Qing, Y.; Jiang, J.; Yang, C.; Xu, T.; Wang, P.; Liu, J.; et al. Serum fatty acid patterns in patients with schizophrenia: A targeted metabonomics study. *Transl. Psychiatry* **2017**, *7*, e1176. [CrossRef]
37. Martins, J.G. EPA but Not DHA Appears to Be Responsible for the Efficacy of Omega-3 Long Chain Polyunsaturated Fatty Acid Supplementation in Depression: Evidence from a Meta-Analysis of Randomized Controlled Trials. *J. Am. Coll. Nutr.* **2009**, *28*, 525–542. [CrossRef]
38. Peet, M.; Brind, J.; Ramchand, C.N.; Shah, S.; Vankar, G.K. Two double-blind placebo-controlled pilot studies of eicosapentaenoic acid in the treatment of schizophrenia. *Schizophr. Res.* **2001**, *49*, 243–251. [CrossRef]
39. Saini, R.K.; Keum, Y.-S. Omega-3 and omega-6 polyunsaturated fatty acids: Dietary sources, metabolism, and significance—A review. *Life Sci.* **2018**, *203*, 255–267. [CrossRef]
40. Messamore, E.; McNamara, R.K. Detection and treatment of omega-3 fatty acid deficiency in psychiatric practice: Rationale and implementation. *Lipids Health Dis.* **2016**, *15*, 25. [CrossRef]

41. Thompson, F.E.; Subar, A.F. Dietary Assessment Methodology. In *Nutrition in the Prevention and Treatment of Disease*; Elsevier: Amsterdam, The Netherlands, 2017; pp. 5–48.
42. Metherel, A.H.; Stark, K.D. The stability of blood fatty acids during storage and potential mechanisms of degradation: A review. *Prostaglandins Leukot. Essent. Fatty Acids* **2016**, *104*, 33–43. [CrossRef]
43. Van Der Burg, K.P.; Cribb, L.; Firth, J.; Karmacoska, D.; Sarris, J. Nutrient and genetic biomarkers of nutraceutical treatment response in mood and psychotic disorders: A systematic review. *Nutr. Neurosci.* **2019**. [CrossRef]

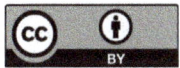

© 2020 by the authors. Licensee MDPI, Basel, Switzerland. This article is an open access article distributed under the terms and conditions of the Creative Commons Attribution (CC BY) license (http://creativecommons.org/licenses/by/4.0/).

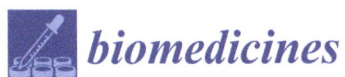

Review

The Biomedical Uses of Inositols: A Nutraceutical Approach to Metabolic Dysfunction in Aging and Neurodegenerative Diseases

Antonio J. López-Gambero [1,2], Carlos Sanjuan [3], Pedro Jesús Serrano-Castro [4], Juan Suárez [2,*] and Fernando Rodríguez de Fonseca [2,*]

1. Departamento de Biología Celular, Genética y Fisiología, Campus de Teatinos s/n, Universidad de Málaga, Andalucia Tech, 29071 Málaga, Spain; antonio.lopez@ibima.eu
2. UGC Salud Mental, Instituto de Investigación Biomédica de Málaga (IBIMA), Hospital Universitario Regional de Málaga, 29010 Málaga, Spain
3. EURONUTRA S.L., 29590 Málaga, Spain; euronutra@euronutra.eu
4. UGC Neurología, Instituto de Investigación Biomédica de Málaga (IBIMA), Hospital Universitario Regional de Málaga, 29010 Málaga, Spain; pedro.serrano.c@gmail.com
* Correspondence: juan.suarez@ibima.eu (J.S.); fernando.rodriguez@ibima.eu (F.R.d.F.); Tel.: +34-952614012 (J.S.)

Received: 22 July 2020; Accepted: 18 August 2020; Published: 20 August 2020

Abstract: Inositols are sugar-like compounds that are widely distributed in nature and are a part of membrane molecules, participating as second messengers in several cell-signaling processes. Isolation and characterization of inositol phosphoglycans containing myo- or D-chiro-inositol have been milestones for understanding the physiological regulation of insulin signaling. Other functions of inositols have been derived from the existence of multiple stereoisomers, which may confer antioxidant properties. In the brain, fluctuation of inositols in extracellular and intracellular compartments regulates neuronal and glial activity. Myo-inositol imbalance is observed in psychiatric diseases and its use shows efficacy for treatment of depression, anxiety, and compulsive disorders. Epi- and scyllo-inositol isomers are capable of stabilizing non-toxic forms of β-amyloid proteins, which are characteristic of Alzheimer's disease and cognitive dementia in Down's syndrome, both associated with brain insulin resistance. However, uncertainties of the intrinsic mechanisms of inositols regarding their biology are still unsolved. This work presents a critical review of inositol actions on insulin signaling, oxidative stress, and endothelial dysfunction, and its potential for either preventing or delaying cognitive impairment in aging and neurodegenerative diseases. The biomedical uses of inositols may represent a paradigm in the industrial approach perspective, which has generated growing interest for two decades, accompanied by clinical trials for Alzheimer's disease.

Keywords: Alzheimer's disease; psychiatric disease; depression; anxiety; Down's syndrome; inositol; nutraceutical; insulin signaling; antioxidant; aging

1. Introduction: Human Brain Aging and Inositols

The aging process in humans is associated with physical decline and impairment of metabolic homeostasis [1]. The dysregulation of the metabolic network leads to an age-related elevated risk of suffering from chronic metabolic disorders, especially insulin resistance-related pathologies. In addition to the well-known peripheral role of insulin on glucose and energy storage, insulin also regulates a series of cognitive processes, such as memory formation, through its effects on glial–neuronal metabolic coupling. Central insulin resistance is a common feature linked to premature aging and is observed in neurological disorders, including early stages of Alzheimer's disease (AD) and Down's syndrome (DS) [2].

Currently, 16% of the EU population is over 65, and this figure is expected to rise to 25% by 2030. Taking this trend into consideration and the prevalence of dementia, including AD, the World Health Organization estimates that population aging will lead to a dramatic increase in dementia prevalence. By 2050, more than 131.5 million people are expected to be affected. AD leads to a loss of memory and neurodegenerative cognitive functions and affects 10% of the population aged over 65 years. Delaying a cognitive decline in AD is a major research challenge and a clinical need, considering the incidence of this disease in the elderly. Common features of AD are the aggregation of β-amyloid (Aβ) plaques and tau protein hyperphosphorylation, leading to neural damage. An approach for slowing down the progress of the disease is targeting the factors that might accelerate neural damage. Present results suggest that unhealthy dietary habits, microbiota changes, and oxidative stress favor the development of brain insulin resistance, which could contribute to a neuroinflammatory profile, directly activating both the resident immune cells of the brain (microglia) and astrocytes, promoting an adverse environment for neuronal survival in the context of AD [3,4]. Accordingly, a more detailed in-depth analysis of central insulin resistance contribution to cognitive impairment is discussed later in this review. A relevant issue on the clinical approach to AD and related pathologies that lead to cognitive impairment is the fact that most of the research efforts on therapeutics have focused on either fighting the symptoms by boosting certain deteriorated transmission pathways (e.g., anti-acetylcholinesterase drugs to enhance cholinergic transmission) or reducing Aβ load via immunotherapy. However, there is a clear lack of therapeutic development designed to restore metabolic impairments associated with these neurodegenerative disorders.

The lack of a "metabolic approach to AD therapeutics" might offer an opportunity to inositols, since in the past years they have gained close attention regarding treatment of pathologies associated with altered insulin signaling. Inositols are sugar-like cyclic alcohols constituent of cells, which are normally incorporated as part of the human diet. Given their structure, there are at least eight isomers of inositols that occur in nature (*myo-*, *muco-*, *neo-*, *scyllo-*, L-*chiro-*, D-*chiro-*, *epi-*, and *allo*-inositol) and one non-occurring in nature (*cis*-inositol) (Figure 1A) [5]. Inositols act as second messengers of the insulin-signaling pathway and their administration exerts insulin-sensitizing and mimetic effects, lowering blood glucose and promoting hepatic glycogen synthesis. D-chiro-inositol has been widely used as a treatment for pathologies associated with insulin resistance, e.g., polycystic ovary syndrome (PCOS) and diabetes [6,7]. Given their polar structure, other inositols show different properties, such as scyllo-inositol, which stabilizes soluble Aβ oligomers and is being tested under clinical trials as a promising therapy for AD [8]. The use of inositols for medical purposes is closely related to their "nutraceutical" nature, although the definition of the term is still debated. Since inositols are acquired through the diet, inositol extracts can be considered a nutraceutical under the definition of an isolated or purified product from natural sources, with specific health benefits against diseases or medical conditions or a protective effect against chronic diseases. Hence, these natural compounds arise as alternatives to treatments for central and peripheral insulin resistance-related disorders.

In the present review, we provide a short description of the structure and pharmacology of inositols. However, it is not the scope of this review to describe the particular chemical characteristics of inositols or to compile their application for metabolic disorders in peripheral tissues, since several works have already elegantly described these concepts previously [5,9–11]. The further sections herein try to establish a descriptive line, detailing the importance of inositols and their derivatives, such as inositol-(phospho)glycans (IPGs or simply IGs) in physiological processes, highlighting their role in insulin signaling, as well as their function in the central nervous system and the perspective of their use in the treatment of neurodegenerative diseases, with a special emphasis on AD and behavioral disorders here.

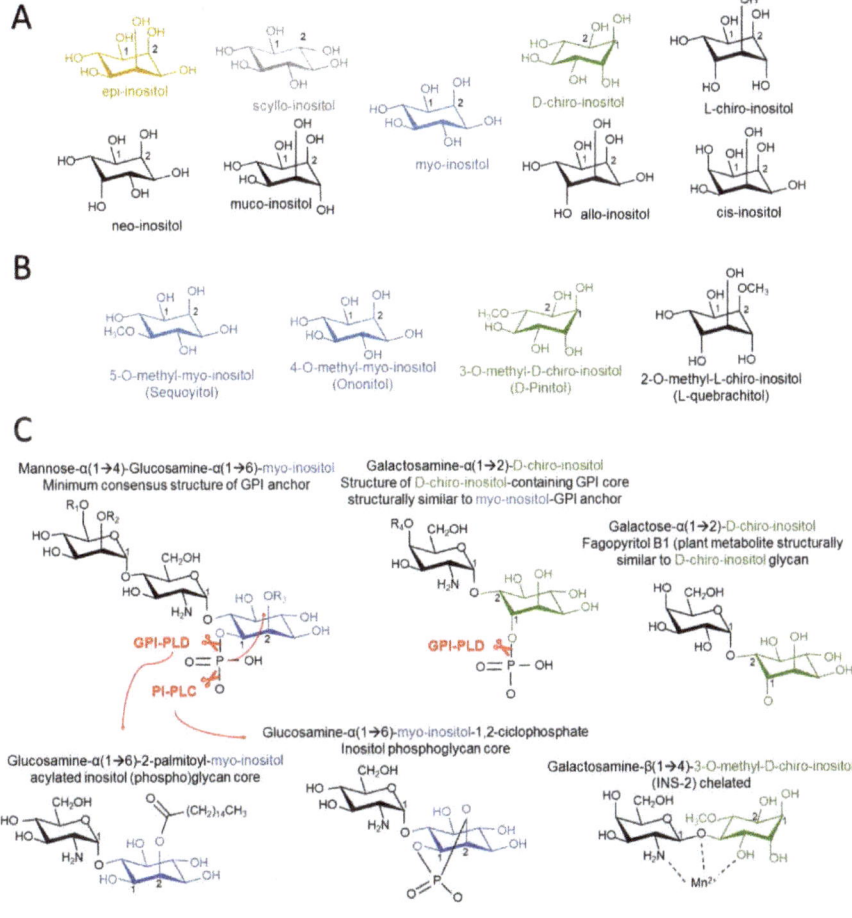

Figure 1. Structure in the chair conformation of inositol stereoisomers (**A**), inositol methyl derivatives (**B**), natural and synthetic inositol phosphoglycan cores, and insulin-mimicking inositol phosphoglycans (**C**). Glycophosphatidyl inositol phospholipase D (GPI-PLC) hydrolyzes phosphate inositol-lipid linkage, releasing unphosphorylated inositol. Phosphatidylinositol phospholipase C (PI-PLC) hydrolyzes phosphate inositol-lipid linkage in α(1→6) myo-inositol (but not α(1→2) D-chiro-inositol) structures when the C2 position is not occupied by an acyl-lipid chain, promoting cyclic (1,2) phosphate linkage to myo-inositol.

2. Inositols in Organisms

2.1. Structure of Inositol Isomers and Inositol Phospholipids

Inositols are naturally occurring substances that resemble simple sugars. They have a cyclic structure of six carbons and six alcohols, being classified as sugar alcohols (polyols with one hydroxyl group attached to each carbon atom). In addition, both inositols and methyl-derived inositols are also classified as cyclitols (cycloalkanes containing at least three hydroxyl groups attached to the carbon atoms).

Thus far, the role of inositols on the body is both structural, as constituents of complex phospholipids in plasma membrane, and functional, since they act on metabolic pathways as second messengers of insulin signaling. Regarding their structural function, in mammalian tissues, inositols are found in the external part of the membrane of phosphoglycerides. The attachment of sugar residues to inositols constitutes the glycosylphosphatidylinositols (GPIs), which are elements of the outer leaflet of the plasma membrane that may serve as anchors for extracellular proteins attached to the membrane. As second messengers, inositols are a well-known part of signal transduction, as they form phosphatidylinositols (PIs) and their phosphorylated forms, phosphoinositides (PIPs) and inositol phosphates (IPs), which are responsible for membrane trafficking and cell signaling as substrates for other protein kinases. The most important members of this family are phosphatidylinositol (4,5)-bisphosphate (PI(4,5)P$_2$, simplified as PIP$_2$), a substrate for the phosphoinositide 3-kinase (PI3K), whose phosphorylation and conversion into phosphatidylinositol (3,4,5)-trisphosphate (PI(3,4,5)P$_3$, simplified as PIP$_3$) is a key step in the insulin/IGF-1 pathway. PIP$_2$ is also a substrate for phospholipase C and the formation of inositol 1,4,5-trisphosphate (IP$_3$), a second messenger mainly involved in intracellular Ca^{2+} trafficking in the endoplasmic reticulum.

2.2. Inositol Incorporation in Organisms

Despite eight out of the nine inositol isomers occurring naturally, only myo-inositol (MI; *cis*-1,2,3,5-*trans*-4,6-cyclohexanehexol), scyllo-inositol (SI; *cis*-1,3,5-*trans*-2,4,6-cyclohexanehexol), and D-chiro-inositol (DCI; *cis*-1,2,4-*trans*-3,5,6-cyclohexanehexol) have been detected as major inositols present in mammalian tissue. Some studies have reported the possible presence of neo-inositol (NI; *cis*-1,2,3-*trans*-4-5-6-cyclohexanehexol) in bovine brains [12] and also epi-inositol (EI; *cis*-1-*trans*-2,3,4,5,6-cyclohexanehexol) and muco-inositol (*cis*-1,4-*trans*-2,3,5,6-cyclohexanehexol) in the liver, muscle, blood, brain, and several other rat tissues with a rate of isomerization from MI of 0.6% [13]. MI interconverts to other inositols via an specific epimerase [13,14] that differs from the epimerase catalyzing the conversion from MI to DCI [15,16]. MI and SI are the most abundant forms of inositols in organisms, representing over 90% of the total inositol content of mammalian cells. SI has been reported to be incorporated into lipids in plants [17]. However, SI is not incorporated into PI lipids at detectable levels, even under SI administration in mammalian tissue [18]. The other inositol found in great levels in mammals is DCI, which acts as a second messenger for insulin signaling, presumably as IG, as will be depicted later. A summary of the current knowledge on inositol stereoisomers sources, distribution, and pharmacological properties can be found in Table 1.

Table 1. Biological sources of inositol stereoisomers, distribution in mammalian tissue, and current pharmacological applications for the treatment of human diseases. PIs: Phosphatidylinositols; IP$_3$: Inositol 1,4,5-trisphosphate; GPIs: Glycosylphosphatidylinositols.

Inositol Stereoisomer	Mainly Found in	Distribution and Function in Mammals	Pharmacological Properties
Myo-inositol	• Plants • Mammals • Bacteria	• Found in all tissues. • Part of membrane PIs. • MI in PIP$_2$ and PIP$_3$ acts in several intracellular signaling pathways. • MI in IP$_3$ regulates metabolic flux, intracellular Ca^{2+}, and membrane excitability. • Acts as an osmolyte.	• Treatment of polycystic ovary syndrome (PCOS) related to insulin resistance and hyperandrogenism in combination with DCI [6,7]. • Prevention of gestational diabetes mellitus in combination with DCI [19]. • Treatment of obsessive-compulsive disorder, panic disorder, and depression [20–22].

Table 1. Cont.

Inositol Stereoisomer	Mainly Found in	Distribution and Function in Mammals	Pharmacological Properties
Epi-inositol	• Plants	• Found in brain, liver, muscle, blood, and other tissues, epimerized from myo-inositol [13]. • Biological function unknown.	• Decreases the aggregation of toxic forms of β-amyloid protein in Alzheimer's disease [23,24].
Scyllo-inositol	• Plants • Mammals • Bacteria	• Found preeminently in the brain [12,13,25]. • Acts as an osmolyte. • Competes with MI for active transport into the cell.	• Decreases the aggregation of toxic forms of β-amyloid protein in Alzheimer's disease [23,24]. • Inhibits the aggregation of α-synuclein in Parkinson's disease [26].
Neo-inositol	• Plants	• Detected in brain [12]. • Biological function unknown.	• No pharmacological properties described.
Muco-inositol	• Plants	• Found in brain, liver, muscle, blood, and other tissues, epimerized from myo-inositol [13]. • Biological function unknown.	• No pharmacological properties described.
D-chiro-inositol	• Plants • Mammals • Bacteria	• Mainly found in insulin-responsive tissues. • Acts as a second messenger in insulin signaling pathway, likely as a part of GPIs.	• Treatment of polycystic ovary syndrome (PCOS) related to insulin resistance and hyperandrogenism in combination with MI [6,7]. • Prevention of gestational diabetes mellitus in combination with MI [27].
L-chiro-inositol	• Plants	• Not detected in mammalian tissue.	• No pharmacological properties described.
Allo-inositol	• Plants • Mammals • Bacteria	• Not detected in mammalian tissue.	• Non-potent inhibitor of the aggregation of toxic forms of β-amyloid protein in Alzheimer's disease [28]
Cis-inositol	• Non-naturally occurring	• Not detected in mammalian tissue.	• No pharmacological properties described.

Inositols can be obtained from the diet as they are abundant components of the cell membrane in plants and animals. The most abundant form of MI incorporation is either free, or in the form of (myo)-inositol hexaphosphate or IP_6 (1,2,3,4,5,6-hexayl hexakis (dihydrogen (phosphate))), also known as phytic acid. Major sources of IP_6 are plants, as IP_6 is a major reservoir of phosphorus, energy, and a source of cations and MI in the cell wall. However, IP_6 cannot be obtained from dietetic sources because its bioavailability is very limited. This is due to its negative charge density, being necessary to be dephosphorylated via bacterial phytases and phosphatases, providing free MI or other IPs before entering bloodstream [29,30]. The only animals that can carry out this transformation belong to the ruminant mammal group. Western diets can provide around 0.5–1 g/day of MI [31,32]. DCI is mainly obtained as the methylated form D-pinitol (DPIN; 3-o-methyl-D-chiro-inositol), which is demethylated to DCI under acidic conditions in the gastrointestinal tract. DPIN acts as an osmolyte in plants, allowing tolerance to heat, high salinity, and drought stress [33]. The *Leguminosae* family is a major source of DPIN, especially carob pods, which provide 10–80 g/kg of DPIN [34]. Many herbal extracts contain methyl-inositol derivatives like sequoyitol (5-o-methyl-myo-inositol) or L-quebrachitol (2-o-methyl-L-chiro-inositol) (Figure 1B) [35,36]. Dietary supply of other inositols seems to be scarce, as evidenced by their low presence in organisms.

Although inositols can be obtained from diet, the main inositol isomer, MI, is also synthesized in the body in great enough quantities for the whole supply required, as kidneys produce 2 g/day each of

MI (4 g total) and other tissues contribute to a small extent to MI synthesis, like the brain and testis [37]. De novo MI synthesis occurs primarily from glucose into cytosol. The process follows glucose phosphorylation into glucose-6-phosphate (G6P) via hexokinase. D-3-*myo*-inositol-phosphate synthase (MIPS) catalyzes the conversion from G6P into myo-inositol 3-phosphate (MIP), and dephosphorylation occurs with inositol monophosphatase (IMPase), rendering free MI. MIPS is a phosphoprotein whose activity is regulated by the glycogen synthase kinase 3 (GSK3) homolog MCK1 in yeast [38,39]. Although this may suggest GSK3 regulation of MIPS activity in humans, there are no data of this proposed mechanism in mammalian cells. Expression of inositol-3-phosphate synthase 1 (Isyna1), a gene encoder for IMPase transcription, is tightly regulated by the disposal of phosphatidic acid (PA) and inositol hexakisphosphate synthase 1 (IP6K1). PA is considered a "metabolic sensor", as its synthesis is upregulated by high levels of glucose or the presence of growth factors and promotes cell growth via a mammalian target of rapamycin (mTOR) [40,41]. Interaction of PA with IP6K1 leads to its translocation into the nucleus and synthesis of IP7, which negatively regulates *Isyna1* via DNA methylation [42].

The transport of inositol isomers into cells is regulated by the sodium-myo-inositol co-transporters (SMIT1 and SMIT2) with a 2 Na^+ to 1 myo-inositol stoichiometric ratio, similar to that of the sodium-glucose co-transporter SGLT1 [43–45]. SMIT1 and SMIT2 both have a different affinity for inositol isomers, which are competitors for inositol transport, and are differentially regulated by monosaccharides. DCI and MI are both effectively transported into cells via SMIT2 with a similar affinity, whereas DPIN, a methyl derivative of DCI, binds to SMIT2 with lower affinity and is a competitor for MI/DCI transport [46]. SI has also a high affinity for the SMIT1 and SMIT2 transporters, whereas other inositol derivatives like sequoyitol, D-ononitol (4-o-methyl-D-chiro-inositol), or viburnitol (1-deoxy-L-chiro-inositol) are also transported with lower affinity [47]. Inositol transport is inhibited in the presence of L-fructose and D-glucose, as they are also competitors of SMIT1 and SMIT2 [46,47]. SMIT2 is highly expressed in mammalian kidneys and is responsible for the reabsorption of inositols into the bloodstream [48,49]. DCI uptake via SMIT2 is highly upregulated in the presence of insulin in human L6 myoblasts, which could explain the lower concentration of DCI in insulin-sensitive tissues and lower DCI re-uptake in the renal tubes in cases of hyperglycemia and insulin resistance [46,50,51], along with decreased epimerase activity [15,16]. The fact that inositol transport is highly dependent on glucose concentrations and insulin signaling limits its potential use in association with food (i.e., as an ingredient), where it would be necessary to adjust the timing, dose, and number of doses to the given metabolic profile of the user.

Inositols may also be transported by a described H^+/myo-inositol transporter (HMIT) in a 1 H^+ to 1 myo-inositol stoichiometric ratio [43,52]. Inositol HMIT transport is pH-dependent and phlorizin-sensitive [52]. HMIT is highly expressed in the brain, but its transcript is also detected in white, brown, and epididymal adipose tissues, and also in the kidney in rats [52]. HMIT is reported to transport MI, SI, DCI, and muco-inositol, but not allo-inositol, and is blocked by phloretin and phlorizin, which are well-described inhibitors of the Na^+/glucose transporters SGLT1 and SGLT2. [52]. There are not many reports about the physiological role of HMIT in inositol transport in the peripheral tissues. HMIT differently controls inositol transport and signaling in the neurons and astrocytes along with SMIT1 and SMIT2, which may stand for a specific role of inositols in osmoregulation, insulin signaling, Ca^{2+} mobilization, and membrane composition in the brain [52–55]. A more detailed mechanism of inositol transport in the brain will be discussed in the other sections of this review.

MI, when available in the cell, is incorporated into PI. All MI-containing phospholipids are derived from PI, which is the most abundant form throughout the cell, constituting 10–15% of mammalian membrane phospholipids [56]. PI synthesis is performed next to the endoplasmic reticulum via PI synthase (PIS). This process requires cytidine diphosphate diacylglycerol (CDP-DAG) and MI. PIS has a low affinity for MI, hence MI availability is the rate-limiting factor for PI synthesis (ref). Some PI is channeled to the luminal face of the endoplasmic reticulum to later derive glycan PI or GPIs, which are acylated and transported to plasma membrane, serving as "anchors" for proteins in the external surface of the plasma membrane [57]. PIs may also be substrate for PI kinases, deriving PI-3, -4, and -5 monophosphate (PI(3)P, PI(4)P, and PI(5)P), which may suffer posterior phosphorylation and be converted into PI-3,5, -3,4, and -4,5 biphosphate (PI(3,5)P$_2$, PI(3,4)P$_2$, and PI(4,5)P$_2$), the latter also rendering the triphosphate form PI(3,4,5)P$_3$, as reviewed in [57,58]. Phospholipase C may cleave PI(4,5)P$_2$ and form inositol (3,4,5) phosphate or IP$_3$, which is subsequently derived into other IPs or recycled back to MI [58].

3. Insulin-Mimetic and Insulin-Sensitizing Properties of Inositols

3.1. Revisiting the Proposed Role of Inositols in Insulin Signaling

Two complementary mechanisms by which inositols modulate the insulin signaling pathway have been proposed [10,59,60] and revised [61,62]. Some questions regarding these models (depicted later) have been addressed, yet there are no clear answers. Recent findings may shed light on some of these unknowns and add other interactors in the signaling mechanism.

3.1.1. Canonical Insulin Signaling

The classical mechanism of action in insulin signaling has been extensively described and reviewed [63–65]. Briefly, the binding of insulin to its receptor (IR) in target tissues promotes tyrosine autophosphorylation, recruiting IR substrates as the IRS and Shc proteins. Shc activates the Ras/MEK/ERK pathway, which accounts for mostly the growth-promoting effects of insulin. On the other hand, IRS1 and IRS2 continue the PI3K/Akt/mTOR pathway. IRS proteins recruit the p85 regulatory domain of phosphatidylinositol 3 kinase (PI3K), leading to phosphatidylinositol-3,4,5-triphosphate (PIP$_3$), and activating the phosphorylation of Akt (also known as PKB). Full activation of Akt needs complementary phosphorylation by mammalian target of rapamycin (mTOR) complex 2 (mTORC2). Akt then mediates most of the insulin effects, as it phosphorylates and inhibits glycogen synthase kinase 3-β (GSK3-β), preventing the inhibition of glycogen synthase (GS) and leading to increased glycogen synthesis. Akt also promotes glucose uptake by the mobilization of glucose transporter 4 (GLUT4) and activates the mTOR complex 1 (mTORC1) via inhibition of tuberous sclerosis 1 (TSC1) and 2 (TSC1), leading to protein and lipid synthesis. Insulin signaling is a more complex process that involves major proteins that participate in the glucogenic pathway, such as fructose 2,6-bisphosphatase (FBPase-2), or the lipogenic pathway, like hormone-sensitive lipase (HSL), which are negatively regulated by protein kinase A (PKA) and also inactivated by Akt.

3.1.2. Non-Canonical Insulin Signaling and the Role of IPGs

The role for inositols in insulin signaling has long been presumed, as early experiments showed the capacity of inositols to promote glycogen synthesis in the liver or as lipid synthesis in adipocytes. The paradigm of insulin signaling changed upon the discovery of insulin modulators that were produced upon phospholipase activity in GPIs, enhancing pyruvate dehydrogenase (PDH) activity and decreasing cAMP production [66,67]. Further research lead to the description of two types of IPGs based on their structure and activity. Type A IPGs (IPG-A) contain myo-inositol and D-glucosamine and inhibit cAMP production and AMPK activity, promoting lipogenesis. The others, named as type G IPGs (IPG-G), consist of a 3-o-methyl-D-chiro-inositol (D-pinitol) and galactosamine, promoting glycogenesis via mitochondrial PDH activation [68–70]. Larner et al. carried out isolation from beef livers and later confirmed the structure of an insulin second messenger (INS-2) with a molar ratio of 1:1 of 3-o-methyl-D-chiro-inositol (D-pinitol) and galactosamine linked by a β-1,4 bond [71] (Figure 1C). INS-2 that contains an inositol glycan structure of the so-called IPG-Ps is an allosteric modulator of PP2Cα [72], which is known to dephosphorylate and activate GS [73], PI3K [74], and inactivate AMPK [75]. INS-2 might also be present under the chelated form with Mn^{2+}. Chelated INS-2 is an allosteric modulator of mitochondrial PDH phosphatase (PDHP) activity and promotes PDH-mediated glycogen synthesis [71]. It should be remarked that the structures of DCI-GPIs are still unknown and may not share structural similarity with MI-GPIs and differ in terms of the axial orientation of the phosphatidyl moiety, as reported by cleavage studies with synthetic DCI-GPIs (Figure 1C) [76].

Larner and colleagues described the role of a $G_{q/11}$ protein as a putative pathway of insulin signaling [77], hence linking the activity of a phospholipase that could explain the release of IPGs from GPI and explain the crucial role for IPGs in insulin signaling. However, the exact structures of circulating inositols released by insulin stimulus are still unknown. This model proposed by Larner [10] raised some questions that were later added to new uncertainties in the review by Croze and Soulage [61]. Deep revision and the current data may help address some of these uncertainties.

The less widespread Müller's theory [59,60] describes the role of IPGs in activating insulin signaling externally. This may be sustained by the observation that IPG internalization is not necessary to stimulate lipogenesis in rat epididymal adipocytes with a maximal activity of 47% of the maximum insulin response [78]. This theory is based on the existence of membrane detergent/carbonate-insoluble glycolipid-enriched raft microdomains (DIGs), which are formed by the high presence of cholesterol (hcDIG) or the low presence of cholesterol (lcDIG) in the plasma membrane. Some portion of insulin receptors seem to be associated with caveolins, mainly located in "caveolae", which are structures in hcDIGs. GPI-anchored proteins would have a natural tendency to move to lcDIGs but are retained in hcDIGs by binding to a membrane protein, presumably p115. Insulin stimulus would lead to the activation of a GPI-PLC, which would release the IPGs. These IPGs may interfere in the binding of the GPI-anchored proteins to the receptor, allowing their displacement to the lcDIGs. This would also lead to a displacement of a protein kinase, $pp59^{Lyn}$, previously attached to caveolin, which would mediate tyrosine phosphorylation on IRS1 or IRS2.

This theory would involve recognizing the existence of a GPI-PLC whose gene has not been identified in mammals, in addition to assuming that cholesterol microdomains are present in all cell types where insulin activity is shown, and this does not explain why IPGs may allosterically modulate intracellular elements of the insulin pathway. While this model cannot be ruled out, this may not represent a generalized mechanism and would serve as an additional route of complementary insulin signaling, but is not strictly necessary for insulin activity, rather than describing the main mechanism of action of the IPGs.

Whether there might be different IPGs contributing to insulin signaling depending on tissue or cell type might depend on the species and tissue proportion of inositol accumulation. Insulin markedly promotes the biosynthesis of DCI-GPIs after 15 min of addition to rat fibroblasts expressing the human IR, whereas a decrease in MI-GPI content is observed after 5 min of insulin treatment, which suggests that insulin promotes epimerase activity and conversion of MI to DCI [15]. DCI-containing IPGs might be the main mediators of insulin signaling, especially those involving glycogen synthesis. MI and SI are more prominent in the brain than DCI, whereas conversion of MI to DCI is far more prominent in fat, liver, muscle, or gonadal tissues [79]. It is foreseeable that DCI-IPGs would exert more important control over insulin signaling, effectively depending on the place of action.

Other debate has been raised between the intracellular or extracellular release of IPGs. The answer implies the interplay of three different proteins. Early experiments showed that IPGs are more likely to be extracellularly formed after GPI cleaving and are later actively transported in the cell. The presence of anti-IPG antibody blocks the activation of intracellular PDH, hence presuming that binding to extracellularly-generated IPGs to the antibody prevents access to the cell interior [80]. As such, some authors have described the existence of an ATP-dependent inositol glycan transporter that is stimulated upon insulin signaling. This plasmatic membrane transporter was first discovered in hepatocytes and has been well described [81]. Thus, it is a putative IPG transporter that would support the extracellular release of IPGs.

Since IPGs are part of the polar head of GPIs, their release relies on phospholipase activity. The proposed mechanism implies an alternate pathway to tyrosine phosphorylation or IRs, with IRs also coupling to a heteromeric protein G_q and the activation of a GPI-phospholipase [10]. Both GPI-PLC and GPI-PLD have been proposed as candidates. Early experiments have determined the generation of IPGs under the activity of bacterial GPI-PLC and GPI-PLD [60,68,71,82]. However, gene encoding for a mammalian GPI-PLC has not been identified yet. Presumably, insulin mediates the generation of IPGs through a GPI-PLD, as has been described [83,84]. GPI-PLD expression is ubiquitous throughout all tissues and is especially prevalent in the liver and circulating in plasma [85]. Current studies appoint the relevance of GPI-PLD in insulin resistance. Significantly increased levels of GPI-PLD have been identified as a novel biomarker of early prediabetes in humans [86] and early stages of latent autoimmune diabetes in adults and those with type 2 diabetes [87]. It has been observed that both insulin and glucose stimulate the secretion of GPI-PLD in rat pancreatic islets [88]. GPI-PLD levels also seem to be higher in the pancreas under islet hyperactivity and lower in the liver from insulin-resistant (ob/ob) mice [88].

In relation to the above, despite the fact that there is no evidence of the mammalian gene for GPI-PLC in humans, this possibility cannot be ruled out yet due to identification of a GPI-PLC-like protein in bovine brains and rat intestines [89,90], but also to the lack of knowledge of the chemical structure of the various IPGs that can be generated in the body. These doubts are raised by the experiments carried out with synthetic IPGs. In one study, it was observed that the phosphate group that binds carbon 1 of inositol to the membrane lipid needs to be maintained after cleavage of phospholipase and forms a cyclic linkage with carbons 1 and 2 of inositol for certain synthetic IPGs that have an insulin-mimetic activity [70]. This is only achieved through the action of a PI-PLC, since the hydrolysis of the phosphate is carried out on the O^- radical bound to the membrane lipid, whereas a GPI-PLC performs a cleavage on the O^- radical of inositol, maintaining the phosphate group in the lipid after the release of the IPG (Figure 1C) [76]. In addition to this, synthetic DCI-GPI anchors with $\alpha(1\rightarrow 2)$ linkage of glucosamine and DCI cannot be a substrate for PI-PLC hydrolysis, but this can be mediated by GPI-PLD (Figure 1C) [76]. This suggests that possible DCI-GPIs are structurally similar to MI-GPI anchors with $\alpha(1\rightarrow 6)$ linkage of glucosamine and that MI relies on GPI-PLD activity. Fagopyritols are galactose and DCI analogs found in plants and are classified according to the binding (type A with galactose-$\alpha(1\rightarrow 3)$-DCI linkage and type B with galactose-$\alpha(1\rightarrow 2)$-DCI linkage). Fagopyritol B1, a galactose-$\alpha(1\rightarrow 2)$-DCI, is a structural analog of the core of the proposed DCI-GPI anchors and has a more powerful insulin-mimetic effect than free DCI, highlighting the possible role of DCI-IPGs in insulin signaling (Figure 1C) [91].

PI-PLC cannot hydrolyze and release IPGs with cyclic phosphate when inositol carbon 2 is palmitoyl-acylated, which is often the case for non-anchored protein-free GPIs [92]. In contrast, GPI-PLD may be cleaved when inositol groups are acylated, supposedly releasing acylated IPGs (A-IPGs) (Figure 1C) [92]. Synthetic A-IPGs also show a strong insulin-mimetic activity [93]. Non-protein linked GPIs are intermediate GPIs, as they quickly bind proteins when reaching the plasma membrane surface. However, non-protein-linked GPIs have been observed to reside both in the inner and outer leaflets of the plasma membrane [94]. GPI-PLD release of acylated IPGs (A-IPGs) is speculated to occur in the intracellular compartment, yet this has not been corroborated [94]. The fact that anti-IPGs block some of the insulin-mediated actions suggests that intracellularly-released A-IPGs have a minor, yet complementary, role in inulin signaling [80]. Besides insulin, GPI-PLD expression is associated with lipid levels [95–97] and its activity is also associated with triglyceride [98] and lipid metabolism in the liver [99], which may be somehow related to the improved lipid profiles of patients suffering from metabolic diseases after supplementation with inositols like DCI [100].

Assuming this approach, inositol supplementation may restore pathologically low levels of IPGs, given that the rate-limiting aspect of GPI synthesis is cytosolic-free inositol supply, as phosphoinositol synthase has a relatively low affinity [57]. Thus, a higher concentration of inositols, especially DCI, which is much more scarce than MI and has a more prominent role in insulin signaling, supports the idea that inositol supplementation would help the synthesis of DCI-GPIs and later form DCI-IPGs when insulin epimerase's activity is diminished in insulin resistance.

Albeit that this model seems to be a fairly close approach to the true role for inositols as insulin-sensitizers (Figure 2), data on supplementation with inositol derivatives might question whether IPGs are the only way for inositols to modulate insulin signaling.

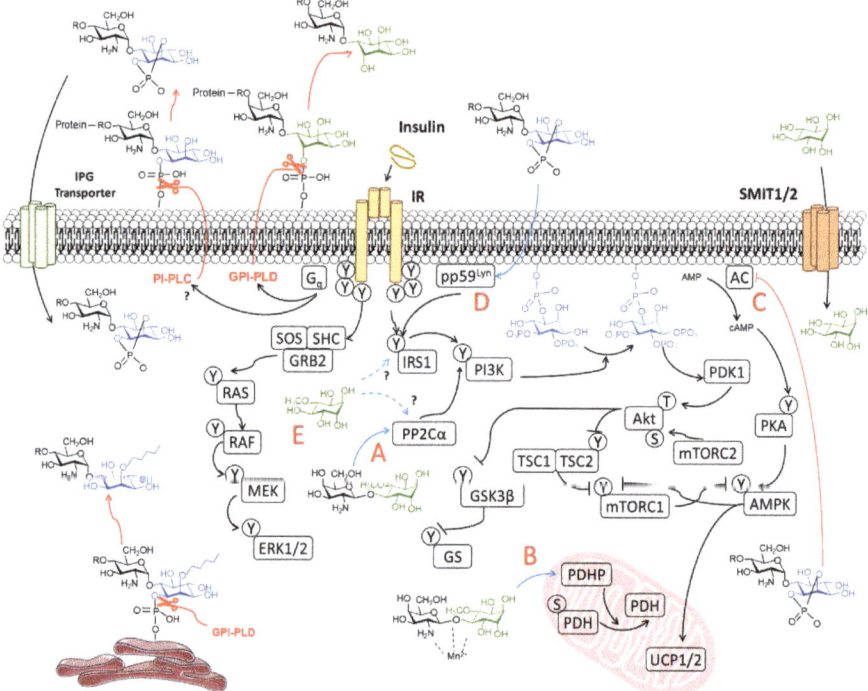

Figure 2. Proposed mechanism of action of inositols in insulin signaling. Non-canonical insulin signaling through the G_q protein presumably stimulates glycophosphatidylinositol phospholipase D (GPI-PLD) and/or (glycol)phosphatidylinositol phospholipase C (PI-PLC), mediating the hydrolysis of phosphate linkage between inositol and membrane lipids, leading to the release of inositol phosphoglycans (IPGs). Acylated-IPGs are formed in the plasma membrane and endoplasmic reticulum. IPGs are internalized via an IPG transporter. Insulin-sensitizing properties of inositols correspond to (**A**) allosteric modulation of protein phosphatase 1A (PP2Cα) and (**B**) pyruvate dehydrogenase phosphatase (PDHP), as observed by D-chiro-inositol glycan (INS-2), and (**C**) the inhibition of adenylate cyclase (AC) and protein kinase A (PKA) activity (observed with myo-inositol glycans). IPGs may also upregulate IRS1 signaling by (**D**) activating the upstream modulator pp59^{Lyn} localized in lipid rafts. Free inositols such as D-pinitol also exert (**E**) insulin-mimetic properties in the absence of an insulin stimulus.

3.2. Are Inositols Direct Insulin Mimetics Rather than Insulin Sensitizers?

Apart from the proposed model of IPGs in insulin signaling, some early in vitro studies of inositol supplementation have shown the direct effect of inositol isomers in insulin signaling apart from IPG activity. It was shown that a 1 mM dose of DCI, DPIN, L-*chiro*-inositol (LCI; *cis*-1,2,4-*trans*-3,5,6-ciclohexanehexol), EI, and muco-I stimulated glucose uptake in rat L6 myotubes in vitro and also promoted that translocation of GLUT4 to the plasma membrane in L6 myotubes in vitro and the skeletal muscles of rats ex vivo to a similar extent as 100 nM of insulin [101]. It should be noted that cells were grown in a medium supplemented with fetal bovine serum (FBS) and starved 18 h prior to the glucose uptake assay with a medium containing 0.2% FBS, so the possibility of insulin traces remaining in the cell culture media should not be ruled out, as these could account for the inositol effect on GLUT4 translocation and glucose uptake at the given concentrations. MI was also supplemented at same concentrations and did not elicit any insulin-mediated response on glucose uptake [101].

When administered to endothelial cells in vitro, both 1 mM of MI and DCI promoted an increased phosphorylation of Akt, ERK1, and ERK2 in human vascular endothelial cells (HUVEC) to a greater extent than 100 nM of insulin [102]. Since cells were serum-starved before MI and DCI treatment, MI and DCI induced kinase phosphorylation in the absence of insulin. It is noteworthy that the Ras/MEK/ERK signaling pathway was also involved, as inositols are regarded to exert insulin-sensitizing effects on the PI3K/Akt/mTOR signaling pathway.

Our recent study has shown that the administration of DPIN to fasting rats promotes a significant reduction of circulating insulin without affecting plasma glucose levels [103]. These results may imply a direct action of DPIN on insulin signaling. An increase in ghrelin levels was also observed upon DPIN administration, which could account for the decreased secretion of insulin in pancreatic β cells [103].

These results show that inositols may act on upstream regulators of insulin signaling. Some experiments agree with this hypothesis. Sequoyitol pretreatment enhances insulin signaling with increased phosphorylation of IRS1 and Akt in HepG2 hepatocytes and 3T3-L1 adipocytes [104]. Interestingly, sequoyitol pretreatment also reverses decreased IR autophosphorylation in the presence of tumor necrosis factor (TNF-α), a well described inhibitor of IR activity [104,105]. TNF-α is known to also inhibit SMIT expression in cultured endothelial cells [106]. Inositol depletion might partially explain the insulin-sensitizing effect of sequoyitol on insulin-resistant cells but does not account for enhanced IR autophosphorylation.

Increased IR autophosphorylation has also been observed in primary hippocampal neurons from rats when administered 100 μM of DCI, DPIN, or INS-2 in a similar way to 1 μM insulin treatment [107]. Moreover, after media replacement with a serum-free HEPES buffer, DCI administration has been shown to promote IR internalization, a mechanism required for ERK activation, in a similar way to insulin [107]. Given that insulin was depleted from the media, again, this mechanism of IR trafficking from dendrites to soma elicits a direct effect of DCI as a free inositol in insulin signaling.

The way free inositols participate in the insulin signaling pathway remains unknown. Given that PLD levels are relatively high in all tissues, insulin stimulation of GPI-PLD might not be crucial for its activity. Somehow, a stimulus would be needed to increase IPG production, which would rely on the basal activity of GPI-PLD [108]. Based on the results obtained both in vitro and in vivo, the group of Ashida suggested an insulin-independent mechanism, implying the activation of PI3K and/or AMPK [101,109]. It has been described that INS-2 allosterically modulates PP2Cα [72], which is known to dephosphorylate and activate PI3K [74] and inactivate AMPK [75]. IPG production could account for GLUT4 translocation and enhanced glucose uptake in muscles. However, inositol supply and increased IPG production does not account for the direct actions of inositols regarding IR autophosphorylation, since their target starts insulin signaling downstream of PI3K and possibly IRS1.

Although unlikely, some hypotheses have arisen regarding the means of IR activity. One of them is the possible allosteric modulation of IR by inositols. A study has identified the molecular docking of MI with active sites of PPARγ, GLUT4, and IR [108]. However, contrasting docking analysis requires specific studies of protein–molecule inhibition or inhibition of the protein target to determine the correlation of effective interactions in a biological system and in silico predictions. Moreover, the fact that MI is predicted to interact with different molecules of the same signaling pathway undermines the reliability of this mechanism. Another possibility could involve the repression of negative regulators of IR. Protein tyrosine phosphatase 1B (PTP1B) is a well-described inhibitor of IR tyrosine kinase activity. PTP1B is activated under different stimuli, including the presence of TNF-α [110]. Other known inhibitors of IR are c-Jun N-terminal protein kinase (JNK) or suppressor of cytokine signaling 3 (SOCS3). It is still unknown if inositols may interact and downregulate one of the inhibitory pathways of IR autophosphorylation,

Mechanisms of the insulin signaling pathway may involve different downstream elements, but they all share a common activation of IRS1/2, PI3K, and Akt. In order to elucidate the target for free inositols, we propose an in vitro study of cultured hepatocytes or myocytes, as highly-responsive cells to insulin stimulus, and the blockade, one by one, of elements composing the cascade of the insulin signaling pathway (IR, IRS1, PI3K, PDK, Akt, mTOR, and AMPK) in a top-down manner. This could be easily achieved via the use of small interfering RNA (siRNA) and transient siRNA-mediated knockdown of IR and their downstream elements [111,112]. Measuring the GLUT4-translocation response of insulin-depleted cells to inositol addition could determine the exact point at which inositols enhance IR signaling in the absence of insulin. In vitro studies let us control medium conditions and eliminate external elements that could interfere with the insulin sensitivity. Alternatively, the use of specific inhibitors for each element could be considered. Identification of inositol targets would make way for further analysis of the exact mechanism of interaction, as well cyclitols, regarding their specificity.

3.3. Putative Role of Inositols in IGF-1 Signaling

Insulin and insulin-like growth factor 1 (IGF-1) are both hormones with a high structural similarity and share some cross-reactivity due to the low-affinity binding of insulin to the IGF-1 receptor (IGF-1R) and from IGF-1 to IR. The existence of active IGF-1/IR heterodimers has also been demonstrated, although their physiological role has not been fully described. In contrast to insulin, IGF-1 is released in the liver and is stimulated by the growth hormone and its function is strongly anabolic. IGF-1 circulates as a ternary complex consisting of IGF-1, IGF binding protein 3 (IGFBP-3) or 5 (IGFBP-5), and the acid labile subunit (ALS), avoiding IGF-1 non-specific insulin-like hypoglycemic activity. The metalloproteinase pregnancy-associated plasma protein A2 (PAPP-A2) is involved in the proteolysis of the IGF-1 ternary complex, releasing free and active IGF-1 on target tissues [113].

Like insulin, IGF-1 is also able to stimulate GPI cleavage and IPG formation, as seen in vitro in 3T3 fibroblasts, BC3H-1 myocytes, and Chinese hamster ovary (CHO) cell lines [114–116]. Moreover, antibody binding to IPGs formed after the addition of IGF-1 blocks the growth-promoting effect on the ears of chicken embryos [117]. However, the addition IPGs without the presence of IGF-1 has a negligible effect on growth, which suggests that IPG formation is necessary, but not necessarily able to promote an IGF-1-mediated growth effect [117]. This effect is likely mediated by IPG-A, since IPG activity has been measured by its capacity of inhibiting PKA [117]. Another study showed that the addition of antibodies against IPG-P blocked the stimulatory effects of both IGF-1 on progesterone synthesis by swine ovary granulosa cells [118]. However, in adult rat hepatocytes, insulin mediates GPI cleavage and IPG formation, and it has been observed that fetal hepatocyte formation of IPGs is dependent on IGF-1 but not insulin activity. Furthermore, the addition of isolated IPG-P, but not insulin, has reduced the activity of glycogen phosphorylase (the rate limiting enzyme for glycogen hydrolysis) [119].

The results mentioned earlier suggest a role for IPGs as putative mediators of IGF-1 signaling. The involvement of IPGs on IGF-1 activity seems to be complementary to the canonical IGF-1 activation of the PI3K/Akt/mTOR and Ras/MEK/ERK pathways during development, acquiring a more prominent role for insulin signaling in adulthood. Despite these results, the study of inositols for IGF-1-like properties has long been neglected and no more recent data are available, including a lack of complementary in vivo results. It is yet to be unveiled whether inositol deficiencies may cause growth and development problems due to poor IGF-1 signaling. The addition of free inositols as compared to inositol glycans during postnatal growth may provide deeper insight inositol mechanisms of action for insulin/IGF-1 signaling.

4. The Antioxidant Capacity of Inositols

In addition to the modulation of insulin signaling, inositols are polyols that might act as modulators of oxidative metabolism, helping to decrease the burden of oxidative stress. Oxidative stress is the most common factor responsible for metabolic disturbances caused by insulin resistance. Under normal reduction-oxidation conditions, physiological metabolism, especially via aerobic processes, produces a series of sub-products called reactive oxygen species (ROS) that include superoxides (O_2^-), hydrogen peroxides (H_2O_2), and hydroxyl radicals (OH^-) as part of the oxidation of metabolites. Normally, antioxidants present in organisms can compensate the generation of ROS, as they accept electrons of negatively charged oxygen molecules, deriving them into H_2O.

A common feature of insulin resistance is the elevated production of cytokines such as TNF-α and interleukin-6. A pro-inflammatory state contributes, along with hyperglycemia and decreased insulin signaling, to a deregulated metabolism and excessive generation of ROS. Oxidative stress in adipose tissue, along with an exacerbated release of cytokines, also promotes a pro-inflammatory state that contributes to the development of insulin resistance, diabetes, and concomitantly increases the risk of obesity-associated metabolic syndrome. In presence of nitric oxide (NO), a quick cross-reaction with O_2^- produces cytotoxic peroxynitrite ($ONOO^-$) as part of the reactive nitrogen species (RNS). Both ROS and RNS attack biological components of cells, including DNA, RNA, protein, or lipid peroxidation, causing severe damage to plasma and organelle membranes [120]. Oxidative/nitrosative stress during insulin resistance causes endothelial dysfunction and vascular complications or atherosclerosis. Endothelial cell production of NO is promoted by insulin via PI3K/Akt signaling, which leads to the activation of endothelial nitric oxide synthase (eNOS) [121,122]. However, decreased insulin signaling, along with elevated NADPH oxidase activity and increased generation of O_2^-, leads to a low bioavailability and bioactivity of NO [123].

In phenolic compounds, hydroxyl groups can transfer their hydrogen to negatively charged free radicals (R^-) in order to be stabilized as neutrally charged radicals (RH). As inositols are polyalcohol molecules, it has long been presumed that they possess antioxidant potential due to the presence of hydroxyl groups. The first approaches to inositol derivative molecules focused on the antioxidant potential of the inositol phosphorylated derivative phytic acid (IP_6) as an iron (Fe^{3+}) chelator. In normal conditions, free radicals are generated in the Fenton reaction by the oxidation of Fe^{2+} as follows: $Fe^{2+} + H_2O_2 \rightarrow Fe^{3+} + HO\bullet + OH^-$. However, the sequestering of Fe^{3+} by IP_6 leads to a rapid depletion of Fe^{2+}, which is oxidized by molecular oxygen (O_2), but not by H_2O_2, hence blocking free radical formation [124,125]. Antioxidant activity of IP_6 is seen to be especially relevant for the xanthine/xanthine oxidase system, which generates H_2O_2 by consecutive hypoxanthine to xanthine and xanthine to uric acid oxidation reactions [126].

The beneficial effects of free inositols in oxidative stress have also been related to radical scavenging properties. An in vitro study showed that the addition of DPIN exhibited dose-dependent inhibition of superoxide and nitric oxide formation [127]. In endothelial cell cultures under high glucose conditions, the addition of DPIN, DCI, and synthetic 3,4-dibutyryl-DCI (db-DCI) has been shown to dose-dependently scavenge superoxide in an xanthine/xanthine oxidase system [128]. It was shown that db-DCI was most effective at reducing ROS levels and exhibited an Fe^{3+}-related mechanism of action, suggesting that db-DCI acts similarly to IP_6, although the detailed mechanism of this has not been determined yet [128]. Interestingly, quebrachitol has also been described as an active component displaying a $ONOO^-$ scavenging activity [36].

The efficacy of inositols as antioxidants may also be attributed to an enhanced activity of antioxidant enzymes. Recent studies on Jian carp have shown that MI supplementation increased the activities of catalase (CAT), glutathione peroxidase (GPx), and glutathione reductase (GR) in copper (Cu)-induced toxicity, but also superoxide dismutase (SOD) and glutathione-S-transferase (GST), both in normal and Cu-induced damage conditions [129,130]. DPIN has also showed an enhancement of endogenous antioxidant activity. DPIN at a dose of 200 mg/kg inhibits oxidative stress caused by 7,12-dimethylbenz(a)anthracene (DMBA) in rats, along with an increased activity of the antioxidant enzymes SOD, CAT, GPx, and GST [127]. In a mouse model of cisplatin-induced oxidative stress, the administration of DPIN increased GSH, SOD, and CAT activities [131]. The administration of an DCI-enriched extract to streptozotocin-induced diabetic mice significantly increased glutathione (GSH) and decreased malondialdehyde (MDA) in the liver, accompanied by decreased pro-inflammatory TNF-α and increased anti-inflammatory IL-6 and interferon gamma (IFN-γ) in the sera [132].

As described previously, endothelial dysfunction is a common pathology derived from insulin resistance. Regarding this, use of inositols yields a synergistic effect for both antioxidant and insulin-sensitizing activities. The administration of MI and DCI in HUVEC cells promotes Akt phosphorylation [106]. The in vitro addition of DPIN, DCI, and db-DCI impaired contraction by the eNOS inhibitor L-NAME and increased NO effectiveness [128]. It has also been shown that db-DCI decreases reduced PKC activation, hexosamine pathway activity, and advanced glycation end products to basal levels in high glucose conditions [128].

Given the increasing problems arising from an unhealthy diet and living conditions, dietary use of inositols should be considered because of their antioxidant and insulin-sensitizing properties (Figure 3). It is still necessary to determine the exact mechanism of free radical scavenging in inositols. Structure differences are likely to contribute to the net antioxidant capacity, as differences have been observed between the sugar alcohols MI and DCI and methyl derivatives DPIN or db-DCI. There are no available research data on the antioxidant activity of IPGs, since PI-derivative structures like IP_6 could be active compounds of inositol activity.

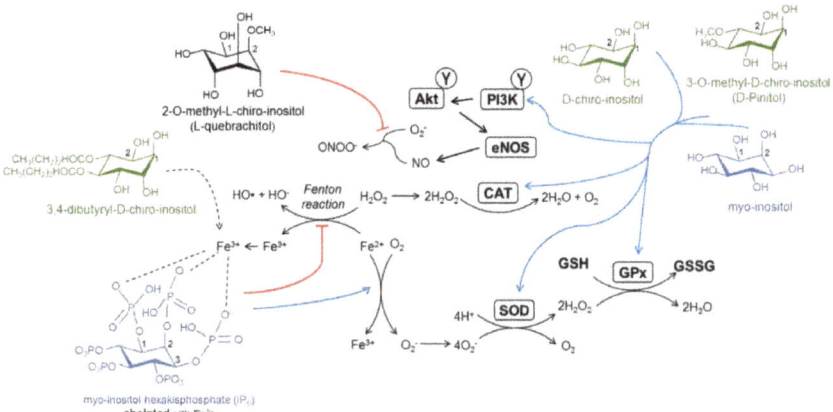

Figure 3. Proposed antioxidant mechanisms of inositol derivatives. Phytic acid (IP$_6$) chelates and sequesters Fe^{3+}, redirecting Fe^{2+} via the Fenton reaction to oxidation with O$_2$. Four molecules of Fe^{2+} are necessary to oxidize one molecule of O$_2$, which generates O$_2^-$, which is later converted in H$_2$O$_2$, and finally inactive H$_2$O. Reactive oxygen species (ROS) are scavenged by the antioxidant enzymes superoxide dismutase (SOD), catalase (CAT), and glutathione peroxidase (GPx). Inositols upregulate antioxidant enzyme levels and activity. The activation of insulin signaling in the endothelium results in increased NO production. L-quebrachitol and 3,4-dibutyryl-D-chiro-inositol scavenge peroxynitrite (ONOO$^-$) and ROS species, respectively, although the mechanisms of this have not been unveiled yet.

5. Inositols in the Brain

5.1. Sources and Distribution of Inositols in the Brain

For many years, inositol disposition in the brain has gained much attention due to the observation that inositol levels are 7-fold higher in the cerebrospinal fluid relative to plasma, and some 50- to 200-fold higher in the brain, in addition to several reports of altered MI and SI levels with different neuropathologies [133]. As in the rest of the body, MI is the main inositol present in mammalian brain tissue, followed by SI and small traces of DCI, NI, EI, or muco-I [12,13,25].

Inositol supply in the brain comes from three major sources, namely, the recycling of PI derivatives, de novo synthesis, and inositol active transport from the peripheral tissues. The synthesis of inositols produced in the brain occurs to a lesser extent relative to the peripheral tissues [37]. The activity of MIPS has been detected in the microvasculature of mammalian brains [134]. In vitro studies with neuroblastoma cells have shown that the expression of the inositol synthesis enzyme IMPase is necessary for GSK3-α but not GSK3-β activity [135]. However, other previous results did not detect IMPase activity in vitro in NT2-N neurons [136]. There are still some discrepancies regarding whether de novo synthesis and inositol recycling are major sources of free inositol for normal neuronal and glial activities without the need for active transport from peripheral sources of inositols. Homozygous SMIT1 KO animals show remarkedly decreased MI levels in the whole brain, especially in the frontal cortex (55% reduction) and hippocampus (60% reduction), but normal levels of PI, IP$_5$, and IP$_6$, which may suggest de novo MI synthesis maintains PI-derivative levels in the brain [137–139]. However, IMPase KO mice show a 65% decrease in IMPase activity but normal MI levels in the hippocampus [140]. We suspect these differences may rely on compensatory mechanisms of inositol replenishment, a pool of inositol reserves as PI, or differences in inositol content and metabolism in neurons versus glia. Although PI intracellular levels do not change in SMIT KO mice, overexpression of SMIT in transfected cells has shown the same PI levels as the control cells and intracellular PIP and PIP$_2$ levels increased, which may suggest a different or minor pool for PI-derived signaling molecules responsive to SMIT or MI levels and these are not sensitive enough to contribute to the total PI pool in the cell [141,142].

The distribution of MI in the brain is unequal and may be representative of particularities in regional activity. MI levels are higher in hypothalamus relative to the hippocampus, as detected by ^{1}H-magnetic resonance spectroscopy (MRS) in mouse brains [143]. MI uptake is also produced at a higher rate when compared to the hippocampus, cortex, caudate, or cerebellum [144] in rat brains. The hypothalamus is adjacent to the third ventricle, where the blood–brain barrier permeabilizes and provides access to metabolic signals from the peripheral tissues like insulin, glucagon, leptin, gherlin, or glucose itself [145]. Variation in regional MI might be due to different expressions of the inositol transporters SMIT1 and SMIT2. Cerebellar mRNA expression of SMIT1 and SMIT2 is higher than hippocampal and cortical expression in mice [47]. Apart from SMIT1 and SMIT2, HMIT has gained relevance as it is expressed predominantly in the brain, especially in the neuronal population of the human hippocampus and cortex, as determined by immunocytochemistry [52,54]. Analysis of RNA expression of HMIT in rat brains has shown that the HMIT transcript is expressed predominantly in the brain, with higher expression found in the cerebral cortex, hippocampus, hypothalamus, cerebellum, and brainstem [52]. Inositol HMIT transport is pH-dependent and phlorizin-sensitive [52].

Importantly, different presences of SMIT1, SMIT2, and HMIT have been detected in astrocytes and neurons. A study in cultured astrocytes and neurons showed that HMIT and SMIT1 are more present in astroglia than SMIT2 and may contribute to a higher uptake of MI due to their affinity [55]. On the other hand, SMIT1, SMIT2, and HMIT are all expressed in neuronal cells, where SMIT2 is expressed at higher levels [55]. Even though HMIT has been suggested to be relocated actively between plasma membrane and vesicles via exocytosis in regions of nerve growth, further studies have shown that HMIT is not actively expressed in the cell membrane of human neurons and does not participate in inositol internalization [53,54]. HMIT is co-stained with Golgi markers in neurons, indicating that it could participate in vesicular inositol trafficking. Since IP$_3$ is a substrate for HMIT transport, it has been speculated that the role of HMIT would be more committed to the regulation of intracellular IP$_3$ levels and Ca^{2+} signaling instead of participating in inositol internalization in neurons [54]. The expression of HMIT has also been detected in astrocytes and it seems to be localized both in intracellular and plasma membrane, as depicted by immunochemistry [52]. HMIT shows high capacity/low affinity transport kinetics and is relevant for MI transport under physiologically relevant MI concentrations, whereas under intracellular acidic conditions or lower extracellular MI conditions, SMIT1 and SMIT2 (to a lesser extent) are the main mediators of inositol uptake in primary cultures of mouse astrocytes [55]. This suggests that inositol transport in neurons and astrocytes is regionalized and mediated by different transport systems, which could be associated with a specific role of inositols in the intracellular signaling mechanism.

When incorporated into phospholipids, PI derivatives show specific functions in the nervous system, as reviewed [146]. Briefly, PI(3)P is important for the hippocampal regulation of GABAergic inhibitory transmission, PI(5)P regulates Notch cell signaling, PI(4,5)P$_2$ is involved in different processes of neuronal excitability, PI(3,5)P$_2$ affect glutamatergic signaling, and both PI(3,4)P$_2$ and PI(3,4,5)P$_3$ have a role in dendrite development.

The recent interest of the inositol derivative lysophosphatidylinositol (LPI) as a central regulator of memory and inflammatory processes should also be highlighted. LPI is formed by the action of phospholipases A1 (PLA1) and A2 (PLA2) on PI and serves as an intermediate for the synthesis of endocannabinoid 2-arachidonoylglycerol (2-AG). However, LPI has an important role in controlling neuronal excitability and responsivity to external stimuli, as it acts as a putative ligand for cannabinoid G protein-coupled receptor 55 (GPR55). In the periphery, GPR55 is known to modulate and increase insulin secretion in beta-pancreatic islets via a mechanism involving the mobilization of intracellular Ca^{2+} [147]. GPR55 is also known to be involved in energy metabolism and pain sensation [148,149]. Specifically in the brain, GPR55 has been shown to be expressed in the hippocampi of mice and rats and is localized in the CA1 and CA3 layers of pyramidal cells [150]. The application of LPI to hippocampal mouse slices enhances the long-term potentiation of CA1 neurons [150]. Moreover, central administration of LPI and GPR55 agonists promotes procedural memory and provokes changes in spatial memory [151,152]. Central actions of GPR55 seem to rely on its ability to modulate intracellular Ca^{2+} presynaptically and boost neurotransmitter release, as observed in the hippocampal CA1 to CA3 subregions of mice brain slices [153]. These results suggest that the inositol derivative LPI is able to regulate cognitive processes through the activation of GPR55. A summary of inositol distribution in the brain and the main activities can be found in Table 2.

Table 2. Distribution of inositols in the brain and the main functions of inositol derivatives. LPI: Lysophosphatidylinositol; GPR55: Cannabinoid G protein-coupled receptor 55; HMIT: H^+/myo-inositol transporter; PIP_2: Phosphatidylinositol (4,5)-bisphosphate; GIRK: G protein-gated inwardly rectifying potassium.

Inositol Sources in the Brain	Inositol Isoform	Main Brain Target	Described Mechanism
De novo synthesis from active transport from peripheral tissues. SMIT1: A 2 Na^+:1 myo-inositol co-transporter, present in microglia and neurons [55]. Expressed in the cerebellum, hippocampus, and cortex [47]. SMIT2: A 2 Na^+:1 myo-inositol co-transporter predominantly present in neurons [55]. Expressed in the cerebellum, hippocampus, and cortex [47]. HMIT: H^+/myo-inositol co-transporter, present in neurons and microglia [52,54]. Expression found in the cerebral cortex, hippocampus, hypothalamus, cerebellum, and brainstem. Participates in the regulation of intracellular IP3 levels [52,54].	Myo-inositol	Astrocytes.	• Acts as an osmolyte in astrocytes. • Alterations in brain MI levels are commonly observed in traumatic and neurodegenerative diseases [154–157].
	LPI	GPR55 in the hippocampus.	• Binding of LPI to GPR55 enhances long-term potentiation and stimulates memory formation [151,152] via the mobilization of intracellular Ca^{2+} [153].
	IP_3	Endoplasmic reticulum in neurons.	• Mobilization of intracellular Ca^{2+} deposits in neurons, modulating membrane excitability in a mechanism associated with HMIT transport [54].
	PIP_2	Potassium channels GIRK and KCNQ2/3, mainly found in the hippocampus.	• PIP_2 bioavailability modulates neuronal excitability in a SMIT1-KCNQ2/3-dependent mechanism [158]. • PIP_2 stimulates the opening of GIRK and KCNQ2/3 channels, promoting M-current [159,160].
	PI(3)P	GABA neurons in the hippocampus.	• Promotes postsynaptic GABA receptor clustering [161].
	$PI(4,5)P_2$	Ion channels found in neurons.	• Regulation of neuronal excitability, as a substrate for normal function of ion channels in neurons [146,162].
	$PI(3,5)P_2$	NMDA and GluA1 channels in neurons.	• Altered $PI(3,5)P_2$ impairs recycling of NMDA and GluA1 channels, affecting glutamatergic transmission [163,164].
	$PI(3,4)P_2$	Neurites.	• $PI(3,4)P_2$ clustering is necessary for neurite initiation [165].

A more detailed description of the role of inositols in the brain could clarify the possibilities of their use as nutraceutical treatments. Nevertheless, when considering the external supply of inositols in the brain, it should be considered that the administration of inositol derivatives like SI decreases the concentration of MI, which may represent a shift in the inositol equilibrium, promoting MI degradation to stabilize brain homeostasis [18]. Hence, the administration of inositol derivatives should be tightly regulated in order to avoid an imbalance in inositol homeostasis.

5.2. Inositols as Osmolytes in Astrocytes

Inositols are described as osmolytes in plants, protecting them from heat, high salinity, and drought stress [33]. In mammals, higher concentrations of inositols in the brain, with respect to the peripheral tissues, stand mainly for their osmoregulatory role in astrocytes, as multinuclear NMR studies have suggested [166]. SMIT gene expression is increased under osmotic stress conditions and rapidly decreased when iso-osmolarity is reestablished [167]. This mechanism allows astrocytes to adapt their size in order to reduce the impact of an ionic imbalance in extracellular media. In hypotonic conditions, the volume-sensitive organic osmolyte anion channel (VSOAC) mediates the rapid efflux of inositol along with other osmolytes, leading to cell shrinkage [168].

This property of MI fluctuation in glial cells has led to its correlation as a widely accepted marker for astrogliosis. An ^{1}H-MRS study in brains showed reduced MI levels after a traumatic brain injury, which was later normalized over time [169]. This decrease in brain MI may be a result of astrocyte cell death or either a mechanism of osmoregulation to prevent the development of brain swelling [170]. However, the activation of microglia and astrocytes leads to the accumulation of osmolytes and increased cell size, reflecting a higher MI content [171]. MI accumulation in astrogliosis is also a common feature observed during aging in the hippocampus and cortex [172], which seems to reflect changes in astroglia cell metabolism, a chronic inflammatory state, and oxidative stress [173,174].

As observed during aging, elevated MI levels in the brain are also observed during previous stages of mild cognitive impairment (MCI), AD, and pre-AD patients with Down's syndrome (DS), with a negative correlation between MI levels and cognitive performance [154–157]. Altered MI levels are also observed with bipolar disorder [175]. Changes observed in MI levels localized in the hippocampus and frontal cortex, involved several functions, including memory and task decision, make MI a valuable biomarker of early stages of cognitive decline as it can be detected in vivo in early stages of cognitive decline and correlates time-dependently with its development.

5.3. Changes in Inositol Derivatives and Excitability in Neurons

It is well established that inositols are osmoregulators in astrocytes. Since this may also be true for neuronal populations, an important role of SMIT transporters and inositol transfer within the cell has been found as intrinsic modulators of neuronal excitability.

Membrane potential is highly influenced by the efflux of K$^+$ through ion-, voltage-, or metabolic-dependent channels, which are responsible for the inhibition of cell excitability. As a substrate, the inositol derivative PIP$_2$ acts as a "metabolic sensor" and interacts with the Kir6.2 and SUR1 subunits of ATP-sensitive K$^+$ channels (K$_{ATP}$), stabilizing the open state of the channel (as opposed to ATP, which stabilizes the closed state of the channel), which is an important mechanism of the pancreatic release of insulin [176–179]. In neurons, excitability is tightly controlled by G protein-gated inwardly rectifying potassium (GIRK) channels and muscarine-sensitive voltage-gated potassium (Kv) channels, where KCNQ2 and KCNQ3, forming the heteromer KCNQ2/3, are major contributors in the hippocampus for M-current, a non-inactivating K$^+$ that defines phasic versus tonic firing [159,160]. As an intracellular signaling molecule, PIP$_2$ promotes the opening of GIRK [180] and KCNQ2/3 [181,182]. According to this, the KCNQ2/3 current is inhibited when PIP$_2$ is depleted via the activation of Gq-coupled receptors and the subsequent PLC cleavage of PIP$_2$ [181].

Regarding the later information, PIP2 is necessary for the modulation of KCNQ2/3 heteromer activity, but recent data point to a SMIT-mediated control of channel function. SMIT1 and SMIT2 interact physically and colocalize with KCNQ2/3 in sciatic nerve nodes of Ranvier and in axon initial segments [158,183]. In the absence of MI, SMIT1 co-expression with KCNQ2/3 modulates channel ion selectivity, gating, and pharmacology, making KCNQ2/3 less sensitive to extracellular K+ and promoting M-current [183]. However, when MI is added, KCNQ2/3 currents augment with a seemingly increased PIP$_2$ synthesis [158]. This fact is supported by increased PIP and PIP2 levels in hypertonic medium and faster cell recovery after drug-mediated suppression of KCNQ2/3 current [141]. Thus, both SMIT and MI synergistically promote hyperpolarizing currents mediated by KCNQ2/3. Interestingly,

GABA modulates KCNQ2/3 in a similar way as SMIT1. The activation of KCNQ2/3 seems to be mediated by SMIT1 through KCNQ2, whereas GABA communicates with KCNQ3. GABA binds to a S5 residue in both KCNQ2 and KCNQ3, mediating a conformational change that leads to loss of SMIT1 influence over KCNQ2/3. Since SMIT1 also binds the same S5 residues, its co-expression reduces GABA potentiation with respect to KCNQ2/3. Thereby, the presence of GABA decreases SMIT1 influence over KCNQ2/3 and vice versa as a negative feedback mechanism [160].

The finding that inositol regulates neuronal excitability is especially relevant regarding correlations of altered KCNQ conductance in several models of neurodegenerative diseases. Alzheimer's disease (AD) has been correlated to a reduced expression of the GirK2, GirK3, GirK4, KCNQ2, and KCNQ3 subunits and genes encoding for the antioxidants SOD, 8-oxoguanine DNA glycosylase (OGG1), and monoamine oxidase A (MAO-A) in rats [184]. Familial-inherited epilepsy has also been associated with mutations in KCNQ2 and KCNQ3 [185–187]. The expression and function of KCNQ2 [188] and KCNQ3 [189] are both also altered in cases of bipolar disorder. Crosstalk between SMIT/MI and KCNQ channels is an important issue, as changing intracellular levels of MI and thus PIP_2 levels may modulate neuronal excitability in the hippocampus. The fact that many neuropathologies are related to either SMIT- or KCNQ2/3-altered function highlights the importance of inositol in normal neuronal function.

6. Neurodegenerative Diseases: Perspectives for the Use of Inositols

6.1. Alzheimer's Disease

6.1.1. Inositols and the Amyloid Pathology

AD dementia is the main clinical entity contributing to the increased prevalence of dementia. In the absence of effective therapies to avoid the deposition of β-amyloid (Aβ) plaques, the main pathogenic factor studied in AD, efforts are also focusing on procedures to delay the cognitive decline associated with this anomalous protein accumulation.

One of the most characteristic features of AD development is the aberrant production and deposition of Aβ peptides, either in $Aβ_{40}$ or $Aβ_{42}$ fragments. Amyloid precursor protein is subject to protease activity by β-secretase (BACE1) and γ-secretase. Presenilin-1, the catalytic subunit of γ-secretase, is regarded as a major contributor of increased Aβ production. Notably, γ-secretase also contributes to the cleavage of other substrates like Notch, which is important for cell differentiation in embryogenesis and adulthood [190]. The accumulation of Aβ oligomers extracellularly leads to the appearance of Aβ-derived diffusible ligands (ADDLs), which are highly neurotoxic and mediate the disruption of neuronal synapses, the depression of signaling, tau hyperphosphorylation (another well studied factor in AD), the disruption of normal autophagic processes, the generation of ROS and RNS, and cell death [107]. The combination of the above factors is seen to be the cause for cognitive impairment and memory loss.

The tendency of Aβ accumulation seems to be facilitated by binding to peroxidized PI lipids as a consequence of oxidative stress, inducing the conformational secondary structure of the β-sheet [191]. Based on this, it was hypothesized that free myo-inositol and inositol stereoisomers might interfere with Aβ aggregation and fibril formation competing for Aβ-PI lipid binding and stabilizing soluble forms of Aβ [23,24]. Early studies in vitro proved that MI, SI, and EI induced formations of stable β-structures of $Aβ_{42}$, but these structures did not result in $Aβ_{42}$ progression to fibrillar structures at a 1:1 ratio (by weight). The same studies showed that non-fibrillar $Aβ_{42}$ oligomers, which may cause neuronal toxicity as well, were non-toxic in the presence of EI and SI at a ratio of 1:20 [24]. DCI, however, was unable to avoid $Aβ_{42}$ fibrillar conformation and toxicity, which is suggested to be due to the necessity of the hydroxyl groups to be oriented at positions 1, 3, and 5 or alternatively 2, 4, and 6 in order to stabilize the inositol-$Aβ_{42}$ complex structure [24].

Further studies in vivo have shown that the prophylactic administration of SI and EI is effective for preventing cognitive decline and Aβ aggregation at early stages in a mouse model of AD (TgCRND8) and 1-month treatment of SI, but EI could not also reverse disease development [192]. Positive effects with SI were corroborated with decreased astrogliosis and an improvement of synaptic transmission, observed by increased levels of synaptophysin [192]. A later study corroborated higher levels of SI in the brain after ad libitum administration to TgCRND8 mice, with reduced A$β_{40}$ and A$β_{42}$ brain levels and decreased plaque formation [18]. Moreover, Aβ cerebroventricular-injected rats with ad libitum access to SI in drinking water had improved performance for learning tasks than non-SI treated rats [193]. Since SI showed better results than EI and other inositol stereoisomers, later studies focused on the SI effect in the same and other murine models of AD, showing improvements in damaged cortical microvasculature caused by Aβ accumulation and improved spatial learning [194–196].

These studies have been substantially reviewed and have raised the not-so-feasible properties of SI (and, to a lesser extent, EI) and its ability to decrease Aβ aggregation and neuronal damage. Some complaints have arisen from the concentration of SI or EI required for interaction with Aβ and the disruption of fibril formation [197]. Other studies have shown the inefficacy of SI at a ratio of 1:10 for inhibiting Aβ aggregation and toxicity, as well as cell death for PC-12 cells and mixed primary rat hippocampal neurons mixed with glial cells [198]. Others have reported that SI binds weakly to other minor-contributing amyloid fragments like A$β_{25-35}$ (formed in aging brains after A$β_{40}$ cleavage) [199,200]. Despite these concerns, SI levels are dramatically increased in the brain after ad libitum access, thus being able to interfere in Aβ toxicity, as observed in animal models [18].

These results led to a phase II clinical study of SI (named as ELND005) for mild-to-moderate AD. The administration of SI at a 250 mg dose resulted, after 78 weeks of treatment, in a slight improvement in neurological performance, increased brain ventricle volume, and lower levels of CFS A$β_{42}$, accompanied by higher levels of SI in CSF, as observed in animal models [201]. Further clinical trials have focused on SI effects on agitation and aggression in AD. Despite these results, higher doses of SI resulted in early deaths (4 deceased for 1000 mg SI dose and 5 deceased for 2000 mg SI dose) [201]. SI toxicity may have been caused by renal failure, as uric acid was decreased dose-dependently in SI-treated patients [201]. However, in young healthy subjects, 10-day administration of 2000 mg SI every 12 h also resulted in higher SI levels in blood and CSF with no adverse effects [202]. Further concerns about SI safety have led to the development of SI derivatives, aiming to increase brain penetration, allowing for better efficacy with lower doses of SI for treating AD. A recent report has highlighted AAD-66, a guanidine-appended SI derivative that has improved cognitive performance in a 5xFAD mouse model of AD, concomitant with a reduction in Aβ deposition and glial reactivity as compared to free SI when both were administered ad libitum at the same dose [203].

Although high doses of SI have not been approved for clinical use due to the adverse effects, the search for inositol derivatives, especially those from SI, represent a promising reality in the use of substances derived from natural compounds for the treatment of AD. Along with SI, DPIN is also being tested in clinical trials for AD pathology treatments. DPIN has shown to be a γ-secretase inhibitor that is Notch-sparing (that is, it does not affect Notch cleavage) in vitro [204]. These results show that inositols can directly intervene in the Aβ pathology of different targets (Figure 4).

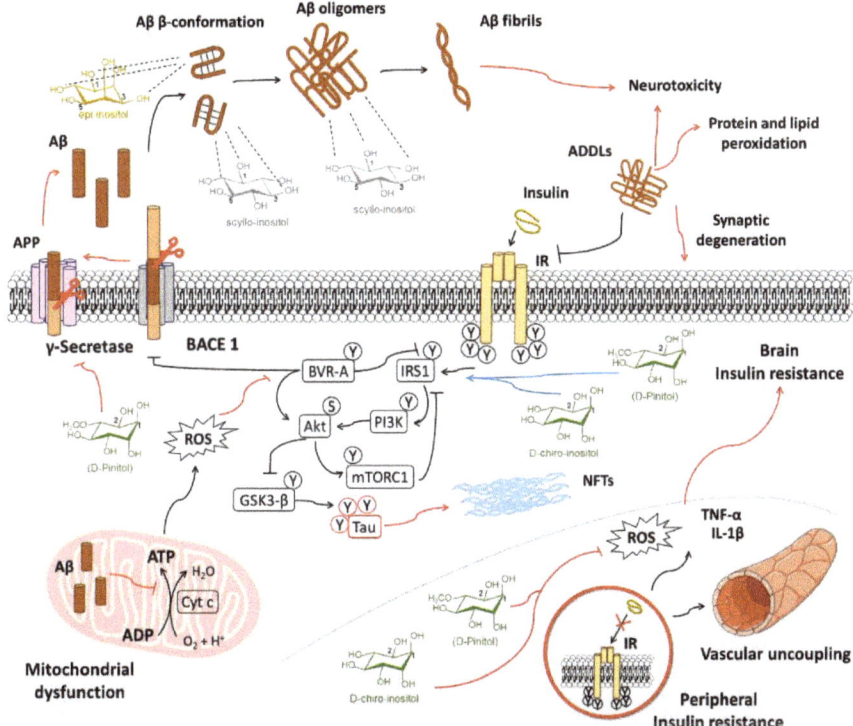

Figure 4. Schematic view of inositol interplay in mechanisms leading to progression of Alzheimer's disease. Epi- and scyllo-inositol stabilize β-sheet conformation of β amyloid (Aβ) products of aberrant APP hydrolysis by β-secretase (BACE1) and γ-secretase. Scyllo-inositol also prevents fibril formation from Aβ oligomers. Pinitol is seen to inhibit γ-secretase cleavage of APP but not Notch products. Brain insulin resistance contributes to amyloid pathology and ultimately to tau hyperphosphorylation, forming toxic microtubule neurofibrillary tangles (NFTs). Mitochondrial dysfunction and presence of Aβ-derived diffusible ligands (ADDLs) worsen the insulin response. D-chiro-inositol and D-pinitol improve insulin sensitivity in the brain, counteracting the development of brain insulin resistance. Inositols prevent early impairment in insulin signaling and the development of vascular dysfunction, which promotes oxidative stress and the release of pro-inflammatory cytokines, ultimately contributing to amyloid pathology in the context of brain insulin resistance in Alzheimer's disease.

6.1.2. Inositol Use for Brain Insulin Resistance in Alzheimer's Disease

Insulin resistance has emerged as one cause–effect of AD [205]. Recent studies have shown that cognitive impairment and AD progression are related to a dysfunction in insulin signaling in the hippocampus and frontal cortex. Postmortem analysis of human hippocampal tissue shows a correlation between high serine-inhibitory phosphorylation of IRS1 and oligomeric Aβ plaques, which were negatively associated with working memory and episodic memory [206]. The same study observed that GSK3-β activity was correlated with insulin resistance and tau hyperphosphorylation [206]. Further studies have shown that early hyperactivation of insulin signaling may cause negative feedback mediated by mTOR and decreased biliverdin-A reductase (BVR-A) activity, an oxidative stress-sensitive antioxidant enzyme and second messenger in insulin signaling, controlling IRS1 and Akt serine phosphorylation [207,208]. Brain insulin resistance and increased oxidative stress lead to overall carbonyl and peroxynitrite protein modifications, leading to signaling dysfunction and a decrease in cognitive performance [209]. An in vitro study showed that the accumulation of ADDLs caused a loss of surface IRs, and ADDL-induced oxidative stress and synaptic spine deterioration could be completely prevented by insulin treatment [209].

Since insulin resistance is an accepted contributor to a worsening AD condition, some strategies have been designed in order to restore insulin signaling in the brain. A proposed strategy is the use of intranasal insulin [210], as it has been proven to be effective at restoring cognitive function, decreasing Aβ aggregation, tau hyperphosphorylation, and nitrosative stress in a 3xTg mouse model of AD [211]. Intranasal insulin has been part of clinical trials, with minimal safety concerns reported so far [212]. Moreover, insulin is a short-life acting molecule, and some derivatives are currently under development [212,213]. Although it is beyond the scope of this review to focus on the insulin molecule itself as a potential treatment for brain insulin resistance-related pathologies, this short summary paves the way for the use of naturally occurring insulin-mimetic compounds, the safety of which has been tested in humans.

The potent stimulatory effect of DCI on insulin signaling is highly likely to contribute to an insulin neuroprotective effect on AD. DCI is effectively transported through the blood–brain barrier and stimulates insulin signaling, as seen in the hypothalamus [214]. An in vitro study showed that DCI, its methyl derivative DPIN, and DCI-GPI INS-2 increased IR autophosphorylation at a dose of 100 μM in primary rat hippocampal neurons [107]. Moreover, the same dose of DCI potentiated insulin-mediated inhibition of ADDL binding to neuron spines and neurites and ADDL-induced synapse damage to neurons [107]. This effect was not observed for MI and was suppressed after addition to PI3K, ERKm, and IGF1R inhibitors, blocking insulin DCI-potentiated signaling [107]. Although these results suggest inositols such as DCI or DPIN are an effective treatment for preserving insulin-deficient signaling in the brain, there are few data on the use of insulin-mimetic inositols in vivo. This is likely due to biased use of SI amongst all inositol derivatives, given its direct interaction with Aβ aggregates.

The use of strong insulin-sensitizers like DCI and their derivatives could serve as an alternative treatment, based on compounds easily obtained from natural sources, whose use in high doses in humans has proven to be safe and effective in other pathologies caused by insulin resistance [27,215]. Moreover, increasing evidence suggesting that peripheral type 2 diabetes exacerbates AD development raises the interest for combinational therapies. The possible protective role of inositols in T2D and AD comorbidity will be summarized in the next section.

6.1.3. Unhealthy Dietary Habits and Microvascular Damage in Alzheimer's Disease: Preventive Inositol Supplementation

Since brain insulin resistance contributes to AD development, increasing evidence suggests that peripheral type 2 diabetes mellitus (T2DM) may overlap and exacerbate AD-related cognitive impairment, neuroinflammation, oxidative stress, Aβ aggregation, tau hyperphosphorylation, and synaptic dysfunction [216–218]. A meta-analysis has shown a 56% increased risk of AD in diabetic patients, and a high prevalence of mixed pathologies [219].

A high fat diet in experimental models, leading to development of T2DM, produces Aβ deposition through altered mechanisms of autophagy and apoptosis, as well as neuroinflammation though alteration in the metabolism and the production of ROS and pro-inflammatory mediators [220–223]. Middle-aged patients with insulin resistance share common features with AD as the uncoupling of macrovascular blood flow and microvascular perfusion, which is likely due to coupling through the metabolic alterations derived from metabolic shifts induced by the oxidation of fatty acids [224,225]. In addition, high fat diets can modify microbiota compositions, altering the reaction of the intestinal immune barrier. These events might result in changes in circulating levels of pro-inflammatory mediators (cytokines, chemokines, endotoxin) produced at the intestinal levels [226].

The concomitant combination of insulin resistance, a chronic pro-inflammatory state, oxidative stress, and vascular endothelial dysfunction might directly promote an adverse environment for neuronal survival in the context of AD, thus worsening AD-related features. As we have previously described, inositols have been effectively used for treatment of insulin resistance-related pathologies.

Regarding insulin-based therapies in AD, the use of intranasal insulin has no cognitive benefits in prediabetic animals compared to non-diabetic animals [227].

In this perspective, the fact that inositols exert an insulin sensitizing effect, but also directly improve endothelial function and act as antioxidant molecules, suggests its use as a supplement in a preventive way. Although no publication exists on the use of Alzheimer's-associated inositols in the context of insulin resistance, some patents have covered this issue. Pasinetti showed that treatment with 100 mg/kg DPIN administered ad libitum in a Tg2576 mouse model of AD exposed to a high fat diet reduced Aβ levels in the hippocampus, neocortex, and serum through the restoration in the brain of insulin receptor signal transduction [204].

Because inositols are insulin-sensitizers that restore deficient insulin signaling without hyperactivation of insulin signaling, avoiding insulin side-effects, their preventive use as prophylactic agents has emerged as a powerful strategy to delay or lessen the impact of cognitive decline, protecting from synaptic dysfunction. Therefore, we suggest a combination of inositol supplementation with healthy dietary intervention, which is able to modulate microbial production of inositols like SI for the pre-treatment and treatment of AD pathology [228].

6.2. Down's Syndrome

DS is a high-risk factor for the early development of AD. Cognitive impairment in adults with DS resembles that of AD patients [229]. As observed in AD, adults with DS present greater brain MI levels, increasing with age [156]. This may be due to an extra copy of the SMIT1 gene in chromosome 21 [230]. Moreover, the overexpression of amyloid precursor APP due to its presence on chromosome 21 is likely the cause for the increased production of Aβ fragments [231]. Brain insulin resistance is also observed to be developed early in DS subjects, as seen in the inhibition of IRS1 and the uncoupling of downstream elements of insulin signaling [232,233]. These alterations are a major factor for triggering early AD in DS.

Given the prevalence of AD in DS, SI (ELND005) has been tested in a phase II clinical trial in subjects with DS. Both doses of 250 mg/day and 250 mg/twice a day of SI resulted in no serious adverse events, and increased SI concentration in plasma. Interestingly, although a small sample group was tested, the subjects with double dose of 250 mg SI showed improvements in their "neuropsychiatric inventory", a behavioral measure that assesses symptoms like irritability and agitation [234]. A phase III clinical trial with SI in DS is expected to start.

6.3. Anxiety, Compulsive, and Depressive Disorders

Anxiety or closely related disorders are characterized by fear and anxiety related to behavioral disturbances, including panic disorder or obsessive-compulsive disorder (OCD). The search for new treatments for anxiety disorders has long led to an analysis of the effect of MI administration. It has been shown by ^{1}H-MRS that frontal cortex MI levels are reduced in patients with depressive and sleep disorders, and MI levels are negatively correlated with depression severity [235,236]. Despite a mechanism of action that is partially unknown, many clinical trials in humans have probed MI at a dose ranging from 12–18 g/day, finding that the dosage is effective for the treatment of panic disorders, OCD, and depression, which are included in the broad spectrum of disorders mainly treated with selective serotonin reuptake inhibitors (SSRIs) [20–22].

Since serotonin receptors (5-HTs) are G-protein-coupled receptors, the net effect of MI was thought to be mediated by the replenishment of PI and PIP_2 availability, avoiding receptor desensitization [237]. In a forced swim test in rats, MI administration reduced depressive behavior, which was abolished by the addition of the specific $5\text{-}HT_{2A}/5\text{-}HT_{2C}$ antagonist ritanserin, but not the $5\text{-}HT_{1A}/5\text{-}HT_{1B}/\beta$ adrenergic antagonist pindolol, which suggests that the MI anti-depressant mechanism specifically involves $5\text{-}HT_2$ subtype receptors [238]. Moreover, the administration of 1.2 g/kg MI for 12 weeks significantly increased type 2 dopamine (D_2) and slightly increased $5\text{-}HT_2$ receptor density in the striatum of guinea pigs, a region involved in locomotor and stereotype behavior [239]. Although the

MI mechanism has not been fully elucidated, its use for anxiety and depressive disorders is still under evaluation. It should also be noted that MI has no additive effect with SSRI treatment, which suggests that somehow both families of compounds intersect regarding their mechanism of action [240,241].

7. From Patents to Clinical Trials of Inositols

The industrialized market for nutritional products, such as dietary supplements, has experienced spectacular growth during the late 1990s and the last decade, and has been focused on the development of functional and nutraceutical food products. One of the reasons for the expansion has been the change in the trend of consumers towards the use of supplements with a natural origin. Because there is no worldwide legislation that establishes a precise definition of nutraceuticals, their protection and marketing have both raised certain doubts. Generally, an updated term for nutraceuticals is a product of natural origin that possesses study-based beneficial effects on health.

As we have described throughout this review, inositols fall within these characteristics. The fact that they are molecules with multiple beneficial functions for health (i.e., via their antioxidant capacity, improvement of insulin resistance, and treatment of cardiovascular problems) has led to a high competitiveness to patent their use in an ambit where effective treatments are not available. This is the figure associated with the Alzheimer's market. Since the mid-2000s, there has been a significant increase in the number of patents related to the use of inositols in AD. To document this, we have performed an advanced search on the World Intellectual Property Organization (WIPO) database, combining results for all nine inositol stereoisomers and derivatives, excluding phosphate-linked forms of inositols and Alzheimer's disease. After compiling all the results that contained the terms described in the title, abstract, or claims, we carried out a refinement process (elimination of duplicates, exclusion of "inositol derivatives" if not specified) and obtained a total of 26 patents distributed according to the mentioned compounds (Figure 5).

In this race to patent publication, however, it should be kept in mind that while some justify the substantiated use of a specific compound, others rely on general formulations of inositols. On the other hand, some of the studies that support the claims include AD either as the main objective in a set of common diseases, or secondarily due to the overlap of previous patents or the lack of consistency for results in an AD model. Despite the tendency slowing, the number of patents has continued to increase during 2020s, with the search for functional radical-substituted inositol derivatives prioritized over inositol stereoisomers. Although not depicted, many patents have emerged regarding the use of inositols as "carriers" of other substances, allowing them to access targets in the brain.

The late goal of nutraceutical compounds is to be approved in clinical trials. The importance of this resides in the definition of an adequate dose and the approval for use as adjuvant therapies, as in the case of AD. Since nutraceuticals are generally marketed for safe human use, this results in an advantage over synthetic drugs. From 2007 on, at least five phase II clinical trials for SI and two phase II clinical trials for DPIN have been completed for AD and AD-like dementia (Table 3). As mentioned earlier, some concerns have arisen regarding high dosages of SI. Nevertheless, a 250 mg dose of SI results in some significant improvements in the biochemical and cognitive parameters of subjects. Moreover, given the outcome of SI in prevention of AD in DS patients, it is expected that a phase III trial will begin, as the phase II trial mentioned here only enrolled 23 participants. It should also be expected that clinical trials for DPIN and DCI will be extended in the following years, as these are the most promising candidates for the palliation of AD development.

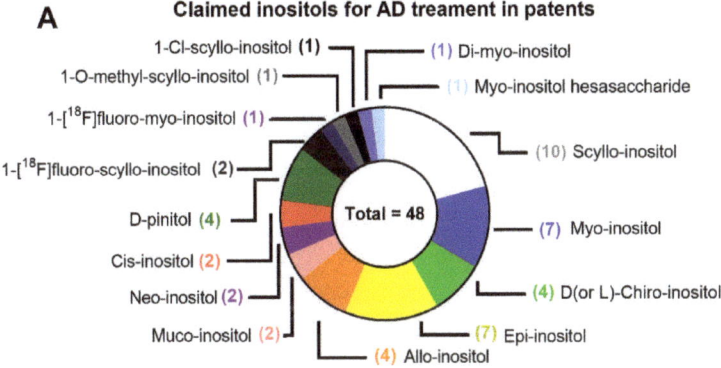

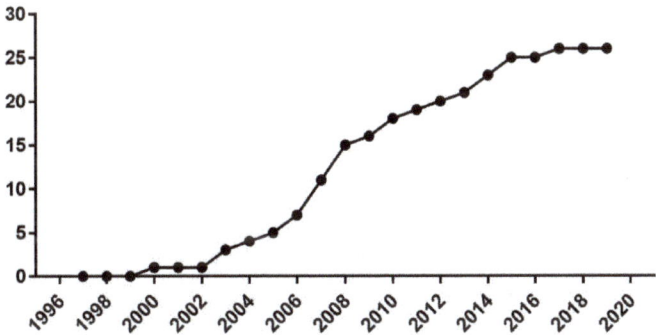

Figure 5. (**A**) Graphical illustration of patents claiming the use of inositols for Alzheimer's disease, including patents mentioning more than one inositol stereoisomer and/or derivative. (**B**) Number of patents mentioning and claiming use of inositols for AD treatment in the last two decades.

Table 3. Clinical trials of scyllo-inositol and D-pinitol in Alzheimer's disease-related patients. Alzheimer's Disease Cooperative Study-Activities of Daily Living (ADCS-ADL), Alzheimer's Disease Cooperative Study Clinician's Global Impression of Change (ADCS-CCGIC), Alzheimer's Disease Assessment Scale-Cognitive Subscale (ADAS-Cog), Clinical Dementia Rating-Sum of Boxes (CDR-SB), Mini-Mental State Examination (MMSE), Neuropsychiatric Inventory (NPI), NPI-C Combined Agitation and Aggression Subscores (NPI-C A+A), Neuropsychological Test Battery (NTB), Treatment Emergent Adverse Events (TEAEs).

Inositol	Title, NCT Number, and Date	Dose	Population	Outcome Measures	Published Results
Scyllo-inositol (ELND005)	• ELND005 in Patients with Mild to Moderate Alzheimer's Disease • Study Start: December 2007 • Study Completion: May 2010 • NCT00568776	Placebo, 250 mg/kg; 1000 mg/kg; 2000 mg/kg at 78 weeks	• Enrollment: 353 • Age: 50 Years to 85 Years (Adult, Older Adult)	• ADCS-ADL • ADAS-Cog • CDR-SB • NPI • NTB	[201]

Table 3. Cont.

Inositol	Title, NCT Number, and Date	Dose	Population	Outcome Measures	Published Results
	• ELND005 Long-Term Follow-up Study in Subjects With Alzheimer's Disease • Study Start: June 2009 • Study Completion: June 2011 • NCT00934050	Placebo, 250 mg/kg; post-Dec 2009, 2000 mg/kg; pre-Dec 2009, 48 weeks	• Enrollment: 103 • Age: Child, Adult, Older Adult	• TEAEs	Confidence agreement
	• Efficacy and Safety Study of ELND005 as a Treatment for Agitation and Aggression in Alzheimer's Disease • Study Start: November 2012 • Study Completion: May 2015 • NCT01735630	Placebo, film coated tablets, twice a day for 12 weeks	• Enrollment: 350 • Age: 50 Years to 95 Years (Adult, Older Adult)	• ADCS-ADL • ADCS-CGIC • MMSE • NPI-C A+A	Confidence agreement
	• A 36-Week Safety Extension Study of ELND005 as a Treatment for Agitation and Aggression in Alzheimer's Disease • Study Start: January 2013 • Study Completion: August 2015 • NCT01766336	Continue at same dose as previous clinical trial for 36 weeks	• Enrollment: 296 • Age: 50 Years to 95 Years (Adult, Older Adult)	• TEAEs	Confidence agreement
	• A 4-Week Safety Study of Oral ELND005 in Young Adults With Down Syndrome Without Dementia • Study Start: September 2013 • Study Completion: June 2014 • NCT01791725	Placebo, 250 mg/kg once a day; 250 mg/kg twice a day, 4 weeks	• Enrollment: 23 • Age: 18 Years to 45 Years (Adult)	• TEAEs	[234]
D-pinitol (NIC5-15)	• Development of NIC5-15 in The Treatment of Alzheimer's Disease • Study Start: January 2007 • Study Completion: March 2010 • NCT00470418	Placebo; dose not specified, 7 weeks	• Enrollment: 15 • Age: Child, Adult, Older Adult	• TEAEs • Clinical Measures of Cognition at Terminal Visit	[242]
	• A Single Site, Randomized, Double-blind, Placebo Controlled Trial of NIC5-15 in Subjects With Alzheimer's Disease • Study Start: April 2007 • Study Completion: June 2014 • NCT01928420	Placebo; dose not specified, 24 weeks	• Enrollment: 30 • Age: 40 Years to 95 Years (Adult, Older Adult)	• ADCS-ADL • ADCS-CGIC • ADAS-Cog • MMSE • NPI • Changes in AD biomarkers, APO-E genotyping	N/A

8. Concluding Remarks

In this work, we have assessed the use of nutraceuticals such as inositols, which are mostly components of human organisms and are generally acquired through diet. The nutraceutical industry is booming due to the change in the perception of pharmacological drugs and the search for alternatives based on natural compounds. These molecules can be derived from extraction processes in plants or fermentation in bioreactors, which is an advantage over chemical synthesis processes.

Inositols, essentially MI and DCI, are usually a part of membrane structures like phospholipids. As such, the study of inositols has been instrumental in understanding the mechanism of insulin resistance. At a given concentration, inositol stereoisomers can stimulate insulin signaling, preferably as IGs, but also show antioxidant capacity. However, after revising the proposed models for inositols in insulin signaling, it is still uncertain whether inositols per se are capable of displaying these characteristics. In addition to supporting insulin signaling, the importance of inositols in the brain appears to lie in their ability to control neuron and glia responses to external environments. In this regard, psychiatric disorders such as depression and anxiety were associated with imbalances in MI content in brain. Treatment with MI has been shown to improve behavioral outcomes in depression, anxiety, panic, and obsessive-compulsive disorders in a mechanism of action related to serotonin receptor activation. Albeit not fully elucidated, MI role may imply PI availability, standing out the importance of MI in physiological regulation of serotonin signaling in behavior.

Inositols are solid candidates for developing new approaches for the treatment or improvement of chronic diseases associated with aging, especially those linked to insulin resistance and oxidative stress. Aging of the population is a challenge for developed countries due to the increasing incidence of dementia. Amongst all types of dementia, sporadic AD represents a heavy burden for patients, their families, and society. AD treatment is considered a high risk, high reward market. Different strategies have been approached in an attempt to merge effective therapy when the disease is clinically diagnosable. This process generally renders unsuccessful results due to the complexity and partial lack of knowledge of the progression of AD development. We have approached AD from the point of view of the initial stages of the disease, as the aging process is closely related to the development of metabolic dysregulations leading to insulin resistance, where inositols might have a potential beneficial use.

This exhaustive review of the physiological role of inositols helps us to understand what benefits can result from external administration, either to compensate for their deficiency or as an adjuvant in oxidative stress processes. The specific position of the hydroxyl radicals gives certain stereoisomers such as SI or EI specific characteristic to limit the aggregation of Aβ, one of the main pathophysiological characteristics of AD and cognitive dementia observed in DS.

The different inositols offer complementary strategies for the preventive treatment of AD. Research of inositols, especially those with a remarkable insulin-sensitizing capacity, such as DCI or its derivative DPIN, may offer a different perspective on how insulin resistance develops in the brain and its contribution to improving cognitive outcomes for AD. The fact that clinical studies on neurological disorders with inositols have been carried out in the last decade meets a necessity and opens a way to the expansion in the use of inositols, whose perspective is not that of being a therapeutic replacement, but a bioactive compound that helps to prevent or suppress decline in neurodegenerative diseases.

Author Contributions: Conceptualization: C.S. and F.R.d.F.; writing—original draft preparation: A.J.L.-G. and J.S.; writing—review and editing: P.J.S.-C. and F.R.d.F. All authors have read and agreed to the published version of the manuscript.

Funding: This research was funded by the Agencia Estatal de Investigación, Ministerio de Economía y Competitividad or Ministerio de Ciencia e Innovación, and European Regional Development Funds-European Union (ERDF-EU), grant numbers RTC-2016-4983-1 and RTC-2019-007329-1; Instituto de Salud Carlos III (ISCIII) and ERDF-EU, grant numbers DTS16/00115, PI19/00343, and COV20/00157; Consejería de Economía, Conocimiento, Empresas y Universidad and ERDF-EU, grant number P18-TP-5194, and Consejería de Salud y Familia de la Junta de Andalucía (NeuroRECA), grant number RIC-0111-2019. J.S. holds a "Miguel Servet II" research contract from the National System of Health, ISCIII, ERDF-EU, FIMABIS, grant number CPII17/00024. A.J.L.-G. holds an "i-PFIS" predoctoral research contract from the ISCIII, ERDF-EU, grant number IFI18/00042.

Conflicts of Interest: Carlos SanJuan declares he receives salary and has share from Euronutra company. The remaining authors declare that they have no known competing financial interests or personal relationships that could have appeared to influence the work reported in this paper. The funders had no role in the design of the study; in the collection, analyses, or interpretation of data; in the writing of the manuscript, or in the decision to publish the results.

References

1. Azzu, V.; Valencak, T.G. Energy metabolism and ageing in the mouse: A mini-review. *Gerontology* **2017**, *63*, 327–336. [CrossRef]
2. Surguchov, A. Caveolin: A new link between diabetes and ad. *Cell. Mol. Neurobiol.* **2020**. [CrossRef] [PubMed]
3. Verdile, G.; Keane, K.N.; Cruzat, V.F.; Medic, S.; Sabale, M.; Rowles, J.; Wijesekara, N.; Martins, R.N.; Fraser, P.E.; Newsholme, P. Inflammation and oxidative stress: The molecular connectivity between insulin resistance, obesity, and alzheimer's disease. *Mediat. Inflamm.* **2015**, *105828*. [CrossRef] [PubMed]

4. Askarova, S.; Umbayev, B.; Masoud, A.-R.; Kaiyrlykyzy, A.; Safarova, Y.; Tsoy, A.; Olzhayev, F.; Kushugulova, A. The links between the gut microbiome, aging, modern lifestyle and alzheimer's disease. *Front. Cell Infect. Microbiol.* **2020**, *10*, 104. [CrossRef] [PubMed]
5. Thomas, M.P.; Mills, S.J.; Potter, B.V. The "other" inositols and their phosphates: Synthesis, biology, and medicine (with Recent Advances in myo-Inositol Chemistry). *Angew. Chem.* **2016**, *55*, 1614–1650. [CrossRef] [PubMed]
6. Mancini, M.; Andreassi, A.; Salvioni, M.; Pelliccione, F.; Mantellassi, G.; Banderali, G. Myoinositol and d-chiro inositol in improving insulin resistance in obese male children: Preliminary data. *Int. J. Endocrinol.* **2016**, 8720342. [CrossRef]
7. Kalra, B.; Kalra, S.; Sharma, J.B. The inositols and polycystic ovary syndrome. *Indian J. Endocrinol. Metab.* **2016**, *20*, 720–724. [CrossRef]
8. Jin, M.; Selkoe, D.J. Systematic analysis of time-dependent neural effects of soluble amyloid β oligomers in culture and in vivo: Prevention by scyllo-inositol. *Neurobiol. Dis.* **2015**, *82*, 152–163. [CrossRef]
9. Chhetri, D.R. Myo-Inositol and its derivatives: Their emerging role in the treatment of human diseases. *Front. Pharmacol.* **2019**, *10*, 1172. [CrossRef]
10. Larner, J.; Brautigan, D.L.; Thorner, M.O. D-chiro-inositol glycans in insulin signaling and insulin resistance. *Mol. Med.* **2010**, *16*, 543–552. [CrossRef]
11. Owczarczyk-Saczonek, A.; Lahuta, L.B.; Ligor, M.; Placek, W.; Górecki, R.J.; Buszewski, B. The healing-promoting properties of selected cyclitols—A review. *Nutrients* **2018**, *10*, 1891. [CrossRef] [PubMed]
12. Hipps, P.P.; Holland, W.H.; Sherman, W.R. Interconversion of myo- and scyllo-inositol with simultaneous formation of neo-inositol by an NADP+ dependent epimerase from bovine brain. *Biochem. Biophys. Res. Commun.* **1977**, *77*, 340–346. [CrossRef]
13. Pak, Y.; Huang, L.C.; Lilley, K.J.; Larner, J. In vivo conversion of [3H]myoinositol to [3H]chiroinositol in rat tissues. *J. Biol. Chem.* **1992**, *267*, 16904–16910. [PubMed]
14. Hipps, P.P.; Ackermann, K.E.; Sherman, W.R. Inositol epimerase–inosose reductase from bovine brain. *Methods Enzymol.* **1982**, *89*, 593–598. [CrossRef]
15. Pak, Y.; Paule, C.R.; Bao, Y.D.; Huang, L.C.; Larner, J. Insulin Stimulates The Biosynthesis of Chiro-Inositol-Containing Phospholipids in a Rat Fibroblast Line Expressing the Human Insulin Receptor. *Proc. Natl. Acad. Sci. USA* **1993**, *90*, 7759–7763. [CrossRef]
16. Sun, T.H.; Heimark, D.B.; Nguygen, T.; Nadler, J.L.; Larner, J. Both myo-inositol to chiro-inositol epimerase activities and chiro-inositol to myo-inositol ratios are decreased in tissues of GK type 2 diabetic rats compared to Wistar controls. *Biochem. Biophys. Res. Commun.* **2002**, *293*, 1092–1098. [CrossRef]
17. Ryals, P.E.; Kersting, M.C. Sodium-dependent uptake of [3H]scyllo-inositol by Tetrahymena: Incorporation into phosphatidylinositol, phosphatidylinositol-linked glycans, and polyphosphoinositols. *Arch. Biochem. Biophys.* **1999**, *366*, 261–266. [CrossRef]
18. Fenili, D.; Brown, M.; Rappaport, R.; McLaurin, J. Properties of scyllo–inositol as a therapeutic treatment of AD-like pathology. *J. Mol. Med.* **2007**, *85*, 603–611. [CrossRef]
19. Santamaria, A.; Di Benedetto, A.; Petrella, E.; Pintaudi, B.; Corrado, F.; D'Anna, R.; Neri, I.; Facchinetti, F. Myo-inositol may prevent gestational diabetes onset in overweight women: A randomized, controlled trial. *J. Matern. Fetal Neonatal Med.* **2016**, *29*, 3234–3237. [CrossRef]
20. Benjamin, J.; Levine, J.; Fux, M.; Aviv, A.; Levy, D.; Belmaker, R.H. Double-blind, placebo-controlled, crossover trial of inositol treatment for panic disorder. *J. Clin. Psychopharmacol.* **1995**, *152*, 1084–1086. [CrossRef]
21. Fux, M.; Levine, J.; Aviv, A.; Belmaker, R.H. Inositol treatment of obsessive-compulsive disorder. *Am. J. Psychiatry* **1996**, *153*, 1219–1221. [CrossRef] [PubMed]
22. Chengappa, K.N.; Levine, J.; Gershon, S.; Mallinger, A.G.; Hardan, A.; Vagnucci, A.; Pollock, B.; Luther, J.; Buttenfield, J.; Verfaille, S.; et al. Inositol as an add-on treatment for bipolar depression. *Bipolar Disord.* **2000**, *2*, 47–55. [CrossRef] [PubMed]
23. McLaurin, J.; Franklin, T.; Chakrabartty, A.; Fraser, P.E. Phosphatidylinositol and inositol involvement in Alzheimer amyloid-beta fibril growth and arrest. *J. Mol. Biol.* **1998**, *278*, 183–194. [CrossRef] [PubMed]
24. McLaurin, J.; Golomb, R.; Jurewicz, A.; Antel, J.P.; Fraser, P.E. Inositol stereoisomers stabilize an oligomeric aggregate of Alzheimer amyloid beta peptide and inhibit abeta -induced toxicity. *J. Biol. Chem.* **2000**, *275*, 18495–18502. [CrossRef] [PubMed]

25. Kaiser, L.G.; Schuff, N.; Cashdollar, N.; Weiner, M.W. Scyllo-inositol in normal aging human brain: 1H magnetic resonance spectroscopy study at 4 Tesla. *NMR Biomed.* **2005**, *18*, 51–55. [CrossRef] [PubMed]
26. Vekrellis, K.; Xilouri, M.; Emmanouilidou, E.; Stefanis, L. Inducible over-expression of wild type alpha-synuclein in human neuronal cells leads to caspase-dependent non-apoptotic death. *J. Neurochem.* **2009**, *109*, 1348–1362. [CrossRef]
27. Fraticelli, F.; Celentano, C.; Zecca, I.A.; Di Vieste, G.; Pintaudi, B.; Liberati, M.; Franzago, M.; Di Nicola, M.; Vitacolonna, E. Effect of inositol stereoisomers at different dosages in gestational diabetes: An open-label, parallel, randomized controlled trial. *Acta Diabetol.* **2018**, *55*, 805–812. [CrossRef]
28. Nitz, M.; Fenili, D.; Darabie, A.A.; Wu, L.; Cousins, J.E.; McLaurin, J. Modulation of amyloid-beta aggregation and toxicity by inosose stereoisomers. *FEBS J.* **2008**, *275*, 1663–1674. [CrossRef]
29. Dersjant-Li, Y.; Awati, A.; Schulze, H.; Partridge, G. Phytase in non-ruminant animal nutrition: A critical review on phytase activities in the gastrointestinal tract and influencing factors. *J. Sci. Food Agric.* **2015**, *95*, 878–896. [CrossRef]
30. Schlemmer, U.; Jany, K.D.; Berk, A.; Schulz, E.; Rechkemmer, G. Degradation of phytate in the gut of pigs–pathway of gastro-intestinal inositol phosphate hydrolysis and enzymes involved. *Arch. Fur. Tierernahr.* **2001**, *55*, 255–280. [CrossRef]
31. Goodhart, R.S.; Shils, M. *Modern Nutrition in Health and Disease*; Lea & Febiger: Philadelphia, PA, USA, 1980.
32. Clements, R.S., Jr.; Darnell, B. Myo-inositol content of common foods: Development of a high-myo-inositol diet. *Am. J. Clin. Nutr.* **1980**, *33*, 1954–1967. [CrossRef] [PubMed]
33. Ahn, C.-H.; Hossain, M.A.; Lee, E.; Kanth, B.K.; Park, P.B. Increased salt and drought tolerance by D-pinitol production in transgenic Arabidopsis thaliana. *Biochem. Biophys. Res. Commun.* **2018**, *504*, 315–320. [CrossRef] [PubMed]
34. Turhan, I. Relationship between sugar profile and d-pinitol content of pods of wild and cultivated types of carob bean (Ceratonia siliqua L.). *Int. J. Food Prop.* **2014**, *17*, 363–370. [CrossRef]
35. Yang, X.W.; Zou, L.; Wu, Q.; Fu, D.X. Studies on chemical constituents from whole plants of Crossostephium chinense. *China J. Chin. Mater. Med.* **2008**, *33*, 905–908.
36. Kim, A.R.; Zou, Y.N.; Park, T.H.; Shim, K.H.; Kim, M.S.; Kim, N.D.; Kim, J.D.; Bae, S.J.; Choi, J.S.; Chung, H.Y. Active components from artemisia iwayomogi displaying ONOO− scavenging activity. *Phytother. Res.* **2004**, *18*, 1–7. [CrossRef]
37. Beemster, P.; Groenen, P.; Steegers-Theunissen, R. Involvement of inositol in reproduction. *Nutr. Rev.* **2002**, *60*, 80–87. [CrossRef]
38. Parthasarathy, R.N.; Lakshmanan, J.; Thangavel, M.; Seelan, R.S.; Stagner, J.I.; Janckila, A.J.; Vadnal, R.E.; Casanova, M.F.; Parthasarathy, L.K. Rat brain myo-inositol 3-phosphate synthase is a phosphoprotein. *Mol. Cell. Biochem.* **2013**, *378*, 83–89. [CrossRef]
39. Yu, W.; Daniel, J.; Mehta, D.; Maddipati, K.R.; Greenberg, M.L. MCK1 is a novel regulator of myo-inositol phosphate synthase (MIPS) that is required for inhibition of inositol synthesis by the mood stabilizer valproate. *PLoS ONE* **2017**, *12*, e0182534. [CrossRef]
40. Dinicola, S.; Minini, M.; Unfer, V.; Verna, R.; Cucina, A.; Bizzarri, M. Nutritional and Acquired Deficiencies in Inositol Bioavailability. Correlations with Metabolic Disorders. *Int. J. Mol. Sci.* **2017**, *18*, 2187. [CrossRef]
41. Foster, D.A.; Salloum, D.; Menon, D.; Frias, M.A. Phospholipase D and the maintenance of phosphatidic acid levels for regulation of mammalian target of rapamycin (mTOR). *J. Biol. Chem.* **2014**, *289*, 22583–22588. [CrossRef]
42. Yu, W.; Ye, C.; Greenberg, M.L. Inositol Hexakisphosphate Kinase 1 (IP6K1) Regulates Inositol Synthesis in Mammalian Cells. *J. Biol. Chem.* **2016**, *291*, 10437–10444. [CrossRef] [PubMed]
43. Bourgeois, F.; Coady, M.J.; Lapointe, J.Y. Determination of transport stoichiometry for two cation-coupled myo-inositol cotransporters: SMIT2 and HMIT. *J. Physiol.* **2005**, *563*, 333–343. [CrossRef] [PubMed]
44. Ostlund, R.E., Jr.; Seemayer, R.; Gupta, S.; Kimmel, R.; Ostlund, E.L.; Sherman, W.R. A stereospecific myo-inositol/D-chiro-inositol transporter in HepG2 liver cells. Identification with D-chiro-[3-3H]inositol. *J. Biol. Chem.* **1996**, *271*, 10073–10078. [CrossRef] [PubMed]
45. Greene, D.A.; Lattimer, S.A. Sodium- and energy-dependent uptake of myo-inositol by rabbit peripheral nerve. Competitive inhibition by glucose and lack of an insulin effect. *J. Clin. Investig.* **1982**, *70*, 1009–1018. [CrossRef]

46. Lin, X.; Ma, L.; Fitzgerald, R.L.; Ostlund, R.E., Jr. Human sodium/inositol cotransporter 2 (SMIT2) transports inositols but not glucose in L6 cells. *Arch. Biochem. Biophys.* **2009**, *481*, 197–201. [CrossRef]
47. Fenili, D.; Weng, Y.-Q.; Aubert, I.; Nitz, M.; McLaurin, J. Sodium/myo-Inositol transporters: Substrate transport requirements and regional brain expression in the TgCRND8 mouse model of amyloid pathology. *PLoS ONE* **2011**, *6*, e24032. [CrossRef]
48. Lahjouji, K.; Aouameur, R.; Bissonnette, P.; Coady, M.J.; Bichet, D.G.; Lapointe, J.Y. Expression and functionality of the Na+/myo-inositol cotransporter SMIT2 in rabbit kidney. *Biochim. Biophys. Acta Biomembr.* **2007**, *1768*, 1154–1159. [CrossRef]
49. Bissonnette, P.; Coady, M.J.; Lapointe, J.Y. Expression of the sodium-myo-inositol cotransporter SMIT2 at the apical membrane of Madin-Darby canine kidney cells. *J. Physiol.* **2004**, *558*, 759–768. [CrossRef]
50. Ostlund, R.E., Jr.; McGill, J.B.; Herskowitz, I.; Kipnis, D.M.; Santiago, J.V.; Sherman, W.R. D-chiro-inositol Metabolism in Diabetes Mellitus. *Proc. Natl. Acad. Sci. USA* **1993**, *90*, 9988–9992. [CrossRef]
51. Asplin, I.; Galasko, G.; Larner, J. Chiro-inositol deficiency and insulin resistance: A comparison of the chiro-inositol- and the myo-inositol-containing insulin mediators isolated from urine, hemodialysate, and muscle of control and type ii diabetic subjects. *Proc. Natl. Acad. Sci. USA* **1993**, *90*, 5924–5928. [CrossRef]
52. Uldry, M.; Ibberson, M.; Horisberger, J.D.; Chatton, J.Y.; Riederer, B.M.; Thorens, B. Identification of a mammalian H(+)-myo-inositol symporter expressed predominantly in the brain. *EMBO J.* **2001**, *20*, 4467–4477. [CrossRef] [PubMed]
53. Uldry, M.; Steiner, P.; Zurich, M.G.; Beguin, P.; Hirling, H.; Dolci, W.; Thorens, B. Regulated exocytosis of an H+/myo-inositol symporter at synapses and growth cones. *EMBO J.* **2004**, *23*, 531–540. [CrossRef] [PubMed]
54. Di Daniel, E.; Mok, M.H.S.; Mead, E.; Mutinelli, C.; Zambello, E.; Caberlotto, L.L.; Pell, T.J.; Langmead, C.J.; Shah, A.J.; Duddy, G.; et al. Evaluation of expression and function of the H+/myo-inositol transporter HMIT. *BMC Cell Biol.* **2009**, *10*, 54. [CrossRef] [PubMed]
55. Fu, H.; Li, B.; Hertz, L.; Peng, L. Contributions in astrocytes of SMIT1/2 and HMIT to myo-inositol uptake at different concentrations and pH. *Neurochem. Int.* **2012**, *61*, 187–194. [CrossRef]
56. Vance, J.E. Phospholipid synthesis and transport in mammalian cells. *Traffic* **2015**, *16*, 1–18. [CrossRef]
57. Michell, R.H. Do inositol supplements enhance phosphatidylinositol supply and thus support endoplasmic reticulum function? *Br. J. Nutr.* **2018**, 1–16. [CrossRef]
58. Abel, K.; Anderson, R.A.; Shears, S.B. Phosphatidylinositol and inositol phosphate metabolism. *J. Cell Sci.* **2001**, *114*, 2207–2208.
59. Muller, G. Dynamics of plasma membrane microdomains and cross-talk to the insulin signalling cascade. *FEBS Lett.* **2002**, *531*, 81–87. [CrossRef]
60. Müller, G.; Schulz, A.; Wied, S.; Frick, W. Regulation of lipid raft proteins by glimepiride- and insulin-induced glycosylphosphatidylinositol-specific phospholipase C in rat adipocytes. *Biochem. Pharmacol.* **2005**, *69*, 761–780. [CrossRef]
61. Croze, M.L.; Soulage, C.O. Potential role and therapeutic interests of myo-inositol in metabolic diseases. *Biochimie* **2013**, *95*, 1811–1827. [CrossRef]
62. Goel, M.; Azev, V.N.; d'Alarcao, M. The biological activity of structurally defined inositol glycans. *Future Med. Chem.* **2009**, *1*, 95–118. [CrossRef] [PubMed]
63. Boucher, J.; Kleinridders, A.; Kahn, C.R. Insulin receptor signaling in normal and insulin-resistant states. *Cold Spring Harb. Perspect. Biol.* **2014**, *6*, a009191. [CrossRef] [PubMed]
64. Saltiel, A.R.; Pessin, J.E. Insulin signaling pathways in time and space. *Trends Cell Biol.* **2002**, *12*, 65–71. [CrossRef]
65. Lizcano, J.M.; Alessi, D.R. The insulin signalling pathway. *Curr. Biol.* **2002**, *12*, R236–R238. [CrossRef]
66. Saltiel, A.R.; Siegel, M.I.; Jacobs, S.; Cuatrecasas, P. Putative mediators of insulin action: Regulation of pyruvate dehydrogenase and adenylate cyclase activities. *Proc. Natl. Acad. Sci. USA* **1982**, *79*, 3513–3517. [CrossRef]
67. Saltiel, A.R.; Cuatrecasas, P. Insulin Stimulates the Generation From Hepatic Plasma Membranes of Modulators Derived from an Inositol Glycolipid. *Proc. Natl. Acad. Sci. USA* **1986**, *83*, 5793–5797. [CrossRef]
68. Kessler, A.; Muller, G.; Wied, S.; Crecelius, A.; Eckel, J. Signalling pathways of an insulin-mimetic phosphoinositolglycan-peptide in muscle and adipose tissue. *Biochem J.* **1998**, *330 Pt 1*, 277–286. [CrossRef]

69. Kunjara, S.; Wang, D.Y.; Greenbaum, A.L.; McLean, P.; Kurtz, A.; Rademacher, T.W. Inositol phosphoglycans in diabetes and obesity: Urinary levels of IPG A-type and IPG P-type, and relationship to pathophysiological changes. *Mol. Genet. Metab.* **1999**, *68*, 488–502. [CrossRef]
70. Frick, W.; Bauer, A.; Bauer, J.; Wied, S.; Muller, G. Structure-activity relationship of synthetic phosphoinositolglycans mimicking metabolic insulin action. *Biochemistry* **1998**, *37*, 13421–13436. [CrossRef]
71. Larner, J.; Price, J.D.; Heimark, D.; Smith, L.; Rule, G.; Piccariello, T.; Fonteles, M.C.; Pontes, C.; Vale, D.; Huang, L. Isolation, Structure, Synthesis, and Bioactivity of a Novel Putative Insulin Mediator. A Galactosamine chiro-Inositol Pseudo-Disaccharide Mn2+ Chelate with Insulin-like Activity. *J. Med. Chem.* **2003**, *46*, 3283–3291. [CrossRef]
72. Brautigan, D.L.; Brown, M.; Grindrod, S.; Chinigo, G.; Kruszewski, A.; Lukasik, S.M.; Bushweller, J.H.; Horal, M.; Keller, S.; Tamura, S.; et al. Allosteric activation of protein phosphatase 2C by D-chiro-inositol-galactosamine, a putative mediator mimetic of insulin action. *Biochemistry* **2005**, *44*, 11067–11073. [CrossRef] [PubMed]
73. Hiraga, A.; Kikuchi, K.; Tamura, S.; Tsuiki, S. Purification and characterization of Mg2+-dependent glycogen synthase phosphatase (phosphoprotein phosphatase IA) from rat liver. *Eur. J. Biochem.* **1981**, *119*, 503–510. [CrossRef] [PubMed]
74. Yoshizaki, T.; Maegawa, H.; Egawa, K.; Ugi, S.; Nishio, Y.; Imamura, T.; Kobayashi, T.; Tamura, S.; Olefsky, J.M.; Kashiwagi, A. Protein phosphatase-2C alpha as a positive regulator of insulin sensitivity through direct activation of phosphatidylinositol 3-kinase in 3T3-L1 adipocytes. *J. Biol. Chem.* **2004**, *279*, 22715–22726. [CrossRef]
75. Wang, M.Y.; Unger, R.H. Role of PP2C in cardiac lipid accumulation in obese rodents and its prevention by troglitazone. *Am. J. Physiol. Endocrinol. Metab.* **2005**, *288*, E216–E221. [CrossRef] [PubMed]
76. Bonilla, J.B.; Cid, M.B.; Contreras, F.X.; Goni, F.M.; Martin-Lomas, M. Phospholipase cleavage of D- and L-chiro-glycosylphosphoinosities asymmetrically incorporated into liposomal membranes. *Chemistry* **2006**, *12*, 1513–1528. [CrossRef] [PubMed]
77. Sleight, S.; Wilson, B.A.; Heimark, D.B.; Larner, J. G(q/11) is involved in insulin-stimulated inositol phosphoglycan putative mediator generation in rat liver membranes: Co-localization of G(q/11) with the insulin receptor in membrane vesicles. *Biochem. Biophys. Res. Commun.* **2002**, *295*, 561–569. [CrossRef]
78. Turner, D.I.; Chakraborty, N.; d'Alarcao, M. A fluorescent inositol phosphate glycan stimulates lipogenesis in rat adipocytes by extracellular activation alone. *Bioorganic Med. Chem. Lett.* **2005**, *15*, 2023–2025. [CrossRef]
79. Larner, J. D-chiro-inositol–its functional role in insulin action and its deficit in insulin resistance. *Int. J. Exp. Diabetes Res.* **2002**, *3*, 47–60. [CrossRef]
80. Romero, G.; Gamez, G.; Huang, L.C.; Lilley, K.; Luttrell, L. Anti-inositolglycan antibodies selectively block some of the actions of insulin in intact BC3H1 cells. *Proc. Natl. Acad. Sci. USA* **1990**, *87*, 1476–1480. [CrossRef]
81. Alvarez, J.F.; Sánchez-Arias, J.A.; Guadaño, A.; Estévez, F.; Varela, I.; Felíu, J.E.; Mato, J.M. Transport in isolated rat hepatocytes of the phospho-oligosaccharide that mimics insulin action. Effects of adrenalectomy and glucocorticoid treatment. *Biochem J.* **1991**, *274 Pt 2*, 369–374. [CrossRef]
82. Suzuki, S.; Sugawara, K.; Satoh, Y.; Toyota, T. Insulin stimulates the generation of two putative insulin mediators, inositol-glycan and diacylglycerol in BC3H-1 myocytes. *J. Biol. Chem.* **1991**, *266*, 8115–8121. [PubMed]
83. Kristiansen, S.; Richter, E.A. GLUT4-containing vesicles are released from membranes by phospholipase D cleavage of a GPI anchor. *Am. J. Physiol. Endocrinol. Metab.* **2002**, *283*, E374–E382. [CrossRef] [PubMed]
84. Ruiz-Albusac, J.M.; Velazquez, E.; Iglesias, J.; Jimenez, E.; Blazquez, E. Insulin promotes the hydrolysis of a glycosyl phosphatidylinositol in cultured rat astroglial cells. *J. Neurochem.* **1997**, *68*, 10–19. [CrossRef] [PubMed]
85. LeBoeuf, R.C.; Caldwell, M.; Guo, Y.; Metz, C.; Davitz, M.A.; Olson, L.K.; Deeg, M.A. Mouse glycosylphosphatidylinositol-specific phospholipase D (Gpld1) characterization. *Mamm. Genome Off. J. Int. Mamm. Genome Soc.* **1998**, *9*, 710–714. [CrossRef]
86. Von Toerne, C.; Huth, C.; de Las Heras Gala, T.; Kronenberg, F.; Herder, C.; Koenig, W.; Meisinger, C.; Rathmann, W.; Waldenberger, M.; Roden, M.; et al. MASP1, THBS1, GPLD1 and ApoA-IV are novel biomarkers associated with prediabetes: The KORA F4 study. *Diabetologia* **2016**, *59*, 1882–1892. [CrossRef]

87. Qin, W.; Liang, Y.Z.; Qin, B.Y.; Zhang, J.L.; Xia, N. The Clinical Significance of Glycoprotein Phospholipase D Levels in Distinguishing Early Stage Latent Autoimmune Diabetes in Adults and Type 2 Diabetes. *PLoS ONE* **2016**, *11*, e0156959. [CrossRef]
88. Bowen, R.F.; Raikwar, N.S.; Olson, L.K.; Deeg, M.A. Glucose and insulin regulate glycosylphosphatidylinositol-specific phospholipase D expression in islet beta cells. *Metab. Clin. Exp.* **2001**, *50*, 1489–1492. [CrossRef]
89. Suh, P.G.; Ryu, S.H.; Moon, K.H.; Suh, H.W.; Rhee, S.G. Inositol phospholipid-specific phospholipase C: Complete cDNA and protein sequences and sequence homology to tyrosine kinase-related oncogene products. *Proc. Natl. Acad. Sci. USA* **1988**, *85*, 5419–5423. [CrossRef]
90. Eliakim, R.; Becich, M.J.; Green, K.; Alpers, D.H. Both tissue and serum phospholipases release rat intestinal alkaline phosphatase. *Am. J. Physiol.* **1990**, *259*, G618–G625. [CrossRef]
91. Wu, W.; Wang, L.; Qiu, J.; Li, Z. The analysis of fagopyritols from tartary buckwheat and their anti-diabetic effects in KK-Ay type 2 diabetic mice and HepG2 cells. *J. Funct. Foods* **2018**, *50*, 137–146. [CrossRef]
92. Jones, D.R.; Avila, M.A.; Sanz, C.; Varela-Nieto, I. Glycosyl-phosphatidylinositol-phospholipase type D: A possible candidate for the generation of second messengers. *Biochem. Biophys. Res. Commun.* **1997**, *233*, 432–437. [CrossRef] [PubMed]
93. Suzuki, S.; Suzuki, C.; Hinokio, Y.; Ishigaki, Y.; Katagiri, H.; Kanzaki, M.; Azev, V.N.; Chakraborty, N.; d'Alarcao, M. Insulin-mimicking bioactivities of acylated inositol glycans in several mouse models of diabetes with or without obesity. *PLoS ONE* **2014**, *9*, e100466. [CrossRef] [PubMed]
94. Mann, K.J.; Hepworth, M.R.; Raikwar, N.S.; Deeg, M.A.; Sevlever, D. Effect of glycosylphosphatidylinositol (GPI)-phospholipase D overexpression on GPI metabolism. *Biochem. J.* **2004**, *378*, 641–648. [CrossRef] [PubMed]
95. Gray, D.L.; O'Brien, K.D.; D'Alessio, D.A.; Brehm, B.J.; Deeg, M.A. Plasma glycosylphosphatidylinositol-specific phospholipase D predicts the change in insulin sensitivity in response to a low-fat but not a low-carbohydrate diet in obese women. *Metab. Clin. Exp.* **2008**, *57*, 473–478. [CrossRef]
96. Deeg, M.A. GPI-specific phospholipase D as an apolipoprotein. *Braz. J. Med. Biol. Res. Rev. Bras. Pesqui. Med. Biol.* **1994**, *27*, 375–381.
97. Deeg, M.A.; Bierman, E.L.; Cheung, M.C. GPI-specific phospholipase D associates with an apoA-I- and apoA-IV-containing complex. *J. Lipid Res.* **2001**, *42*, 442–451.
98. Raikwar, N.S.; Cho, W.K.; Bowen, R.F.; Deeg, M.A. Glycosylphosphatidylinositol-specific phospholipase D influences triglyceride-rich lipoprotein metabolism. *Am. J. Physiol. Endocrinol. Metab.* **2006**, *290*, E463–E470. [CrossRef]
99. Chalasani, N.; Vuppalanchi, R.; Raikwar, N.S.; Deeg, M.A. Glycosylphosphatidylinositol-specific phospholipase d in nonalcoholic Fatty liver disease: A preliminary study. *J. Clin. Endocrinol. Metab.* **2006**, *91*, 2279–2285. [CrossRef]
100. Tabrizi, R.; Ostadmohammadi, V.; Lankarani, K.B.; Peymani, P.; Akbari, M.; Kolahdooz, F.; Asemi, Z. The effects of inositol supplementation on lipid profiles among patients with metabolic diseases: A systematic review and meta-analysis of randomized controlled trials. *Lipids Health Dis.* **2018**, *17*, 123. [CrossRef]
101. Yap, A.; Nishiumi, S.; Yoshida, K.; Ashida, H. Rat L6 myotubes as an in vitro model system to study GLUT4-dependent glucose uptake stimulated by inositol derivatives. *Cytotechnology* **2007**, *55*, 103–108. [CrossRef]
102. D'Oria, R.; Laviola, L.; Giorgino, F.; Unfer, V.; Bettocchi, S.; Scioscia, M. PKB/Akt and MAPK/ERK phosphorylation is highly induced by inositols: Novel potential insights in endothelial dysfunction in preeclampsia. *Pregnancy Hypertens.* **2017**, *10*, 107–112. [CrossRef] [PubMed]
103. Navarro, J.A.; Decara, J.; Medina-Vera, D.; Tovar, R.; Suarez, J.; Pavon, J.; Serrano, A.; Vida, M.; Gutierrez-Adan, A.; Sanjuan, C.; et al. D-Pinitol from Ceratonia siliqua is an orally active natural inositol that reduces pancreas insulin secretion and increases circulating ghrelin levels in Wistar rats. *Nutrients* **2020**, *12*, 2030. [CrossRef] [PubMed]
104. Shen, H.; Shao, M.; Cho, K.W.; Wang, S.; Chen, Z.; Sheng, L.; Wang, T.; Liu, Y.; Rui, L. Herbal constituent sequoyitol improves hyperglycemia and glucose intolerance by targeting hepatocytes, adipocytes, and β-cells. *Am. J. Physiol. Endocrinol. Metab.* **2012**, *302*, E932–E940. [CrossRef] [PubMed]

105. Hotamisligil, G.S.; Murray, D.L.; Choy, L.N.; Spiegelman, B.M. Tumor necrosis factor alpha inhibits signaling from the insulin receptor. *Proc. Natl. Acad. Sci. USA* **1994**, *91*, 4854–4858. [CrossRef]
106. Yorek, M.A.; Dunlap, J.A.; Thomas, M.J.; Cammarata, P.R.; Zhou, C.; Lowe, W.L., Jr. Effect of TNF-alpha on SMIT mRNA levels and myo-inositol accumulation in cultured endothelial cells. *Am. J. Physiol.* **1998**, *274*, C58–C71. [CrossRef] [PubMed]
107. Pitt, J.; Thorner, M.; Brautigan, D.; Larner, J.; Klein, W.L. Protection against the synaptic targeting and toxicity of Alzheimer's-associated Aβ oligomers by insulin mimetic chiro-inositols. *FASEB J.* **2013**, *27*, 199–207. [CrossRef]
108. Antony, P.J.; Gandhi, G.R.; Stalin, A.; Balakrishna, K.; Toppo, E.; Sivasankaran, K.; Ignacimuthu, S.; Al-Dhabi, N.A. Myoinositol ameliorates high-fat diet and streptozotocin-induced diabetes in rats through promoting insulin receptor signaling. *Biomed. Pharmacother.* **2017**, *88*, 1098–1113. [CrossRef]
109. Dang, N.T.; Mukai, R.; Yoshida, K.; Ashida, H. D-pinitol and myo-inositol stimulate translocation of glucose transporter 4 in skeletal muscle of C57BL/6 mice. *Biosci. Biotechnol. Biochem.* **2010**, *74*, 1062–1067. [CrossRef]
110. Lorenzo, M.; Fernandez-Veledo, S.; Vila-Bedmar, R.; Garcia-Guerra, L.; De Alvaro, C.; Nieto-Vazquez, I. Insulin resistance induced by tumor necrosis factor-alpha in myocytes and brown adipocytes. *J. Anim. Sci.* **2008**, *86*, E94–E104. [CrossRef]
111. Czauderna, F.; Fechtner, M.; Aygün, H.; Arnold, W.; Klippel, A.; Giese, K.; Kaufmann, J. Functional studies of the PI(3)-kinase signalling pathway employing synthetic and expressed siRNA. *Nucleic Acids Res.* **2003**, *31*, 670–682. [CrossRef]
112. Zhou, Q.L.; Park, J.G.; Jiang, Z.Y.; Holik, J.J.; Mitra, P.; Semiz, S.; Guilherme, A.; Powelka, A.M.; Tang, X.; Virbasius, J.; et al. Analysis of insulin signalling by RNAi-based gene silencing. *Biochem. Soc. Trans.* **2004**, *32*, 817–821. [CrossRef] [PubMed]
113. Oxvig, C. The role of PAPP-A in the IGF system: Location, location, location. *J. Cell Commun. Signal.* **2015**, *9*, 177–187. [CrossRef] [PubMed]
114. Farese, R.V.; Nair, G.P.; Standaert, M.L.; Cooper, D.R. Epidermal growth factor and insulin-like growth factor I stimulate the hydrolysis of the insulin-sensitive phosphatidylinositol-glycan in BC3H-1 myocytes. *Biochem. Biophys. Res. Commun.* **1988**, *156*, 1346–1352. [CrossRef]
115. Kojima, I.; Kitaoka, M.; Ogata, E. Insulin-like growth factor-I stimulates diacylglycerol production via multiple pathways in Balb/c 3T3 cells. *J. Biol. Chem.* **1990**, *265*, 16846–16850.
116. Villalba, M.; Alvarez, J.F.; Russell, D.S.; Mato, J.M.; Rosen, O.M. Hydrolysis of glycosyl-phosphatidylinositol in response to insulin is reduced in cells bearing kinase-deficient insulin receptors. *Growth Factors* **1990**, *2*, 91–97. [CrossRef]
117. León, Y.; Vazquez, E.; Sanz, C.; Vega, J.A.; Mato, J.M.; Giraldez, F.; Represa, J.; Varela-Nieto, I. Insulin-like growth factor-I regulates cell proliferation in the developing inner ear, activating glycosyl-phosphatidylinositol hydrolysis and Fos expression. *Endocrinology* **1995**, *136*, 3494–3503. [CrossRef]
118. Romero, G.; Garmey, J.C.; Veldhuis, J.D. The involvement of inositol phosphoglycan mediators in the modulation of steroidogenesis by insulin and insulin-like growth factor-I. *Endocrinology* **1993**, *132*, 1561–1568. [CrossRef]
119. Ruiz-Albusac, J.M.; Zueco, J.A.; Velazquez, E.; Blazquez, E. Insulin does not induce the hydrolysis of a glycosyl phosphatidylinositol in rat fetal hepatocytes. *Diabetes* **1993**, *42*, 1262–1272. [CrossRef]
120. Butterfield, D.A.; Di Domenico, F.; Barone, E. Elevated risk of type 2 diabetes for development of Alzheimer disease: A key role for oxidative stress in brain. *Biochim. Biophys. Acta* **2014**, *1842*, 1693–1706. [CrossRef]
121. Maeno, Y.; Li, Q.; Park, K.; Rask-Madsen, C.; Gao, B.; Matsumoto, M.; Liu, Y.; Wu, I.H.; White, M.F.; Feener, E.P.; et al. Inhibition of insulin signaling in endothelial cells by protein kinase C-induced phosphorylation of p85 subunit of phosphatidylinositol 3-kinase (PI3K). *J. Biol. Chem.* **2012**, *287*, 4518–4530. [CrossRef]
122. Dimmeler, S.; Fleming, I.; Fisslthaler, B.; Hermann, C.; Busse, R.; Zeiher, A.M. Activation of nitric oxide synthase in endothelial cells by Akt-dependent phosphorylation. *Nature* **1999**, *399*, 601–605. [CrossRef] [PubMed]
123. Duncan, E.R.; Crossey, P.A.; Walker, S.; Anilkumar, N.; Poston, L.; Douglas, G.; Ezzat, V.A.; Wheatcroft, S.B.; Shah, A.M.; Kearney, M.T. Effect of endothelium-specific insulin resistance on endothelial function in vivo. *Diabetes* **2008**, *57*, 3307–3314. [CrossRef] [PubMed]
124. Graf, E.; Empson, K.L.; Eaton, J.W. Phytic acid. A natural antioxidant. *J. Biol. Chem.* **1987**, *262*, 11647–11650. [PubMed]

125. Graf, E.; Eaton, J.W. Antioxidant functions of phytic acid. *Free Radic. Biol. Med.* **1990**, *8*, 61–69. [CrossRef]
126. Muraoka, S.; Miura, T. Inhibition of xanthine oxidase by phytic acid and its antioxidative action. *Life Sci.* **2004**, *74*, 1691–1700. [CrossRef]
127. Rengarajan, T.; Rajendran, P.; Nandakumar, N.; Balasubramanian, M.P.; Nishigaki, I. Free radical scavenging and antioxidant activity of D-pinitol against 7, 12 dimethylbenz (a) anthracene induced breast cancer in sprague dawley rats. *Asian Pac. J. Trop. Dis.* **2014**, *4*, 384–390. [CrossRef]
128. Nascimento, N.R.F.; Lessa, L.M.A.; Kerntopf, M.R.; Sousa, C.M.; Alves, R.S.; Queiroz, M.G.R.; Price, J.; Heimark, D.B.; Larner, J.; Du, X.; et al. Inositols prevent and reverse endothelial dysfunction in diabetic rat and rabbit vasculature metabolically and by scavenging superoxide. *Proc. Natl. Acad. Sci. USA* **2006**, *103*, 218–223. [CrossRef]
129. Jiang, W.D.; Wu, P.; Kuang, S.Y.; Liu, Y.; Jiang, J.; Hu, K.; Li, S.H.; Tang, L.; Feng, L.; Zhou, X.Q. Myo-inositol prevents copper-induced oxidative damage and changes in antioxidant capacity in various organs and the enterocytes of juvenile Jian carp (Cyprinus carpio var. Jian). *Aquat. Toxicol.* **2011**, *105*, 543–551. [CrossRef]
130. Jiang, W.-D.; Feng, L.; Liu, Y.; Jiang, J.; Zhou, X.-Q. Myo-inositol prevents oxidative damage, inhibits oxygen radical generation and increases antioxidant enzyme activities of juvenile Jian carp (Cyprinus carpio var. Jian). *Aquac. Res.* **2009**, *40*, 1770–1776. [CrossRef]
131. Vasaikar, N.; Mahajan, U.; Patil, K.R.; Suchal, K.; Patil, C.R.; Ojha, S.; Goyal, S.N. D-pinitol attenuates cisplatin-induced nephrotoxicity in rats: Impact on pro-inflammatory cytokines. *Chem. Biol. Interact.* **2018**, *290*, 6–11. [CrossRef]
132. Roman-Ramos, R.; Almanza-Perez, J.C.; Fortis-Barrera, A.; Angeles-Mejia, S.; Banderas-Dorantes, T.R.; Zamilpa-Alvarez, A.; Diaz-Flores, M.; Jasso, I.; Blancas-Flores, G.; Gomez, J.; et al. Antioxidant and anti-inflammatory effects of a hypoglycemic fraction from Cucurbita ficifolia Bouche in streptozotocin-induced diabetes mice. *Am. J. Chin. Med.* **2012**, *40*, 97–110. [CrossRef] [PubMed]
133. Fisher, S.K.; Novak, J.E.; Agranoff, B.W. Inositol and higher inositol phosphates in neural tissues: Homeostasis, metabolism and functional significance. *J. Neurochem.* **2002**, *82*, 736–754. [CrossRef] [PubMed]
134. Wong, Y.H.; Kalmbach, S.J.; Hartman, B.K.; Sherman, W.R. Immunohistochemical staining and enzyme activity measurements show myo-inositol-1-phosphate synthase to be localized in the vasculature of brain. *J. Neurochem.* **1987**, *48*, 1434–1442. [CrossRef] [PubMed]
135. Mejias-Aponte, C.A.; Ye, C.; Bonci, A.; Kiyatkin, E.A.; Morales, M. A subpopulation of neurochemically-identified ventral tegmental area dopamine neurons is excited by intravenous cocaine. *J. Neurosci. Off. J. Soc. Neurosci.* **2015**, *35*, 1965–1978. [CrossRef]
136. Novak, J.E.; Turner, R.S.; Agranoff, B.W.; Fisher, S.K. Differentiated human NT2-N neurons possess a high intracellular content of myo-inositol. *J. Neurochem.* **1999**, *72*, 1431–1440. [CrossRef] [PubMed]
137. Berry, G.T.; Wu, S.; Buccafusca, R.; Ren, J.; Gonzales, L.W.; Ballard, P.L.; Golden, J.A.; Stevens, M.J.; Greer, J.J. Loss of Murine Na+/myo-Inositol Cotransporter Leads to Brain myo-Inositol Depletion and Central Apnea. *J. Biol. Chem.* **2003**, *278*, 18297–18302. [CrossRef]
138. Buccafusca, R.; Venditti, C.P.; Kenyon, L.C.; Johanson, R.A.; Van Bockstaele, E.; Ren, J.; Pagliardini, S.; Minarcik, J.; Golden, J.A.; Coady, M.J.; et al. Characterization of the null murine sodium/myo-inositol cotransporter 1 (Smit1 or Slc5a3) phenotype: Myo-inositol rescue is independent of expression of its cognate mitochondrial ribosomal protein subunit 6 (Mrps6) gene and of phosphatidylinositol levels in neonatal brain. *Mol. Genet. Metab.* **2008**, *95*, 81–95. [CrossRef]
139. Bersudsky, Y.; Shaldubina, A.; Agam, G.; Berry, G.T.; Belmaker, R.H. Homozygote inositol transporter knockout mice show a lithium-like phenotype. *Bipolar Disord.* **2008**, *10*, 453–459. [CrossRef]
140. Cryns, K.; Shamir, A.; Van Acker, N.; Levi, I.; Daneels, G.; Goris, I.; Bouwknecht, J.A.; Andries, L.; Kass, S.; Agam, G.; et al. IMPA1 is essential for embryonic development and lithium-like pilocarpine sensitivity. *Neuropsychopharmacol. Off. Publ. Am. Coll. Neuropsychopharmacol.* **2008**, *33*, 674–684. [CrossRef]
141. Dai, G.; Yu, H.; Kruse, M.; Traynor-Kaplan, A.; Hille, B. Osmoregulatory inositol transporter SMIT1 modulates electrical activity by adjusting PI(4,5)P2 levels. *Proc. Natl. Acad. Sci. USA* **2016**, *113*, E3290–E3299. [CrossRef]
142. Dickson, E.J.; Jensen, J.B.; Hille, B. Golgi and plasma membrane pools of PI(4)P contribute to plasma membrane PI(4,5)P2 and maintenance of KCNQ2/3 ion channel current. *Proc. Natl. Acad. Sci. USA* **2014**, *111*, E2281–E2290. [CrossRef] [PubMed]
143. Lei, H.; Poitry-Yamate, C.; Preitner, F.; Thorens, B.; Gruetter, R. Neurochemical profile of the mouse hypothalamus using in vivo 1H MRS at 14.1T. *NMR Biomed.* **2010**, *23*, 578–583. [CrossRef] [PubMed]

144. Patishi, Y.; Lubrich, B.; Berger, M.; Kofman, O.; van Calker, D.; Belmaker, R.H. Differential uptake of myo-inositol in vivo into rat brain areas. *Eur. Neuropsychopharmacol.* **1996**, *6*, 73–75. [CrossRef]
145. López-Gambero, A.J.; Martínez, F.; Salazar, K.; Cifuentes, M.; Nualart, F. Brain Glucose-Sensing Mechanism and Energy Homeostasis. *Mol. Neurobiol.* **2019**, *56*, 769–796. [CrossRef] [PubMed]
146. Raghu, P.; Joseph, A.; Krishnan, H.; Singh, P.; Saha, S. Phosphoinositides: Regulators of Nervous System Function in Health and Disease. *Front. Mol. Neurosci.* **2019**, *12*. [CrossRef]
147. Liu, B.; Song, S.; Ruz-Maldonado, I.; Pingitore, A.; Huang, G.C.; Baker, D.; Jones, P.M.; Persaud, S.J. GPR55-dependent stimulation of insulin secretion from isolated mouse and human islets of Langerhans. *Diabetes Obes. Metab.* **2016**, *18*, 1263–1273. [CrossRef]
148. Bjursell, M.; Ryberg, E.; Wu, T.; Greasley, P.J.; Bohlooly-Y., M.; Hjorth, S. Deletion of Gpr55 Results in Subtle Effects on Energy Metabolism, Motor Activity and Thermal Pain Sensation. *PLoS ONE* **2016**, *11*, e0167965. [CrossRef]
149. Deliu, E.; Sperow, M.; Console-Bram, L.; Carter, R.L.; Tilley, D.G.; Kalamarides, D.J.; Kirby, L.G.; Brailoiu, G.C.; Brailoiu, E.; Benamar, K.; et al. The Lysophosphatidylinositol Receptor GPR55 Modulates Pain Perception in the Periaqueductal Gray. *Mol. Pharmacol.* **2015**, *88*, 265–272. [CrossRef]
150. Hurst, K.; Badgley, C.; Ellsworth, T.; Bell, S.; Friend, L.; Prince, B.; Welch, J.; Cowan, Z.; Williamson, R.; Lyon, C.; et al. A putative lysophosphatidylinositol receptor GPR55 modulates hippocampal synaptic plasticity. *Hippocampus* **2017**, *27*, 985–998. [CrossRef]
151. Marichal-Cancino, B.A.; Fajardo-Valdez, A.; Ruiz-Contreras, A.E.; Méndez-Díaz, M.; Prospéro-García, O. Possible role of hippocampal GPR55 in spatial learning and memory in rats. *Acta Neurobiol. Exp.* **2018**, *78*, 41–50. [CrossRef]
152. Marichal-Cancino, B.A.; Sánchez-Fuentes, A.; Méndez-Díaz, M.; Ruiz-Contreras, A.E.; Prospéro-García, O. Blockade of GPR55 in the dorsolateral striatum impairs performance of rats in a T-maze paradigm. *Behav. Pharmacol.* **2016**, *27*, 393–396. [CrossRef] [PubMed]
153. Sylantyev, S.; Jensen, T.P.; Ross, R.A.; Rusakov, D.A. Cannabinoid- and lysophosphatidylinositol-sensitive receptor GPR55 boosts neurotransmitter release at central synapses. *Proc. Natl. Acad. Sci. USA* **2013**, *110*, 5193–5198. [CrossRef] [PubMed]
154. Waragai, M.; Moriya, M.; Nojo, T. Decreased N-Acetyl Aspartate/Myo-Inositol Ratio in the Posterior Cingulate Cortex Shown by Magnetic Resonance Spectroscopy May Be One of the Risk Markers of Preclinical Alzheimer's Disease: A 7-Year Follow-Up Study. *J. Alzheimer's Dis.* **2017**, *60*, 1411–1427. [CrossRef] [PubMed]
155. Mitolo, M.; Stanzani-Maserati, M.; Capellari, S.; Testa, C.; Rucci, P.; Poda, R.; Oppi, F.; Gallassi, R.; Sambati, L.; Rizzo, G.; et al. Predicting conversion from mild cognitive impairment to Alzheimer's disease using brain (1)H-MRS and volumetric changes: A two- year retrospective follow-up study. *Neuroimage Clin.* **2019**, *23*, 101843. [CrossRef] [PubMed]
156. Huang, W.; Alexander, G.E.; Daly, E.M.; Shetty, H.U.; Krasuski, J.S.; Rapoport, S.I.; Schapiro, M.B. High Brain myo-Inositol Levels in the Predementia Phase of Alzheimer's Disease in Adults With Down's Syndrome: A 1H MRS Study. *Am. J. Psychiatry* **1999**, *156*, 1879–1886. [CrossRef]
157. Beacher, F.; Simmons, A.; Daly, E.; Prasher, V.; Adams, C.; Margallo-Lana, M.L.; Morris, R.; Lovestone, S.; Murphy, K.; Murphy, D.G.M. Hippocampal Myo-inositol and Cognitive Ability in Adults With Down Syndrome: An In Vivo Proton Magnetic Resonance Spectroscopy Study. *Arch. Gen. Psychiatry* **2005**, *62*, 1360–1365. [CrossRef]
158. Neverisky, D.L.; Abbott, G.W. KCNQ-SMIT complex formation facilitates ion channel-solute transporter cross talk. *FASEB J.* **2017**, *31*, 2828–2838. [CrossRef]
159. Wang, H.S.; Pan, Z.; Shi, W.; Brown, B.S.; Wymore, R.S.; Cohen, I.S.; Dixon, J.E.; McKinnon, D. KCNQ2 and KCNQ3 potassium channel subunits: Molecular correlates of the M-channel. *Science* **1998**, *282*, 1890–1893. [CrossRef]
160. Manville, R.W.; Abbott, G.W. Potassium channels act as chemosensors for solute transporters. *Commun. Biol.* **2020**, *3*, 90. [CrossRef]
161. Papadopoulos, T.; Rhee, H.J.; Subramanian, D.; Paraskevopoulou, F.; Mueller, R.; Schultz, C.; Brose, N.; Rhee, J.S.; Betz, H. Endosomal Phosphatidylinositol 3-Phosphate Promotes Gephyrin Clustering and GABAergic Neurotransmission at Inhibitory Postsynapses. *J. Biol. Chem.* **2017**, *292*, 1160–1177. [CrossRef]
162. Hille, B.; Dickson, E.J.; Kruse, M.; Vivas, O.; Suh, B.C. Phosphoinositides regulate ion channels. *Biochim. Biophys. Acta* **2015**, *1851*, 844–856. [CrossRef] [PubMed]

163. Tsuruta, F.; Green, E.M.; Rousset, M.; Dolmetsch, R.E. PIKfyve regulates CaV1.2 degradation and prevents excitotoxic cell death. *J. Cell Biol.* **2009**, *187*, 279–294. [CrossRef] [PubMed]
164. Seebohm, G.; Neumann, S.; Theiss, C.; Novkovic, T.; Hill, E.V.; Tavaré, J.M.; Lang, F.; Hollmann, M.; Manahan-Vaughan, D.; Strutz-Seebohm, N. Identification of a novel signaling pathway and its relevance for GluA1 recycling. *PLoS ONE* **2012**, *7*, e33889. [CrossRef] [PubMed]
165. Zhang, S.X.; Duan, L.H.; He, S.J.; Zhuang, G.F.; Yu, X. Phosphatidylinositol 3,4-bisphosphate regulates neurite initiation and dendrite morphogenesis via actin aggregation. *Cell Res.* **2017**, *27*, 253–273. [CrossRef] [PubMed]
166. Brand, A.; Richter-Landsberg, C.; Leibfritz, D. Multinuclear NMR studies on the energy metabolism of glial and neuronal cells. *Dev. Neurosci.* **1993**, *15*, 289–298. [CrossRef] [PubMed]
167. Ibsen, L.; Strange, K. In situ localization and osmotic regulation of the Na(+)-myo-inositol cotransporter in rat brain. *Am. J. Physiol.* **1996**, *271*, F877–F885. [CrossRef]
168. Jackson, P.S.; Morrison, R.; Strange, K. The volume-sensitive organic osmolyte-anion channel VSOAC is regulated by nonhydrolytic ATP binding. *Am. J. Physiol.* **1994**, *267*, C1203–C1209. [CrossRef]
169. Harris, J.L.; Yeh, H.-W.; Choi, I.-Y.; Lee, P.; Berman, N.E.; Swerdlow, R.H.; Craciunas, S.C.; Brooks, W.M. Altered neurochemical profile after traumatic brain injury: (1)H-MRS biomarkers of pathological mechanisms. *J. Cereb. Blood Flow Metab.* **2012**, *32*, 2122–2134. [CrossRef]
170. Cordoba, J.; Gottstein, J.; Blei, A.T. Glutamine, myo-inositol, and organic brain osmolytes after portocaval anastomosis in the rat: Implications for ammonia-induced brain edema. *Hepatology* **1996**, *24*, 919–923. [CrossRef]
171. Filibian, M.; Frasca, A.; Maggioni, D.; Micotti, E.; Vezzani, A.; Ravizza, T. In vivo imaging of glia activation using 1H-magnetic resonance spectroscopy to detect putative biomarkers of tissue epileptogenicity. *Epilepsia* **2012**, *53*, 1907–1916. [CrossRef]
172. Harris, J.L.; Yeh, H.-W.; Swerdlow, R.H.; Choi, I.-Y.; Lee, P.; Brooks, W.M. High-field proton magnetic resonance spectroscopy reveals metabolic effects of normal brain aging. *Neurobiol. Aging* **2014**, *35*, 1686–1694. [CrossRef] [PubMed]
173. Zhang, X.; Liu, H.; Wu, J.; Zhang, X.; Liu, M.; Wang, Y. Metabonomic alterations in hippocampus, temporal and prefrontal cortex with age in rats. *Neurochem. Int.* **2009**, *54*, 481–487. [CrossRef] [PubMed]
174. von Leden, R.E.; Khayrullina, G.; Moritz, K.E.; Byrnes, K.R. Age exacerbates microglial activation, oxidative stress, inflammatory and NOX2 gene expression, and delays functional recovery in a middle-aged rodent model of spinal cord injury. *J. NeuroInflamm.* **2017**, *14*, 161. [CrossRef] [PubMed]
175. Silverstone, P.H.; McGrath, B.M.; Kim, H. Bipolar disorder and myo-inositol: A review of the magnetic resonance spectroscopy findings. *Bipolar Disord.* **2005**, *7*, 1–10. [CrossRef]
176. Shyng, S.L.; Nichols, C.G. Membrane phospholipid control of nucleotide sensitivity of KATP channels. *Science* **1998**, *282*, 1138–1141. [CrossRef]
177. Baukrowitz, T.; Schulte, U.; Oliver, D.; Herlitze, S.; Krauter, T.; Tucker, S.J.; Ruppersberg, J.P.; Fakler, B. PIP2 and PIP as determinants for ATP inhibition of KATP channels. *Science* **1998**, *282*, 1141–1144. [CrossRef]
178. Ribalet, B.; John, S.A.; Weiss, J.N. Regulation of cloned ATP-sensitive K channels by phosphorylation, MgADP, and phosphatidylinositol bisphosphate (PIP(2)): A study of channel rundown and reactivation. *J. Gen. Physiol.* **2000**, *116*, 391–410. [CrossRef]
179. Enkvetchakul, D.; Loussouarn, G.; Makhina, E.; Shyng, S.L.; Nichols, C.G. The kinetic and physical basis of K(ATP) channel gating: Toward a unified molecular understanding. *Biophys. J.* **2000**, *78*, 2334–2348. [CrossRef]
180. Lacin, E.; Aryal, P.; Glaaser, I.W.; Bodhinathan, K.; Tsai, E.; Marsh, N.; Tucker, S.J.; Sansom, M.S.P.; Slesinger, P.A. Dynamic role of the tether helix in PIP(2)-dependent gating of a G protein-gated potassium channel. *J. Gen. Physiol.* **2017**, *149*, 799–811. [CrossRef]
181. Zhang, H.; Craciun, L.C.; Mirshahi, T.; Rohacs, T.; Lopes, C.M.; Jin, T.; Logothetis, D.E. PIP(2) activates KCNQ channels, and its hydrolysis underlies receptor-mediated inhibition of M currents. *Neuron* **2003**, *37*, 963–975. [CrossRef]
182. Suh, B.-C.; Hille, B. Electrostatic interaction of internal Mg2+ with membrane PIP2 Seen with KCNQ K+ channels. *J. Gen. Physiol.* **2007**, *130*, 241–256. [CrossRef] [PubMed]
183. Manville, R.W.; Neverisky, D.L.; Abbott, G.W. SMIT1 Modifies KCNQ Channel Function and Pharmacology by Physical Interaction with the Pore. *Biophys. J.* **2017**, *113*, 613–626. [CrossRef] [PubMed]

184. Mayordomo-Cava, J.; Yajeya, J.; Navarro-López, J.D.; Jiménez-Díaz, L. Amyloid-β(25-35) Modulates the Expression of GirK and KCNQ Channel Genes in the Hippocampus. *PLoS ONE* **2015**, *10*, e0134385. [CrossRef] [PubMed]
185. Charlier, C.; Singh, N.A.; Ryan, S.G.; Lewis, T.B.; Reus, B.E.; Leach, R.J.; Leppert, M. A pore mutation in a novel KQT-like potassium channel gene in an idiopathic epilepsy family. *Nat. Genet.* **1998**, *18*, 53–55. [CrossRef] [PubMed]
186. Singh, N.A.; Charlier, C.; Stauffer, D.; DuPont, B.R.; Leach, R.J.; Melis, R.; Ronen, G.M.; Bjerre, I.; Quattlebaum, T.; Murphy, J.V.; et al. A novel potassium channel gene, KCNQ2, is mutated in an inherited epilepsy of newborns. *Nat. Genet.* **1998**, *18*, 25–29. [CrossRef]
187. Maljevic, S.; Vejzovic, S.; Bernhard, M.K.; Bertsche, A.; Weise, S.; Döcker, M.; Lerche, H.; Lemke, J.R.; Merkenschlager, A.; Syrbe, S. Novel KCNQ3 Mutation in a Large Family with Benign Familial Neonatal Epilepsy: A Rare Cause of Neonatal Seizures. *Mol. Syndr.* **2016**, *7*, 189–196. [CrossRef]
188. Judy, J.T.; Seifuddin, F.; Pirooznia, M.; Mahon, P.B.; Bipolar Genome Study, C.; Jancic, D.; Goes, F.S.; Schulze, T.; Cichon, S.; Noethen, M.; et al. Converging Evidence for Epistasis between ANK3 and Potassium Channel Gene KCNQ2 in Bipolar Disorder. *Front. Genet.* **2013**, *4*, 87. [CrossRef]
189. Kaminsky, Z.; Jones, I.; Verma, R.; Saleh, L.; Trivedi, H.; Guintivano, J.; Akman, R.; Zandi, P.; Lee, R.S.; Potash, J.B. DNA methylation and expression of KCNQ3 in bipolar disorder. *Bipolar Disord.* **2015**, *17*, 150–159. [CrossRef]
190. Augelli-Szafran, C.E.; Wei, H.X.; Lu, D.; Zhang, J.; Gu, Y.; Yang, T.; Osenkowski, P.; Ye, W.; Wolfe, M.S. Discovery of notch-sparing gamma-secretase inhibitors. *Curr. Alzheimer Res.* **2010**, *7*, 207–209. [CrossRef]
191. Koppaka, V.; Axelsen, P.H. Accelerated accumulation of amyloid beta proteins on oxidatively damaged lipid membranes. *Biochemistry* **2000**, *39*, 10011–10016. [CrossRef]
192. McLaurin, J.; Kierstead, M.E.; Brown, M.E.; Hawkes, C.A.; Lambermon, M.H.; Phinney, A.L.; Darabie, A.A.; Cousins, J.E.; French, J.E.; Lan, M.F.; et al. Cyclohexanehexol inhibitors of Abeta aggregation prevent and reverse Alzheimer phenotype in a mouse model. *Nat. Med.* **2006**, *12*, 801–808. [CrossRef] [PubMed]
193. Townsend, M.; Cleary, J.P.; Mehta, T.; Hofmeister, J.; Lesne, S.; O'Hare, E.; Walsh, D.M.; Selkoe, D.J. Orally available compound prevents deficits in memory caused by the Alzheimer amyloid-beta oligomers. *Ann. Neurol.* **2006**, *60*, 668–676. [CrossRef] [PubMed]
194. Morrone, C.D.; Bazzigaluppi, P.; Beckett, T.L.; Hill, M.E.; Koletar, M.M.; Stefanovic, B.; McLaurin, J. Regional differences in Alzheimer's disease pathology confound behavioural rescue after amyloid-β attenuation. *Brain* **2019**, *143*, 359–373. [CrossRef] [PubMed]
195. Aytan, N.; Choi, J.-K.; Carreras, I.; Kowall, N.W.; Jenkins, B.G.; Dedeoglu, A. Combination therapy in a transgenic model of Alzheimer's disease. *Exp. Neurol.* **2013**, *250*, 228–238. [CrossRef] [PubMed]
196. Dorr, A.; Sahota, B.; Chinta, L.V.; Brown, M.E.; Lai, A.Y.; Ma, K.; Hawkes, C.A.; McLaurin, J.; Stefanovic, B. Amyloid-β-dependent compromise of microvascular structure and function in a model of Alzheimer's disease. *Brain* **2012**, *135*, 3039–3050. [CrossRef] [PubMed]
197. Wang, H.; Raleigh, D.P. General amyloid inhibitors? A critical examination of the inhibition of IAPP amyloid formation by inositol stereoisomers. *PLoS ONE* **2014**, *9*, e104023. [CrossRef]
198. Sinha, S.; Du, Z.; Maiti, P.; Klärner, F.-G.; Schrader, T.; Wang, C.; Bitan, G. Comparison of three amyloid assembly inhibitors: The sugar scyllo-inositol, the polyphenol epigallocatechin gallate, and the molecular tweezer CLR01. *ACS Chem. Neurosci.* **2012**, *3*, 451–458. [CrossRef]
199. Wei, G.; Shea, J.E. Effects of solvent on the structure of the Alzheimer amyloid-beta(25-35) peptide. *Biophys. J.* **2006**, *91*, 1638–1647. [CrossRef]
200. Bleiholder, C.; Do, T.D.; Wu, C.; Economou, N.J.; Bernstein, S.S.; Buratto, S.K.; Shea, J.E.; Bowers, M.T. Ion mobility spectrometry reveals the mechanism of amyloid formation of Abeta(25-35) and its modulation by inhibitors at the molecular level: Epigallocatechin gallate and scyllo-inositol. *J. Am. Chem. Soc.* **2013**, *135*, 16926–16937. [CrossRef]
201. Salloway, S.; Sperling, R.; Keren, R.; Porsteinsson, A.P.; van Dyck, C.H.; Tariot, P.N.; Gilman, S.; Arnold, D.; Abushakra, S.; Hernandez, C.; et al. A phase 2 randomized trial of ELND005, scyllo-inositol, in mild to moderate Alzheimer disease. *Neurology* **2011**, *77*, 1253–1262. [CrossRef]

202. Liang, E.; Garzone, P.; Cedarbaum, J.M.; Koller, M.; Tran, T.; Xu, V.; Ross, B.; Jhee, S.S.; Ereshefsky, L.; Pastrak, A.; et al. Pharmacokinetic Profile of Orally Administered Scyllo-Inositol (Elnd005) in Plasma, Cerebrospinal Fluid and Brain, and Corresponding Effect on Amyloid-Beta in Healthy Subjects. *Clin. Pharmacol. Drug Dev.* **2013**, *2*, 186–194. [CrossRef] [PubMed]
203. Lee, D.; Lee, W.-S.; Lim, S.; Kim, Y.K.; Jung, H.-Y.; Das, S.; Lee, J.; Luo, W.; Kim, K.-T.; Chung, S.-K. A guanidine-appended scyllo-inositol derivative AAD-66 enhances brain delivery and ameliorates Alzheimer's phenotypes. *Sci. Rep.* **2017**, *7*, 14125. [CrossRef] [PubMed]
204. Pasinetti, G.M. Compositions and Methods for Treating Alzheimer's Disease and Related Disorders and Promoting A Healthy Nervous System. U.S. Patent 8,921,347, 30 December 2014.
205. De Felice, F.G.; Vieira, M.N.; Bomfim, T.R.; Decker, H.; Velasco, P.T.; Lambert, M.P.; Viola, K.L.; Zhao, W.Q.; Ferreira, S.T.; Klein, W.L. Protection of synapses against Alzheimer's-linked toxins: Insulin signaling prevents the pathogenic binding of Abeta oligomers. *Proc. Natl. Acad. Sci. USA* **2009**, *106*, 1971–1976. [CrossRef]
206. Talbot, K.; Wang, H.-Y.; Kazi, H.; Han, L.-Y.; Bakshi, K.P.; Stucky, A.; Fuino, R.L.; Kawaguchi, K.R.; Samoyedny, A.J.; Wilson, R.S.; et al. Demonstrated brain insulin resistance in Alzheimer's disease patients is associated with IGF-1 resistance, IRS-1 dysregulation, and cognitive decline. *J. Clin. Investig.* **2012**, *122*, 1316–1338. [CrossRef] [PubMed]
207. Barone, E.; Di Domenico, F.; Cassano, T.; Arena, A.; Tramutola, A.; Lavecchia, M.A.; Coccia, R.; Butterfield, D.A.; Perluigi, M. Impairment of biliverdin reductase-A promotes brain insulin resistance in Alzheimer disease: A new paradigm. *Free Radic. Biol. Med.* **2016**, *91*, 127–142. [CrossRef] [PubMed]
208. Barone, E.; Di Domenico, F.; Cenini, G.; Sultana, R.; Cini, C.; Preziosi, P.; Perluigi, M.; Mancuso, C.; Butterfield, D.A. Biliverdin reductase-A protein levels and activity in the brains of subjects with Alzheimer disease and mild cognitive impairment. *Biochim. Biophys. Acta (BBA)-Mol. Basis Dis.* **2011**, *1812*, 480–487. [CrossRef] [PubMed]
209. Butterfield, D.A.; Reed, T.T.; Perluigi, M.; De Marco, C.; Coccia, R.; Keller, J.N.; Markesbery, W.R.; Sultana, R. Elevated levels of 3-nitrotyrosine in brain from subjects with amnestic mild cognitive impairment: Implications for the role of nitration in the progression of Alzheimer's disease. *Brain Res.* **2007**, *1148*, 243–248. [CrossRef]
210. Hanson, L.R.; Frey, W.H. Strategies for Intranasal Delivery of Therapeutics for the Prevention and Treatment of NeuroAIDS. *J. Neuroimmune Pharmacol.* **2007**, *2*, 81–86. [CrossRef]
211. Barone, E.; Tramutola, A.; Triani, F.; Calcagnini, S.; Di Domenico, F.; Ripoli, C.; Gaetani, S.; Grassi, C.; Butterfield, D.A.; Cassano, T.; et al. Biliverdin Reductase-A Mediates the Beneficial Effects of Intranasal Insulin in Alzheimer Disease. *Mol. Neurobiol.* **2019**, *56*, 2922–2943. [CrossRef]
212. Santiago, J.C.P.; Hallschmid, M. Outcomes and clinical implications of intranasal insulin administration to the central nervous system. *Exp. Neurol.* **2019**, *317*, 180–190. [CrossRef]
213. Claxton, A.; Baker, L.D.; Hanson, A.; Trittschuh, E.H.; Cholerton, B.; Morgan, A.; Callaghan, M.; Arbuckle, M.; Behl, C.; Craft, S. Long-acting intranasal insulin detemir improves cognition for adults with mild cognitive impairment or early-stage Alzheimer's disease dementia. *J. Alzheimer's Dis.* **2015**, *44*, 897–906. [CrossRef] [PubMed]
214. Isoda, F.; Shiry, L.; Abergel, J.; Allan, G.; Mobbs, C. D-chiro-Inositol enhances effects of hypothalamic toxin gold-thioglucose. *Brain Res.* **2003**, *993*, 172–176. [CrossRef] [PubMed]
215. Maurizi, A.R.; Menduni, M.; Del Toro, R.; Kyanvash, S.; Maggi, D.; Guglielmi, C.; Pantano, A.L.; Defeudis, G.; Fioriti, E.; Manfrini, S.; et al. A pilot study of D-chiro-inositol plus folic acid in overweight patients with type 1 diabetes. *Acta Diabetol.* **2017**, *54*, 361–365. [CrossRef] [PubMed]
216. Holscher, C. Diabetes as a risk factor for Alzheimer's disease: Insulin signalling impairment in the brain as an alternative model of Alzheimer's disease. *Biochem. Soc. Trans.* **2011**, *39*, 891–897. [CrossRef]
217. Chatterjee, S.; Mudher, A. Alzheimer's Disease and Type 2 Diabetes: A Critical Assessment of the Shared Pathological Traits. *Front. Neurosci.* **2018**, *12*, 383. [CrossRef]
218. De la Monte, S.M.; Wands, J.R. Alzheimer's disease is type 3 diabetes-evidence reviewed. *J. Diabetes Sci. Technol.* **2008**, *2*, 1101–1113. [CrossRef]
219. Wong, C.H.Y.; Wanrooy, B.J.; Bruce, D.G. Chapter 10-Neuroinflammation, Type 2 Diabetes, and Dementia. In *Type 2 Diabetes and Dementia*; Srikanth, V., Arvanitakis, Z., Eds.; Academic Press: London, UK, 2018; pp. 195–209. [CrossRef]

220. Busquets, O.; Ettcheto, M.; Pallas, M.; Beas-Zarate, C.; Verdaguer, E.; Auladell, C.; Folch, J.; Camins, A. Long-term exposition to a high fat diet favors the appearance of beta-amyloid depositions in the brain of C57BL/6J mice. A potential model of sporadic Alzheimer's disease. *Mech. Ageing Dev.* **2017**, *162*, 38–45. [CrossRef]
221. Pistell, P.J.; Morrison, C.D.; Gupta, S.; Knight, A.G.; Keller, J.N.; Ingram, D.K.; Bruce-Keller, A.J. Cognitive impairment following high fat diet consumption is associated with brain inflammation. *J. Neuroimmunol.* **2010**, *219*, 25–32. [CrossRef]
222. Kim, M.S.; Choi, M.-S.; Han, S.N. High fat diet-induced obesity leads to proinflammatory response associated with higher expression of NOD2 protein. *Nutr. Res. Pract.* **2011**, *5*, 219–223. [CrossRef]
223. Ho, L.; Qin, W.; Pompl, P.N.; Xiang, Z.; Wang, J.; Zhao, Z.; Peng, Y.; Cambareri, G.; Rocher, A.; Mobbs, C.V.; et al. Diet-induced insulin resistance promotes amyloidosis in a transgenic mouse model of Alzheimer's disease. *FASEB J.* **2004**, *18*, 902–904. [CrossRef]
224. Hoscheidt, S.M.; Kellawan, J.M.; Berman, S.E.; Rivera-Rivera, L.A.; Krause, R.A.; Oh, J.M.; Beeri, M.S.; Rowley, H.A.; Wieben, O.; Carlsson, C.M.; et al. Insulin resistance is associated with lower arterial blood flow and reduced cortical perfusion in cognitively asymptomatic middle-aged adults. *J. Cereb. Blood Flow Metab.* **2017**, *37*, 2249–2261. [CrossRef] [PubMed]
225. Lourenco, C.F.; Ledo, A.; Barbosa, R.M.; Laranjinha, J. Neurovascular uncoupling in the triple transgenic model of Alzheimer's disease: Impaired cerebral blood flow response to neuronal-derived nitric oxide signaling. *Exp. Neurol.* **2017**, *291*, 36–43. [CrossRef] [PubMed]
226. Duan, Y.; Zeng, L.; Zheng, C.; Song, B.; Li, F.; Kong, X.; Xu, K. Inflammatory Links Between High Fat Diets and Diseases. *Front. Immunol.* **2018**, *9*, 2649. [CrossRef] [PubMed]
227. Marks, D.R.; Tucker, K.; Cavallin, M.A.; Mast, T.G.; Fadool, D.A. Awake intranasal insulin delivery modifies protein complexes and alters memory, anxiety, and olfactory behaviors. *J. Neurosci.* **2009**, *29*, 6734–6751. [CrossRef] [PubMed]
228. Hoffman, J.D.; Yanckello, L.M.; Chlipala, G.; Hammond, T.C.; McCulloch, S.D.; Parikh, I.; Sun, S.; Morganti, J.M.; Green, S.J.; Lin, A.L. Dietary inulin alters the gut microbiome, enhances systemic metabolism and reduces neuroinflammation in an APOE4 mouse model. *PLoS ONE* **2019**, *14*, e0221828. [CrossRef]
229. Oliver, C.; Crayton, L.; Holland, A.; Hall, S.; Bradbury, J. A four year prospective study of age-related cognitive change in adults with Down's syndrome. *Psychol. Med.* **1998**, *28*, 1365–1377. [CrossRef]
230. Cardenas, A.M.; Fernandez-Olivares, P.; Diaz-Franulic, I.; Gonzalez-Jamett, A.M.; Shimahara, T.; Segura-Aguilar, J.; Caviedes, R.; Caviedes, P. Knockdown of Myo-Inositol Transporter SMIT1 Normalizes Cholinergic and Glutamatergic Function in an Immortalized Cell Line Established from the Cerebral Cortex of a Trisomy 16 Fetal Mouse, an Animal Model of Human Trisomy 21 (Down Syndrome). *Neurotox. Res.* **2017**, *32*, 614–623. [CrossRef]
231. Rumble, B.; Retallack, R.; Hilbich, C.; Simms, G.; Multhaup, G.; Martins, R.; Hockey, A.; Montgomery, P.; Beyreuther, K.; Masters, C.L. Amyloid A4 protein and its precursor in Down's syndrome and Alzheimer's disease. *New Engl. J. Med.* **1989**, *320*, 1446–1452. [CrossRef]
232. Perluigi, M.; Pupo, G.; Tramutola, A.; Cini, C.; Coccia, R.; Barone, E.; Head, E.; Butterfield, D.A.; Di Domenico, F. Neuropathological role of PI3K/Akt/mTOR axis in Down syndrome brain. *Biochim. Biophys. Acta* **2014**, *1842*, 1144–1153. [CrossRef]
233. Tramutola, A.; Lanzillotta, C.; Di Domenico, F.; Head, E.; Butterfield, D.A.; Perluigi, M.; Barone, E. Brain insulin resistance triggers early onset Alzheimer disease in Down syndrome. *Neurobiol. Dis.* **2020**, *137*, 104772. [CrossRef]
234. Rafii, M.S.; Skotko, B.G.; McDonough, M.E.; Pulsifer, M.; Evans, C.; Doran, E.; Muranevici, G.; Kesslak, P.; Abushakra, S.; Lott, I.T.; et al. A Randomized, Double-Blind, Placebo-Controlled, Phase II Study of Oral ELND005 (scyllo-Inositol) in Young Adults with Down Syndrome without Dementia. *J. Alzheimer's Dis.* **2017**, *58*, 401–411. [CrossRef] [PubMed]
235. Frey, R.; Metzler, D.; Fischer, P.; Heiden, A.; Scharfetter, J.; Moser, E.; Kasper, S. Myo-inositol in depressive and healthy subjects determined by frontal 1H-magnetic resonance spectroscopy at 1.5 tesla. *J. Psychiatr. Res.* **1998**, *32*, 411–420. [CrossRef]
236. Urrila, A.S.; Hakkarainen, A.; Castaneda, A.; Paunio, T.; Marttunen, M.; Lundbom, N. Frontal Cortex Myo-Inositol Is Associated with Sleep and Depression in Adolescents: A Proton Magnetic Resonance Spectroscopy Study. *Neuropsychobiology* **2017**, *75*, 21–31. [CrossRef] [PubMed]

237. Rahman, S.; Neuman, R.S. Myo-inositol reduces serotonin (5-HT2) receptor induced homologous and heterologous desensitization. *Brain Res.* **1993**, *631*, 349–351. [CrossRef]
238. Einat, H.; Clenet, F.; Shaldubina, A.; Belmaker, R.H.; Bourin, M. The antidepressant activity of inositol in the forced swim test involves 5-HT2 receptors. *Behav. Brain Res.* **2001**, *118*, 77–83. [CrossRef]
239. Harvey, B.H.; Scheepers, A.; Brand, L.; Stein, D.J. Chronic inositol increases striatal D(2) receptors but does not modify dexamphetamine-induced motor behavior. *Relev. Obs. Compuls. Disord. Pharmacol. Biochem. Behav.* **2001**, *68*, 245–253. [CrossRef]
240. Leppink, E.W.; Redden, S.A.; Grant, J.E. A double-blind, placebo-controlled study of inositol in trichotillomania. *Int. Clin. Psychopharmacol.* **2017**, *32*, 107–114. [CrossRef]
241. Seedat, S.; Stein, D.J. Inositol augmentation of serotonin reuptake inhibitors in treatment-refractory obsessive-compulsive disorder: An open trial. *Int. Clin. Psychopharmacol.* **1999**, *14*, 353–356. [CrossRef]
242. Grossman, H.; Marzloff, G.; Luo, X.; LeRoith, D.; Sano, M.; Pasinetti, G. P1-279: NIC5-15 as a treatment for Alzheimer's: Safety, pharmacokinetics and clinical variables. *Alzheimer's Dement.* **2009**, *5*, 259. [CrossRef]

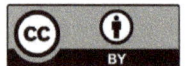

© 2020 by the authors. Licensee MDPI, Basel, Switzerland. This article is an open access article distributed under the terms and conditions of the Creative Commons Attribution (CC BY) license (http://creativecommons.org/licenses/by/4.0/).

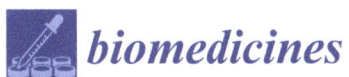

Review

Psilocybin as a New Approach to Treat Depression and Anxiety in the Context of Life-Threatening Diseases—A Systematic Review and Meta-Analysis of Clinical Trials

Ana Sofia Vargas [1], Ângelo Luís [1,2,3], Mário Barroso [4], Eugenia Gallardo [1,3] and Luísa Pereira [2,5,*]

1. Centro de Investigação em Ciências da Saúde (CICS-UBI), Universidade da Beira Interior, Av. Infante D. Henrique, 6200-506 Covilhã, Portugal; anadinisvargas@gmail.com (A.S.V.); angelo.luis@ubi.pt (Â.L.); egallardo@fcsaude.ubi.pt (E.G.)
2. Grupo de Revisões Sistemáticas (GRUBI), Faculdade de Ciências da Saúde, Universidade da Beira Interior, Av. Infante D. Henrique, 6200-506 Covilhã, Portugal
3. Laboratório de Fármaco-Toxicologia, UBIMedical, Universidade da Beira Interior, Estrada Municipal 506, 6200-284 Covilhã, Portugal
4. Serviço de Química e Toxicologia Forenses, Instituto Nacional de Medicina Legal e Ciências Forenses, I.P.—Delegação do Sul, Rua Manuel Bento de Sousa, 3, 1150-219 Lisboa, Portugal; mario.j.barroso@inmlcf.mj.pt
5. Centro de Matemática e Aplicações (CMA-UBI), Universidade da Beira Interior, Rua Marquês d'Ávila e Bolama, 6201-001 Covilhã, Portugal
* Correspondence: lpereira@ubi.pt; Tel.: +351-275-319-700

Received: 9 June 2020; Accepted: 2 September 2020; Published: 5 September 2020

Abstract: Psilocybin is a naturally occurring tryptamine known for its psychedelic properties. Recent research indicates that psilocybin may constitute a valid approach to treat depression and anxiety associated to life-threatening diseases. The aim of this work was to perform a systematic review with meta-analysis of clinical trials to assess the therapeutic effects and safety of psilocybin on those medical conditions. The Beck Depression Inventory (BDI) was used to measure the effects in depression and the State-Trait Anxiety Inventory (STAI) was used to measure the effects in anxiety. For BDI, 11 effect sizes were considered (92 patients) and the intervention group was significantly favored (WMD = −4.589; 95% CI = −4.207 to −0.971; p-value = 0.002). For STAI-Trait, 11 effect sizes were considered (92 patients), being the intervention group significantly favored when compared to the control group (WMD = −5.906; 95% CI = −7.852 to −3.960; p-value < 0.001). For STAI-State, 9 effect sizes were considered (41 patients) and the intervention group was significantly favored (WMD = −6.032; 95% CI = −8.900 to −3.164; p-value < 0.001). The obtained results are promising and emphasize the importance of psilocybin translational research in the management of symptoms of depression and anxiety, since the compound may be effective in reducing symptoms of depression and anxiety in conditions that are either resistant to conventional pharmacotherapy or for which pharmacologic treatment is not yet approved. Moreover, it may be also relevant for first-line treatment, given its safety.

Keywords: psilocybin; depression; anxiety; clinical trials; systematic review; meta-analysis

---

1. Introduction

Major depressive disorder (MDD) is characterized by the persistence of negative thoughts and emotions that disrupt mood, cognition, motivation, and behavior [1]. According to the Diagnostic Statistical Manual V (DSM), symptoms, etiologies and pathophysiologies of MDD are heterogeneous and their subtypes have been already described. Although symptomatic remission increases the probability for recovery in MDD, most patients do not achieve nor sustain a state of full remission [2]. The options for treatment when the patient is resistant to the available standard treatments generally involve combining, augmenting, or switching medications, introducing electroconvulsive therapy (ECT) or other neurostimulation strategies. However, the risk of complications associated with those approaches exists, including increased toxicity with higher medication dosages and combination regimens [1].

Anxiety is a very common psychiatric symptom in terminally ill patients. Factors such as treatment process, disease progression, uncontrolled pain, dying and uncertainty about death have a negative impact on these patients [3]. Anxiety also contributes to poor recovery from medical procedures and lower survival time in terminally-ill patients [4].

Depression and anxiety are independent risk factors of early death in patients with life-threatening diseases, like cancer [5] and most of these individuals develop a chronic syndrome of psychological distress, usually associated with decreased treatment adherence, prolonged hospitalization, decreased quality of life and increased suicidality [6]. Antidepressants and benzodiazepines are used to treat depressed mood and anxiety in patients with life-threatening diseases [7], although there are no Food and Drug Administration (FDA) approved pharmacotherapies for the psychological distress related to those diseases. In addition, the onset of clinical improvement with antidepressants is delayed, relapse rates are high and significant side effects compromise adherence to therapy [8].

Regarding the treatment of severe depression and anxiety, special attention should be paid to the approval of intranasal Spravato® by the FDA in March 2019. Its active compound is esketamine, a ketamine enantiomer, which is a non-competitive N-methyl-D-aspartate (NMDA) glutamate receptor antagonist. The effects of ketamine have made it a popular recreational drug, due to its euphoric and dissociative properties [9]. Nonetheless, esketamine appears to provide significant short-term symptom improvement in severe depression and anxiety and it is considered an innovative and promising therapeutic approach. Moreover, molecules such as 3,4-methylenedioxy-methamphetamine (MDMA) and lysergic acid diethylamide (LSD) are also being studied for the treatment of anxiety conditions, namely, post-traumatic stress disorder (PTSD) and generalized anxiety disorder (GAD). Nevertheless, none of these drugs has been approved by the FDA.

In spite of all studies and therapeutic innovations in this area, further research is needed, notably on classic hallucinogens like psilocybin, to provide patients with depression and anxiety associated with life-threatening diseases better chances of recovery and consequently better quality of life.

Recently, Goldberg et al., 2020 [10] published a meta-analysis concerning the use of psilocybin and symptoms of anxiety and depression. The approach used in their meta-analysis is different from the one we present in several aspects, for instance—it does not include data on previous pathologies of the patients receiving psilocybin and did not analyze physiological effects induced by the drug. Also, the authors did not examine psilocybin dose and administration duration as moderators of treatment effects [10].

In this context, this paper aims to perform a systematic review, complying with the Preferred Reported Items for Systematic Reviews and Meta-Analysis (PRISMA) statement, followed by a meta-analysis of clinical trials on the therapeutic potential of psilocybin in anxiety and depression associated with life-threatening diseases.

2. Methods

2.1. Search Strategy, Study Selection, Inclusion and Exclusion Criteria

The search for this systematic review with meta-analysis was performed on several electronic databases (PubMed, Web of Science, Scopus and SciELO) during January 2020. These databases were queried using the Boolean operator tools with the following search strategy—((((((depression) OR anxiety) OR post-traumatic stress disorder)) AND ((((((hallucinogens) OR entheogens) OR psychedelics)

OR classic hallucinogens) OR serotonergic hallucinogens) OR serotoninergic hallucinogens)) AND (psilocybin) AND ((((((clinical trials) OR human) OR humans) OR man) OR woman) OR patients). The references' lists of the relevant studies were also checked to find further works. Following the PRISMA statement [11], titles and abstracts of the selected articles were initially screened and the full texts of those considered important were subsequently analyzed in detail [12]. The selection process of the studies was performed independently by two authors, with a third being consulted in case of disagreements. The defined inclusion criteria were—studies in humans presenting a true control group; studies in patients with depression and anxiety associated with a life-threatening disease; drug psilocybin; use of Beck Depression Inventory (BDI) to assess depression and/or State-Trait Anxiety Inventory (STAI) to assess anxiety.

BDI was first proposed by Beck et al., 1961 [13] and it is one of the most used scales to assess the severity of depressive symptoms. It is a self-reported questionnaire, consisting on 21 items that measure characteristic attitudes and symptoms of depression. STAI is a self-report questionnaire divided in 2 subscales, called STAI-Trait and STAI-State. STAI allows the detection of the presence and severity of current symptoms of anxiety and a generalized propensity to be anxious. It contains 40 items, 20 of them concerning STAI-State and the remaining 20 concerning STAI-Trait [14].

2.2. Risk of Bias Assessment

The risk of publication bias of each included study was assessed using the "Cochrane Guide for Review Authors on Assessing Study Quality", which is based on "Cochrane Collaboration's tool for assessing risk of bias" [15]. This tool classifies the risk of bias in randomized controlled trials (RCTs) included in reviews as either "High risk", "Unclear" or "Low risk" in accordance with 7 domains—random sequence generation, allocation concealment, blinding of participants and personnel, blinding of outcome assessment, incomplete outcome data, selective reporting and other sources of bias [16]. This classification was independently assigned by 2 authors and discrepancies in assessment were resolved through discussions between the authors or by consultation with a third researcher. The results of the risk of bias assessment were presented in a risk of bias summary and a risk of bias graph, which were sketched using the software Review Manager 5.3 (Version 5.3.5) (http://community.cochrane.org/).

2.3. Data Extraction and Summary

The included studies were carefully analyzed, and the following data were extracted and summarized—publication year, sample size, study design, medical condition, age and gender of participants, conditions of intervention and control groups and study duration. The data extraction was independently performed by two authors using a prespecified procedure with a third reviewer consulted to analyze inconsistencies.

2.4. Statistical Analyses

For the outcomes of interest, an assessment was performed on the pooled effect of the treatment with psilocybin in terms of weighted mean differences (WMD) between the change from pre- and post-treatment mean values of the intervention and control groups. WMD combine measures, where the mean, standard deviation (SD) and sample size are known. The weight given to each study (how much influence each study has on the overall results of the meta-analysis) is determined by the precision of its estimate of effect and corresponds to the inverse of the variance. Statistical data analysis was performed using the Comprehensive Meta-Analysis software (Version 2.0) [17]. Forest plots were generated to illustrate the study-specific effect sizes with a 95% confidence interval (CI). The statistic I^2 of Higgins was used as a measure of the inconsistency across the findings of the included studies. The scale of I^2 has a range of 0 to 100% and values on the order of 25%, 50% and 75% are considered low, moderate, and high heterogeneity, respectively [18]. Subgroup analysis was performed on the primary outcomes, depending on the dose and on the follow-up time after psilocybin administration.

Three different analyses were used to evaluate the potential impact of publication bias on the present meta-analysis—Funnel plots; Egger's regression test; Duval and Tweedie's Trim and Fill approach. The sensitivity analysis was also achieved by eliminating each study one at a time to evaluate the stability of the results.

3. Results

3.1. Search and Selection of Studies

The detailed steps of the article selection process are depicted as a flow-diagram (Figure 1). Initially, the search yielded 722 articles concerning the hypothetical therapeutic use of psilocybin. This initial search included 8 articles obtained through research in other sources. After, duplicates were removed, 670 articles remained and after the screening of titles and abstracts according to PRISMA statement, 32 of them remained and were further evaluated for inclusion and exclusion criteria. Among them, 26 did not meet the inclusion criteria.

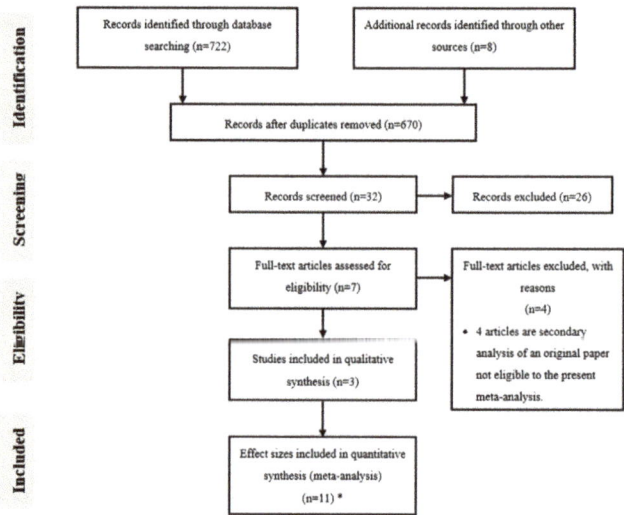

Figure 1. Preferred Reported Items for Systematic Reviews and Meta-Analysis (PRISMA) flow-diagram of database search, study selection and articles included in this systematic review with meta-analysis. * The works from Griffiths et al., 2016 [6], Ross et al., 2016 [19] and Grob et al., 2011 [20] were divided into several effect sizes based on different times of follow-up after psilocybin administration. (The division of each work in several effect sizes is indicated by the letters in unpaired parenthesis in Table 1).

Then, seven articles were assessed for eligibility through full-text evaluation and four of them were excluded (Stroud et al., 2018 [21], Lyons and Carhart-Harris, 2018 [22], Carhart-Harris et al., 2017 [23] and Carhart-Harris et al., 2016 [24]), because they were secondary analyses of the same data, and as such none was eligible since a true control group was not present in either of them. Finally, three articles were included in qualitative synthesis and three of them were divided into several effect sizes based on different times of follow-up after psilocybin administration. In a general view, the three articles studied the effects of psilocybin in the treatment of depression and anxiety associated with a life-threatening disease. The data from Ross et al., 2016 [19] was divided in seven data groups and the data from Griffiths et al., 2016 [6] and from Grob et al., 2011 [20] were divided into two data groups each, considering different times of follow-up after psilocybin administration. In total, 11 effect sizes were included in this meta-analysis.

Table 1. Characteristics of the included studies in this systematic review with meta-analysis.

Study/Year	Sample Size	Study Design	Medical Condition	Mean/Range Age (Years)	Gender (F/M)	Intervention Drug	Control Group	Duration [1]	Primary Outcomes	Secondary Outcomes
Ross et al., 2016 [19]	29	Double-blind, randomized	Depression and anxiety associated with a life-threatening disease (cancer)	56.28	18/11	Psilocybin, 0.3 mg/kg	Niacin, 250 mg	(a) 1 day post-dose 1 (b) 14 days post-dose 1 (c) 42 days post-dose 1 (d) 49 days post-dose 1 (e) 1 day post-dose 2 (f) 42 days post-dose 2 (g) 189 days post-dose 2	BDI, STAI-State, STAI-Trait	-
Griffiths et al., 2016 [6]	51	Double-blind, randomized	Depression and anxiety associated with a life-threatening disease (cancer)	56.3	25/26	Psilocybin, 0.3 or 0.4 mg/kg	Psilocybin, 1 or 3 mg/70 kg	(a) 28 days pre-crossover 35 days pre-crossover (b) 28 days pre-crossover 35 days post-crossover	BDI, STAI-Trait	SBP, DBP, HR
Grob et al., 2011 [20]	12	Pilot	Anxiety associated with a life-threatening disease (advanced-stage cancer)	From 36 to 58	11/1	Psilocybin, 0.2 mg/kg	Niacin, 250 mg	(a) 1 day (b) 14 days	BDI, STAI-State, STAI-Trait	SBP, DBP, HR

[1] The letters in unpaired parenthesis indicate the division of each study in several effect sizes.

3.2. Included Studies and Trials Characteristics

The main characteristics of the included trials are outlined in Table 1. The three included studies were published between 2011 and 2016 and 92 patients received psilocybin with doses ranging from 0.2 to 0.4 mg/kg, depending on the trials. The different units used to measure doses (some of them depending on the weight of the patients) made results standardization difficult. Patients had depression and anxiety associated with life-threatening diseases, namely aggressive oncologic conditions. Although psilocybin is a natural substance found in some mushrooms, it was synthesized (in the laboratory) for the trials and was administered in the form of oral capsules. Concerning the duration of the intervention, results were usually assessed through the scales, days after the administration of psilocybin and in a longer follow-up, in some cases up to three months.

3.3. Risk of Publication Bias

The results found in the assessment of the risk of publication bias from the included studies are summarized in Figure 2. In general, all the studies satisfied the seven domains of bias defined by Cochrane Collaboration. All the included articles had a focused issue and all the patients who entered the trial were properly accounted for at its conclusion. Aside from the experimental intervention, both the control and intervention groups were treated equally, and all clinically important outcomes were considered. The randomization process was applied in the three articles that were also double-blinded.

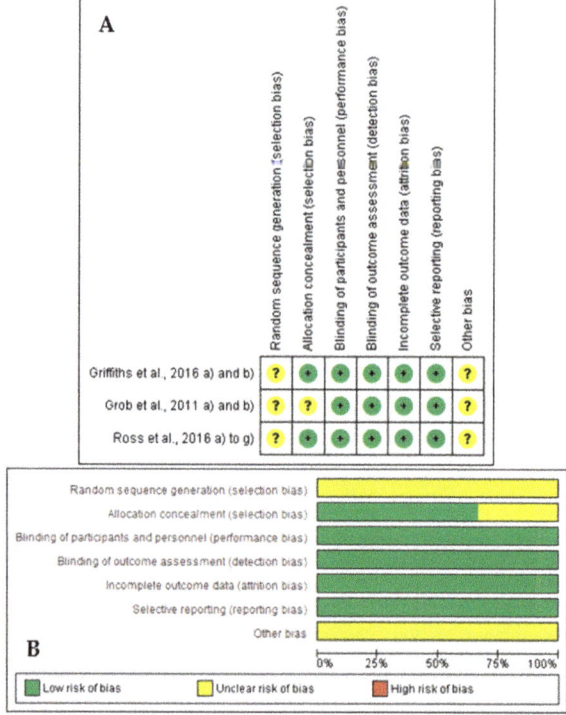

Figure 2. Results of risk of bias assessment regarding the methodological quality of included studies ((**A**) Risk of bias summary: review authors' judgments about each risk of bias item for each included study; (**B**) Risk of bias graph: review authors' judgments about each risk of bias item presented as percentages across all included studies).

3.4. Primary Outcomes: Effects of Psilocybin on Depression and Anxiety

BDI and STAI were considered the psychometric scales for this work since they are the most widely used in clinical settings to quantify symptoms of either depression or anxiety.

The meta-analysis results for the effects of psilocybin in depression through BDI are graphically reported in Figure 3A and Table 2. For BDI, 11 effect sizes were considered, including 92 patients, with a diagnosis of depression and anxiety associated with a life-threatening disease. It was concluded that the intervention group was significantly favored when compared to the control group (WMD = −4.589; 95% CI = −4.207 to −0.971; p-value = 0.002). For these results, a fixed effects model was used, given the homogeneity of the studies ($I^2 = 0$%).

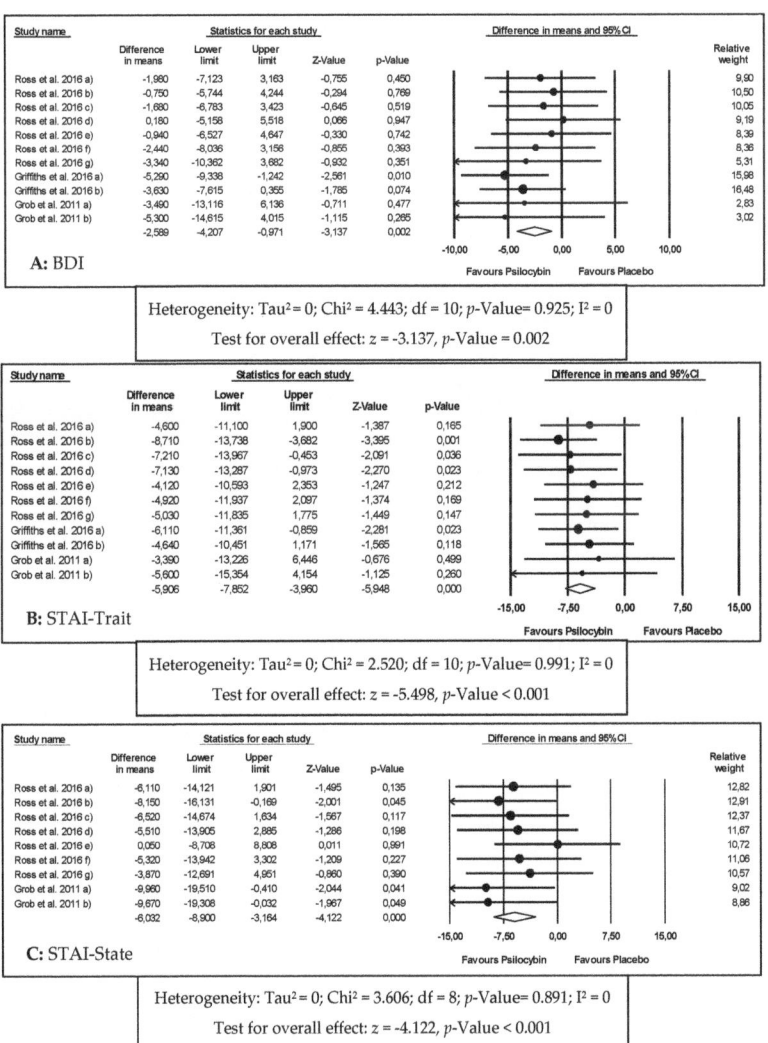

Figure 3. Forest plots of comparisons of the effects of psilocybin on the primary outcomes of this meta-analysis ((**A**) Beck Depression Inventory (BDI); (**B**) State-Trait Anxiety Inventory (STAI)-Trait; (**C**) STAI-State).

Table 2. Effects of psilocybin on depression and anxiety.

Outcome Analyzed	Number of Effect Sizes	WMD Observed (95% CI)	p-Value	I^2 (%)	Model USED	WMD Adjusted (95% CI)
BDI	11	−4.589 (−4.207 to −0.971)	0.002 *	0	Fixed	−4.589 (−4.207 to −0.971)
STAI-Trait	11	−5.906 (−7.852 to −3.960)	<0.001 *	0	Fixed	−6.389 (−8.151 to −4.626)
STAI-State	9	−6.032 (−8.900 to −3.164)	<0.001 *	0	Fixed	−6.032 (−8.900 to −3.164)

WMD—weighted mean differences; CI—confidence interval; * Indicates a significant result.

The meta-analysis results for the effects of psilocybin in anxiety through STAI-Trait and STAI-State are graphically reported in Figure 3B,C, respectively and Table 2.

For STAI-Trait, 11 effect sizes were considered, including 92 patients, with a diagnosis of depression and anxiety associated with a life-threatening disease. Among these, 28 patients had genitourinary cancer, 26 had breast cancer, 16 had digestive cancer, 12 had hematologic malignancies and 10 had other oncologic pathologies. All patients were in advanced stages of their illnesses and some had recurrent metastatic diseases. Apart from that, all patients had also been diagnosed using the DSM V meeting criteria for either chronic adjustment disorder with anxiety, chronic adjustment disorder with mixed anxiety and depressed mood, dysthymic disorder, GAD, MDD or dual diagnosis between GAD and MDD or GAD and dysthymic disorder.

It was concluded that the intervention group was significantly favored when compared to the control group (WMD = −5.906; 95% CI = −7.852 to −3.960; p-value < 0.001). For these results, a fixed effects model was used, given the homogeneity between studies ($I^2 = 0\%$).

For STAI-State, 9 effect sizes were considered, including 41 patients, with a diagnosis of depression and anxiety associated with a life-threatening disease (oncologic conditions). For this outcome, it was concluded that the intervention group was significantly favored when compared to the control group (WMD = −6.032; 95% CI = −8.900 to −3.164; p-value < 0.001). For these results, a fixed effects model was used, given the homogeneity between studies ($I^2 = 0\%$).

3.5. Subgroup and Sensitivity Analyses

A subgroup analysis was performed for each primary outcome of the study, except for STAI-State because of the limited number of studies reporting this outcome (Table 3). Accordingly, the influence of psilocybin in either BDI or STAI-Trait was studied separately depending on the dose and on the follow-up time after psilocybin administration.

It was shown that psilocybin induces reduction in both BDI and STAI-Trait at all the tested doses, but the reduction is not dose-dependent. In fact, compared to the control group, this outcome was only statistically significant at the doses of 0.4 mg/kg for BDI and of 0.3 and 0.4 mg/kg for STAI-Trait.

Concerning the time of the follow-up, psilocybin induces statistically significant results in a period of 38 to 189 days in BDI and in 14 to 189 days in STAI-Trait.

The sensitivity analysis was performed by excluding some studies and evaluating how those studies would affect the results (results not shown). This analysis indicates that the pooled effects of psilocybin in depression and anxiety through BDI, STAI-Trait and STAI-State did not change substantially if a few studies were omitted. The sensitivity analysis proved that the overall results obtained in this meta-analysis are robust.

Table 3. Subgroup analysis of the effects of psilocybin on depression and anxiety.

Variable	BDI				STAI–Trait			
	Number of Effect Sizes	95% CI	p–Value	I² (%)	Number of Effect Sizes	95% CI	p–Value	I² (%)
Total	11	–	–	–	11	–	–	–
WMD observed	–	−2.589 (−4.207 to −0.971)	0.002 *	0	–	−5.906 (−7.852 to −3.960)	<0.001 *	0
WMD adjusted	–	−2.589 (−4.207 to −0.971)	–	–	–	−5.906 (−7.852 to −3.960)	–	–
Dose (mg/kg)	**BDI**				**STAI–Trait**			
	Number of Effect Sizes	95% CI	p–Value	I² (%)	Number of Effect Sizes	95% CI	p–Value	I² (%)
0.2	2	−4.425 (−11.118 to −2.269)	0.195	0	2	−4.509 (−11.430 to 2.422)	0.208	0
0.3	7	−1.438 (−3.498 to 0.622)	0.171	0	7	−6.240 (−8.615 to −3.865)	<0.001 *	0
0.4	2	−4.447 (−7.287 to −1.607)	0.002 *	0	2	−5.449 (−9.345 to −1.553)	0.008 *	0
Time (days) after Psilocybin Administration	**BDI**				**STAI–Trait**			
	Number of Effect Sizes	95% CI	p–Value	I² (%)	Number of Effect Sizes	95% CI	p–Value	I² (%)
1	3	−1.769 (−5.290 to 1.752)	0.325	0	2	−4.359 (−8.946 to 0.228)	0.067	0
14	2	−1.766 (−6.167 to 2.635)	0.432	0	3	−7.258 (−11.330 to −3.184)	0.005 *	39.340
35–189	6	−3.024 (−5.026 to −1.023)	0.003 *	0	6	−5.854 (−8.385 to −3.322)	<0.001 *	0

WMD—weighted mean differences; CI—confidence interval; * Indicates a significant result.

3.6. Publication Bias

Publication bias was examined through funnel plots and statistically using the Trim and Fill method (results not shown). Publication bias evaluation was performed separately considering the 3 scales used to measure the effects of psilocybin in depression, through BDI and anxiety, through STAI. Funnel plots indicate asymmetries in the distribution of studies based on sample sizes. The presence of publication bias was further explored using Egger's regression test. This test indicates evidence of publication bias for the effects of psilocybin on depression and anxiety (p-value > 0.05).

3.7. Secondary Outcomes: Effects of Psilocybin on Systolic Blood Pressure, Diastolic Blood Pressure and Heart Rate

Systolic blood pressure (SBP), diastolic blood pressure (DBP) and heart rate were evaluated in this meta-analysis as secondary outcomes. The obtained results are summarized in Table 4. As noted, psilocybin produced significant increases in SBP and DBP, up to 6 (p-value < 0.017) and 5 h (p-value < 0.001) following administration, respectively. The DBP verified increases between 1.194 and 11.381 mmHg, being the average of the increase 7.741 mmHg. Both SBD and DBP tended to stabilize to normal values after 6 or more hours after administration. Psilocybin also significantly increases the heart rate, this increase being highest on the 3rd and 4th hours following administration. Similarly to what was verified for SBP and DBP, heart rate tended to stabilize after 6 or more hours after the administration.

Table 4. Meta-analysis for secondary outcomes.

Time (Hours) after Psilocybin Administration	WMD (95% CI)	p-Value	I^2 (%)
Systolic blood pressure (SBP)			
1	13.824 (9.433 to 18.216)	<0.001 *	0
2	22.601 (18.075 to 27.128)	<0.001 *	0
3	18.939 (14.893 to 22.986)	<0.001 *	49.577
4	15.252 (10.998 to 19.505)	<0.001 *	0
5	7.978 (4.184 to 11.773)	<0.001 *	0
6	4.222 (0.792 to 7.652)	0.016 *	0
Overall	12.741 (11.100 to 14.382)	<0.001 *	82.280
Diastolic blood pressure (DBP)			
1	11.242 (8.843 to 13.640)	<0.001 *	0
2	11.020 (8.598 to 13.441)	<0.001 *	61.227
3	11.381 (9.020 13.743)	<0.001 *	52.635
4	8.625 (6.080 to 11.170)	<0.001 *	0
5	4.912 (2.374 to 7.450)	<0.001 *	0
6	1.194 (-0.883 to 3.271)	0.260	0
Overall	7.741 (6.722 to 8.710)	<0.001 *	86.350
Heart Rate			
1	5.056 (0.787 to 9.325)	0.020 *	0
2	8.268 (4.115 to 12.421)	<0.001 *	0
3	8.281 (4.288 to 12.275)	<0.001 *	44.279
4	8.520 (4.495 to 12.546)	<0.001 *	64.899
5	5.599 (1.495 to 9.703)	0.008 *	0
6	3.363 (-0.716 to 7.441)	0.106	13.130
Overall	6.549 (4.875 to 8.223)	<0.001 *	24.596

WMD—weighted mean differences; CI—confidence interval; * Indicates a significant result.

4. Discussion

Psilocybin is a molecule with structural similarities to serotonin, an endogenous neurotransmitter. It can be found in some mushrooms and has been widely used to induce hallucinations and altered states of consciousness. Its laboratory synthesis was performed by Albert Hofmann while working at Sandoz Laboratories and it was marketed later under the commercial name Indocybin® for basic psychopharmacology and clinical research [25].

Nonetheless, it was withdrawn in the early 1970s and was classified as a Schedule I drug due to its use outside of medical research and in association with emerging counterculture. Despite withdrawal and criminalization, its potential therapeutic value led many scientists to study the effects and mechanisms of action of the drug. There is preliminary evidence that psilocybin may be useful in the treatment of anxiety and depression in life-threatening diseases, depression, obsessive-compulsive disorder, alcoholism and nicotine addiction, cluster headaches and autism [25]. Although further research is needed to assess the efficacy and safety in the treatment of these conditions, it should be noted that psilocybin is illegal in most countries. Therefore, the illegal status of psilocybin adds complexity and some costs to clinical trials involving its administration to human subjects.

The mechanism of action of psilocybin in depression is still unknown. However, some research suggests that its therapeutic effects in depression may reflect the deactivation of the medial prefrontal cortex (mPFC) that is usually hyperactive in depressed patients [26].

The deactivation of mPFC by psilocybin is detected using functional magnetic resonance imaging (fMRI) and it is correlated with the subjective effects induced by the drug. Other studies with fMRI support that psilocybin attenuates amygdala activation on response to threat-related visual stimuli [27]. This may be one of the mechanisms underlying the therapeutic effectiveness of psilocybin in depression and anxiety, given that the amygdala is extremely important in perception and generation of emotions and amygdala hyperactivity in response to negative stimuli is correlated to negative mood states in depressed patients [28]. Furthermore, the mechanism of action of psilocybin, an agonist of 5-HT(2A) receptors, indicates other evidence of its action in depression, since cortical 5-HT(2A) receptor expression is usually increased in postmortem samples of depressed and suicidal patients [29].

Patients with a potentially life-threatening disease often experience considerable anxiety and psychological distress, depression, anger, loss of perceived self-worth, social isolation, hopelessness, and helplessness [30]. There is no FDA approved pharmacotherapy for psychological distress related with life-threatening diseases and conventional therapy often shows limited efficacy to address symptoms of anxiety and depression. The obtained results in the present work emphasize the importance of psilocybin translational research, when used in the correct environment and with trained professionals and may give clues to future clinical trials.

Psilocybin produces sustained reduction in symptoms of both depression and anxiety. However, a recommendation for its use could only be given under rigorous definition of the conditions and precautions. The efficacy of psychedelic therapy may, unlike conventional pharmacotherapy, be linked to an experiential and meaningful process, responsible for the long-term effects and positive effects in cognition, affect, behavior and spirituality [31]. After psilocybin administration, patients report alleviation from anxiety, reconciliation with death, emotional uncoupling from cancer, spiritual or religious phenomena, reconnection to life and greater confidence [32]. The activation of serotonin receptors 5-HT(2A) mediates perception, attention, and emotional regulation, influencing the waking consciousness, sensory experiences, affectivity, experience of self and dream-like visual imagery [31]. Psilocybin is, therefore, responsible for inducing a profound shift in consciousness, with intensification of affective responses, enhanced ability for introspection, regression to primitive and childlike thinking and activation of vivid memory traces with pronounced emotional processes [33].

The persistence in time of the positive effects of psilocybin suggests that the acute destabilization of brain networks induced by the drug modifies activity in a long-lasting way [34]. Psilocybin may alter acutely brain network activity, decreasing connectivity within the default mode network (DMN) [26].

DMN has a role in consciousness and high-level constructs, such as the self, being essential for the maintenance of cognitive integration and constraint under normal conditions [35].

The increases of both SBP and DBP and heart rate are consistent with the sympathetic effects of psilocybin reported in the literature [36]. The sympathetic effects may also be noticeable through the induction of pupil dilatation [37]. Psilocybin, however, is not likely to cause changes on electrocardiograph or body temperature nor to affect the ionic balance, blood glucose or cholesterol [31].

There were not reported serious adverse effects following psilocybin administration. Besides transient moderate increases in SBD, DBP and heart rate, there are some references to nausea, both physical and psychological discomfort, transient episodes of psychological distress and anxiety. There are, however, no cases of hallucinogen persisting perception disorder (HPPD) neither prolonged psychosis, although literature points these effects to be quite dangerous and life-impairing following hallucinogen consumption [38]. This may occur because in all studies included in the present meta-analysis, patients were carefully monitored in a calm and relaxed environment and had been previously informed about the effects that the drug might have in their bodies and mind. This is known as "set and setting" and it is designed to facilitate a mystical experience and to increase the probability of a positive outcome after the administration of any hallucinogen [25]. In fact, many drug-related and not drug-related variables may influence the adverse effects experienced by patients, namely, age, gender, education, experimental setting, and drug dose [39].

According to the literature, besides the mentioned adverse effects, psilocybin may also cause somatic symptoms such as dizziness, weakness, tremor, drowsiness, yawning, paresthesia, blurred vision, and increased tendon reflexes [40]. Although not applicable to the studies included in this meta-analysis, psilocybin is very likely to induce nausea when consumed through psilocybin-containing mushrooms [41].

Classical hallucinogens are not likely to cause addiction, as it is mainly linked to the dopaminergic system, while classical hallucinogens act mostly on the serotoninergic system. Furthermore, these drugs lead to tachyphylaxis, the rapid decrease in the effect of a drug in consecutive doses, related to their mechanism of action. Thus, the development of addiction by patients after treatment with psilocybin is not of concern. However, authors suggest that if a psilocybin-containing medicines is approved, it should be included in the Schedule IV of Controlled Substance Schedules [42].

5. Conclusions

This work demonstrated that psilocybin may be effective in reducing symptoms of depression and anxiety. The results also showed the presence of publication bias, which, however, do not invalidate the conclusions of this meta-analysis. The obtained results are promising and emphasize the importance of psilocybin translational research that may lead to clinically relevant studies. Mechanistic studies are also needed to clarify the mechanism of action of the drug.

Author Contributions: Conceptualization, A.S.V. and E.G.; methodology, Â.L.; validation, M.B.; formal analysis, A.S.V., Â.L., M.B., E.G. and L.P.; investigation, A.S.V. and L.P.; data curation, L.P.; writing—original draft preparation, A.S.V.; writing—review and editing, Â.L.; supervision, E.G. and L.P.; All authors have read and agreed to the published version of the manuscript.

Funding: Â.L. acknowledges the contract of Scientific Employment in the scientific area of Microbiology financed by Fundação para a Ciência e a Tecnologia (FCT). This work was partially supported by CICS-UBI, which is financed by National Funds from FCT and Community Funds (UIDB/00709/2020). Authors would also like to thank to "Operação Centro-01-0145-FEDER-000019-C4-Centro de Competências em Cloud Computing," co-financed by the CENTRO 2020 (C4 WP3.1-Data mining for systematic reviews and Meta-Analyses in Health Sciences).

Conflicts of Interest: The authors declare no conflict of interest.

References

1. Akil, H.; Gordon, J.; Hen, R.; Javitch, J.; Mayberg, H.; McEwen, B.; Meaney, M.J.; Nestler, E.J. Treatment resistant depression: A multi-scale, systems biology approach. *Neurosci. Biobehav. Rev.* **2018**, *84*, 272–288. [CrossRef] [PubMed]
2. McIntyre, R.S.; Filteau, M.; Martin, L.; Patry, S.; Carvalho, A.; Cha, D.S.; Barakat, M.; Miguelez, M. Treatment-resistant depression: Definitions, review of the evidence, and algorithmic approach. *J. Affect. Disord.* **2014**, *156*, 1–7. [CrossRef] [PubMed]
3. Passik, S.D.; Kirsh, K.L.; Rosenfield, B.; McDonald, M.V.; Theobald, D.E. The changeable nature of patients' fears regarding chemotherapy: Implications for palliative care. *J. Pain Symptom Manag.* **2001**, *21*, 113–120. [CrossRef]
4. Groenvold, M.; Petersen, M.A.; Idler, E.; Bjorner, J.B.; Fayers, P.M.; Mouridsen, H.T. Psychological distress and fatigue predicted recurrence and survival in primary breast cancer patients. *Breast Cancer Res. Treat.* **2007**, *105*, 209–219. [CrossRef] [PubMed]
5. Pinquart, M.; Duberstein, P.R. Depression and cancer mortality: A meta-analysis. *Psychol. Med.* **2010**, *40*, 1797–1810. [CrossRef] [PubMed]
6. Griffiths, R.R.; Johnson, M.W.; Carducci, M.A.; Umbricht, A.; Richards, W.A.; Richards, B.D.; Cosimano, M.P.; Klinedinst, M.A. Psilocybin produces substantial and sustained decreases in depression and anxiety in patients with life-threatening cancer: A randomized double-blind trial. *J. Psychopharmacol.* **2016**, *30*, 1181–1197. [CrossRef] [PubMed]
7. Grassi, L.; Spiegel, D.; Riba, M. Advancing psychosocial care in cancer patients. *F1000Research* **2017**, *6*, 2083. [CrossRef] [PubMed]
8. Freedman, R.A.; Kouri, E.M.; West, D.W.; Lii, J.; Keating, N.L. Association of Breast Cancer Knowledge With Receipt of Guideline-Recommended Breast Cancer Treatment. *J. Oncol. Pract.* **2016**, *12*, e613–e625. [CrossRef]
9. Orhurhu, V.J.; Claus, L.E.; Cohen, S.P. *Ketamine Toxicity*; StatPearls Publishing: Treasure Island, FL, USA, 2019.
10. Goldberg, S.B.; Pace, B.T.; Nicholas, C.R.; Raison, C.L.; Hutson, P.R. The experimental effects of psilocybin on symptoms of anxiety and depression: A meta-analysis. *Psychiatry Res.* **2020**, *284*, 112749. [CrossRef]
11. Moher, D.; Shamseer, L.; Clarke, M.; Ghersi, D.; Liberati, A.; Petticrew, M.; Shekelle, P.; Stewart, L.A. Preferred Reporting Items for Systematic Review and Meta-Analysis Protocols (PRISMA-P) 2015 statement. *Syst. Rev.* **2015**, *4*, 1–9. [CrossRef]
12. Moher, D.; Liberati, A.; Tetzlaff, J.; Altman, D.G. Preferred Reporting Items for Systematic Reviews and Meta-Analyses: The PRISMA Statement. *Ann. Intern. Med.* **2009**, *151*, 264–270. [CrossRef] [PubMed]
13. Beck, A.T.; Ward, C.H.; Mendelson, M.; Mock, J.; Erbaugh, J. An inventory for measuring depression. *Arch. Gen. Psychiatry* **1961**, *4*, 561–571. [CrossRef] [PubMed]
14. Julian, L.J. Measures of anxiety: State-Trait Anxiety Inventory (STAI), Beck Anxiety Inventory (BAI), and Hospital Anxiety and Depression Scale-Anxiety (HADS-A). *Arthritis Care Res.* **2011**, *63*, S467–S472. [CrossRef] [PubMed]
15. Ryan, R.; Hill, S.; Prictor, M.; McKenzie, J. Cochrane Consumers & Communication Review Group Study Quality Guide Guide for Review Authors on Assessing Study Quality. 2013. Available online: https://cccrg.cochrane.org/sites/cccrg.cochrane.org/files/public/uploads/StudyQualityGuide_May%202013.pdf (accessed on 8 February 2020).
16. Higgins, J.P.T.; Altman, D.G.; Gotzsche, P.C.; Juni, P.; Moher, D.; Oxman, A.D.; Savocic, J.; Schilz, K.F.; Weeks, L.; Sterne, J.A.C. The Cochrane Collaboration's tool for assessing risk of bias in randomised trials. *BMJ* **2011**, *343*, d5928. [CrossRef] [PubMed]
17. Borenstein, M.; Hedges, L.; Higgins, J. *Introduction to Meta-Analysis*; John Wiley & Sons: Chichester, UK, 2009.
18. Higgins, J.; Thompson, S.G.; Deeks, J.J.; Altman, D.G. Measuring inconsistency in meta-analyses. *BMJ* **2003**, *327*, 557–560. [CrossRef]
19. Ross, S.; Bossis, A.; Guss, J.; Agin-Liebes, G.; Malone, T.; Cohen, B.; Mennenga, S.E.; Belser, A.; Kalliontzi, K.; Babb, J.; et al. Rapid and sustained symptom reduction following psilocybin treatment for anxiety and depression in patients with life-threatening cancer: A randomized controlled trial. *J. Psychopharmacol.* **2016**, *30*, 1165–1180. [CrossRef]

20. Grob, C.S.; Danforth, A.L.; Chopra, G.S.; Hagerty, M.; McKay, C.R.; Halberstadt, A.L.; Greer, G.R. Pilot Study of Psilocybin Treatment for Anxiety in Patients With Advanced-Stage Cancer. *Arch. Gen. Psychiatry* **2011**, *68*, 71. [CrossRef]
21. Stroud, J.B.; Freeman, T.P.; Leech, R.; Hindocha, C.; Lawn, W.; Nutt, D.J.; Curran, H.V.; Carhart-Harris, R.L. Psilocybin with psychological support improves emotional face recognition in treatment-resistant depression. *Psychopharmacology* **2018**, *235*, 459–466. [CrossRef]
22. Lyons, T.; Carhart-Harris, R.L. More Realistic Forecasting of Future Life Events After Psilocybin for Treatment-Resistant Depression. *Front. Psychol.* **2018**, *9*, 1721. [CrossRef]
23. Carhart-Harris, R.L.; Bolstridge, M.; Day, C.M.J.; Rucker, J.; Watts, R.; Erritzoe, D.E.; Kaelen, M.; Giribaldi, B.; Bloomfield, M.; Pillimg, S.; et al. Psilocybin with psychological support for treatment-resistant depression: Six-month follow-up. *Psychopharmacology* **2018**, *235*, 399–408. [CrossRef]
24. Carhart-Harris, R.L.; Bolstridge, M.; Rucker, J.; Day, C.M.J.; Erritzoe, D.; Kaelen, M.; Bloomfield, M.; Rickard, J.A.; Forbes, B.; Feilding, A.; et al. Psilocybin with psychological support for treatment-resistant depression: An open-label feasibility study. *Lancet* **2016**, *3*, 619–627. [CrossRef]
25. Nichols, D.E. Psychedelics. *Pharmacol. Rev.* **2016**, *68*, 264–355. [CrossRef] [PubMed]
26. Carhart-Harris, R.L.; Erritzoe, D.; Williams, T.; Stone, J.M.; Reed, L.J.; Colasanti, A.; Tyacke, R.J.; Leech, R.; Malizia, A.L.; Murphy, K.; et al. Neural correlates of the psychedelic state as determined by fMRI studies with psilocybin. *Proc. Natl. Acad. Sci. USA* **2012**, *109*, 2138–2143. [CrossRef] [PubMed]
27. Kraehenmann, R.; Preller, K.H.; Scheidegger, M.; Pokorny, T.; Bosch, O.G.; Seifritz, E.; Vollenweider, F.X. Psilocybin-Induced Decrease in Amygdala Reactivity Correlates with Enhanced Positive Mood in Healthy Volunteers. *Biol. Psychiatry* **2015**, *78*, 572–581. [CrossRef] [PubMed]
28. DeRubeis, R.J.; Siegle, G.J.; Hollon, S.D. Cognitive therapy versus medication for depression: Treatment outcomes and neural mechanisms. *Nat. Rev. Neurosci.* **2008**, *9*, 788–796. [CrossRef]
29. Pandey, G.N.; Dwivedi, Y.; Rizavi, H.S.; Ren, X.; Pandey, S.C.; Pesold, C.; Roberts, R.C.; Conley, R.R.; Tamminga, C.A. Higher expression of serotonin 5-HT(2A) receptors in the postmortem brains of teenage suicide victims. *Am. J. Psychiatry* **2002**, *159*, 419–429. [CrossRef]
30. Breitbart, W.; Rosenfeld, B.; Pessin, H.; Kaim, M.; Funesti-Esch, J.; Galietta, M.; Nelson, C.J.; Brescia, R. Depression, Hopelessness, and Desire for Hastened Death in Terminally Ill Patients With Cancer. *JAMA* **2000**, *284*, 2907. [CrossRef]
31. Hasler, F.; Grimberg, U.; Benz, M.A.; Huber, T.; Vollenweider, F.X. Acute psychological and physiological affects of psilocybin in healthy humans: A double-blind, placebo-controlled dose-effect study. *Psychopharmacology* **2004**, *172*, 145–156. [CrossRef]
32. Swift, T.C.; Belser, A.B.; Agin-Liebes, G.; Devenot, N.; Terrana, S.; Friedman, H.L.; Guss, J.; Bossis, A.P.; Ross, S. Cancer at the Dinner Table: Experiences of Psilocybin-Assisted Psychotherapy for the Treatment of Cancer-Related Distress. *J. Humanist. Psychol.* **2017**, *57*, 488–519. [CrossRef]
33. Studerus, E.; Kometer, M.; Hasler, F.; Vollenweider, F.X. Acute, subacute and long-term subjective effects of psilocybin in healthy humans: A pooled analysis of experimental studies. *J. Psychopharmacol.* **2011**, *25*, 1434–1452. [CrossRef]
34. Nichols, D.E.; Johnson, M.W.; Nichols, C.D. Psychedelics as Medicines: An Emerging New Paradigm. *Clin. Pharmacol. Ther.* **2017**, *101*, 209–219. [CrossRef] [PubMed]
35. Raichle, M.E. The neural correlates of consciousness: An analysis of cognitive skill learning. *Philos. Trans. R. Soc. Lond. B. Biol. Sci.* **1998**, *353*, 1889–1901.
36. Passie, T.; Seifert, J.; Schneider, U.; Emrick, H.M. The pharmacology of psilocybin. *Addict. Biol.* **2002**, *7*, 357–364. [CrossRef]
37. Isbell, H. Comparison of the reactions induced by psilocybin and LSD-25 in man. *Psychopharmacologia* **1959**, *1*, 29–38. [CrossRef] [PubMed]
38. Hermle, L.; Simon, M.; Ruchsow, M.; Geppert, M. Hallucinogen-persisting perception disorder. *Ther. Adv. Psychopharmacol.* **2012**, *2*, 199–205. [CrossRef] [PubMed]
39. Studerus, E.; Gamma, A.; Kometer, M.; Vollenweider, F.X. Prediction of psilocybin response in healthy volunteers. *PLoS ONE* **2012**, *7*, e30800. [CrossRef] [PubMed]
40. Johnson, M.; Richards, W.; Griffiths, R. Human hallucinogen research: Guidelines for safety. *J. Psychopharmacol.* **2008**, *22*, 603–620. [CrossRef]

41. Tylš, F.; Páleníček, T.; Horáček, J. Psilocybin—Summary of knowledge and new perspectives. *Eur. Neuropsychopharmacol.* **2014**, *24*, 342–356. [CrossRef] [PubMed]
42. Johnson, M.W.M.; Griffiths, R.R.; Hendricks, P.S.; Henningfield, J.E. The abuse potential of medical psilocybin according to the 8 factors of the Controlled Substances Act. *Neropharmacology* **2018**, *142*, 143–166. [CrossRef]

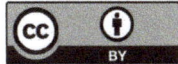

© 2020 by the authors. Licensee MDPI, Basel, Switzerland. This article is an open access article distributed under the terms and conditions of the Creative Commons Attribution (CC BY) license (http://creativecommons.org/licenses/by/4.0/).

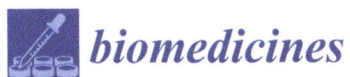

Review

Monitoring the Redox Status in Multiple Sclerosis

Masaru Tanaka [1,2] and László Vécsei [1,2,*]

1. MTA-SZTE, Neuroscience Research Group, Semmelweis u. 6, H-6725 Szeged, Hungary; tanaka.masaru.1@med.u-szeged.hu
2. Department of Neurology, Interdisciplinary Excellence Centre, Faculty of Medicine, University of Szeged, Semmelweis u. 6, H-6725 Szeged, Hungary
* Correspondence: vecsei.laszlo@med.u-szeged.hu; Tel.: +36-62-545-351

Received: 21 September 2020; Accepted: 9 October 2020; Published: 12 October 2020

Abstract: Worldwide, over 2.2 million people suffer from multiple sclerosis (MS), a multifactorial demyelinating disease of the central nervous system. MS is characterized by a wide range of motor, autonomic, and psychobehavioral symptoms, including depression, anxiety, and dementia. The blood, cerebrospinal fluid, and postmortem brain samples of MS patients provide evidence on the disturbance of reduction-oxidation (redox) homeostasis, such as the alterations of oxidative and antioxidative enzyme activities and the presence of degradation products. This review article discusses the components of redox homeostasis, including reactive chemical species, oxidative enzymes, antioxidative enzymes, and degradation products. The reactive chemical species cover frequently discussed reactive oxygen/nitrogen species, infrequently featured reactive chemicals such as sulfur, carbonyl, halogen, selenium, and nucleophilic species that potentially act as reductive, as well as pro-oxidative stressors. The antioxidative enzyme systems cover the nuclear factor erythroid-2-related factor 2 (NRF2)-Kelch-like ECH-associated protein 1 (KEAP1) signaling pathway. The NRF2 and other transcriptional factors potentially become a biomarker sensitive to the initial phase of oxidative stress. Altered components of the redox homeostasis in MS were discussed in search of a diagnostic, prognostic, predictive, and/or therapeutic biomarker. Finally, monitoring the battery of reactive chemical species, oxidative enzymes, antioxidative enzymes, and degradation products helps to evaluate the redox status of MS patients to expedite the building of personalized treatment plans for the sake of a better quality of life.

Keywords: oxidative stress; redox; antioxidant; multiple sclerosis; biomarker; neurodegenerative disease; personalized medicine

1. Introduction

Multiple sclerosis (MS) is an immune-mediated demyelinating disease of the brain and spinal cord, which over 2.2 million people worldwide suffer from; it affects primarily young adults from 20 to 40 years of age. After one to two decades, many MS patients enter a progressive phase of the disease. As survival rates have improved, MS patients suffer throughout the adult life. Years lived with disability begin to increase steeply early in the second decade of life and disability-adjusted life years peak in the sixth decade of life [1]. MS encompasses a wide range of symptoms from motor and autonomic dysfunctions to psychobehavioral disturbances, including gait difficulties, paresthesia, spasticity, vision problems, dizziness and vertigo, incontinence, constipation, sexual disturbances, pain, cognitive and emotional changes, anxiety, and depression [2–5]. Increased risk of depression and painful conditions in chronic illnesses are likely to be mediated by the kynurenine pathway of tryptophan metabolism [6,7].

Several genetic susceptibilities, environmental factors, and the aging process have been proposed to alter the risk of developing MS, but the underlying cause of the disease remains unknown [8,9]. The most typical pathomechanisms involved in MS are simultaneous inflammatory and neurodegenerative processes [10,11]. Main pathological findings of MS include the blood-brain barrier disruption, multifocal inflammation, demyelination, oligodendrocyte loss, reactive gliosis, and axonal degeneration [12]. Multifocal immune-mediated destruction of myelin and oligodendrocytes leading to progressive axonal loss is a main cause of neurological deficits in MS [13–15].

The diagnosis of MS is confirmed by the presence of two or more multifocal inflammatory or demyelinating attacks in the central nervous system (CNS) with objective clinical evidence, a single attack with magnetic resonance imaging (MRI)-detected lesions, and positive cerebrospinal fluid (CSF) analysis, or insidious neurological progression with positive brain MRI or CSF analysis [16]. The symptomatic course classifies MS into four subtypes. Approximately 85% of MS patients have alternating episodes of neurological disability and recovery that last for many years, termed relapsing-remitting MS (RRMS). Almost 90% of RRMS patients progress to steady neurological decline within 25 years, termed secondary progressive MS (SPMS). Nearly 10% of MS patients suffer from steady deterioration of neurological functions without recovery, termed primary progressive MS (PPMS). As few as 5% of MS patients present progressive neurological deficits with acute attacks with or without recovery, termed progressive-relapsing MS (PRMS) [17]. However, PRMS is no longer considered a subtype of MS and is now grouped into PPMS with active disease of new symptoms or changes in the MRI scan [18]. In addition, clinically isolated syndrome (CIS) is a single episode of monofocal or multifocal neurological deficits that lasts at least 24 h. CIS is one of the courses of MS disease [12].

As in other neurodegenerative diseases, MS is a clinically classified disease of CNS in which multifactorial factors, including genetic, environmental, socioeconomic, cultural, personal lifestyle, and aging play an initial role to form a causative complex, eventually converging into similar pathognomonic clinical pictures [4]. Inflammatory and demyelinating attacks are unique manifestations in MS, but different pathomechanisms govern the distinguished clinical courses in each subtype of MS.

Currently there is no cure for MS. Disease-modifying therapy is the mainstay of MS treatment. Immunomodulators, immunosuppressors, and cytotoxic agents are main groups of medicine. Immunomodulators, such as interferon (IFN)-beta (β), glatiramer acetate (GA), and siponimod are used for CIS. Short courses of high-dose corticosteroid methylprednisolone alleviate acute flare-ups of RRMS, indicating that an inflammatory process predominates in RRMS and relapse prevention of RRMS [19,20]. Siponimod is indicated for RRMS [20]. For active RRMS monoclonal antibodies alemtuzumab and ocrelizumab, and immunomodulator dimethyl fumarate, fingolimod, and teriflunomide are prescribed besides IFN-β and GA. For highly active RRMS, cytotoxic agents cladribine and mitoxantrone are indicated, besides immunomodulatory fingolimod, and monoclonal antibodies, natalizumab and ocrelizumab. PPMS and SPMS are characterized by a neurodegenerative process leading to neural death [18]. An immunosuppressive monoclonal antibody ocrelizumab is indicated for treatment of PPMS [21] and diroximel fumarate, siponimod, and ofatumumab were recently licensed for treatment of SPMS [20,22,23] (Table 1).

Table 1. Licensed disease-modifying drugs in multiple sclerosis [19–26].

Class	Drugs	Indications
Immunomodulators	Interferon beta (IFN-β)	CIS Active RRMS
	Methylprednisolone	Acute flare-ups RRMS Relapse prevention
	Glatiramer acetate (GA)	CIS Active RRMS
	Dimethyl fumarate	Active RRMS
	Diroximel fumarate	CIS RRMS Active SPMS
	Fingolimod	Active RRMS High-active RRMS
	Teriflunomide	Active RRMS
	Siponimod	CIS RRMS SPMS
Immunosuppressors	Alemtuzumab	Active RRMS
	Natalizumab	High-active RRMS
	Ocrelizumab	Active RRMS High-active RRMS PPMS
	Ofatumumab	CIS RRMS Active SPMS
Cytotoxic Agents	Cladribine	High-active RRMS
	Mitoxantrone	High-active RRMS

Either causative, accompanying, or resultant events of inflammation and neurodegeneration, disturbance of reduction-oxidation (redox) metabolism have been observed and play a crucial role in pathogenesis of MS [27–29]. The serum proteomics revealed that ceruloplasmin, clusterin, apolipoprotein E, and complement C3 were up-regulated in RRMS patients, compared to healthy controls. Vitamin D-binding protein showed a progressive trend of oxidation and the increased oxidation of apolipoprotein A-IV in progression from remission to relapse of MS [30]. CSF samples of patients in the remission stage of RRMS showed higher purine oxidation product uric acid, reduced antioxidant, and increased intrathecal synthesis of IgG [31]. The observations suggest the presence of redox metabolism disturbance and involvement of inflammatory process in RRMS. Furthermore, higher serum alpha (α)-tocopherol levels were associated with reduced T1 gadolinium (Gd^+)-enhancing lesions and subsequent T2 lesions in MRI of RRMS patients on IFN-β. Antioxidant glutathione (GSH) mapping showed lower GSH concentrations in the frontoparietal region of patients suffering from PPMS and SPMS than RRMS and no significant difference between those of RRMS and controls. Thus, the oxidative stress in CNS was linked to neurodegeneration in progressive types of MS [32].

This review article reviewed participants of redox homeostasis, including reactive chemical species, oxidative and antioxidative enzymes, and resulting degradation products, all of which serve as evidence of biochemical assaults and tissue injuries under redox disequilibrium. Literature research was carried out using PubMed/MEDLINE and Google Scholar, using appropriate search terms, such as: "reactive oxygen species", "oxidative stress", "redox", "biomarker", "neurodegenerative disease", "inflammation", "neurodegeneration", and/or "multiple sclerosis". Meta-analyses, systematic reviews, expert reviews, case-control studies, and cohort studies were included in this review. Selection criteria and a risk of bias assessment are described in Tables A1 and A2 of Appendix A. Alterations of redox components in MS in general, phase-, and treatment-specific components were reviewed in search of a potential diagnostic, prognostic, predictive, and/or therapeutic redox biomarker. Finally, monitoring different redox components, including oxidative enzymes, antioxidative enzymes, and degradation products during the disease progression helps to evaluate the redox status of MS patients, thus expediting the building of the most appropriate personalized treatment plans for MS patients [33].

2. Oxidative Stress

A redox reaction is a type of chemical reaction that involves the transfer of electrons between two molecules. A pair of electrons transfers from a nucleophile to an electrophile, forming a new covalent bond. The redox reaction is common and vital to the basic function of life such as cellular respiration, in which sugar is oxidized to release energy, which is stored in ATP. Redox metabolisms constitute multiple metabolic pathways involved in the series of redox chemical reactions indispensable for sustaining life and, at same time, engaged in removal of electrophilic oxidative species and other harmful nucleophiles. The dynamic activities range from a single electron transfer, enzyme reaction, chemical reaction cascade, to signaling in cells, tissues, organ systems, and whole organismal levels [34]. Oxidative stress is a state caused by an imbalance between the relative levels of production of reactive oxidizing metabolites and their elimination by the enzymatic or non-enzymatic antioxidant system. The oxidative state is induced by oxidative stressors either derived from xenobiotics or produced from the activities of oxidative enzymes and essential cellular constituents [35] (Figure 1a). Oxidative stressors are linked to the aging process, neurologic disease, and psychiatric disorders including Alzheimer's disease (AD), Parkinson's disease (PD), MS, amyotrophic lateral sclerosis (ALS), and depression [36–40].

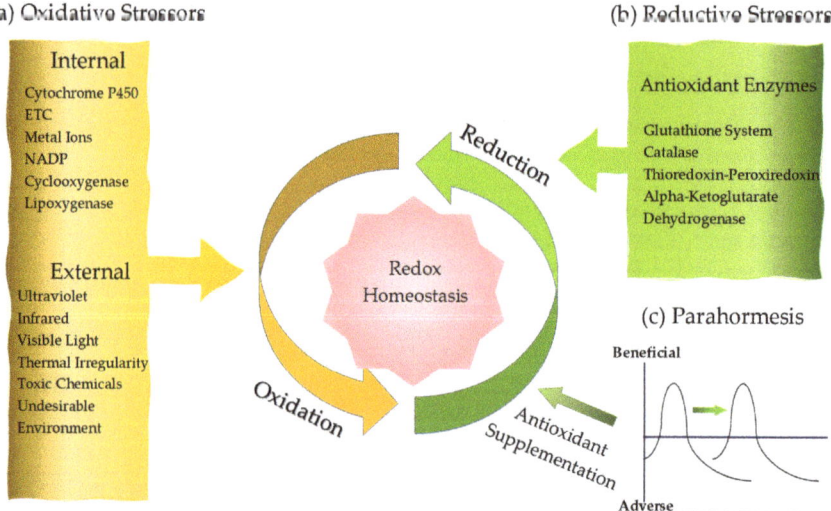

Figure 1. Redox homeostasis and antioxidant supplementation. (**a**) Oxidative stressors comprise of external and internal stressors, exerting oxidative chemical reactions in organism. Oxidation is an indispensable bioenergetic process to sustain life. (**b**) Reductive stressors are products of antioxidative enzymes that generate antioxidants in response to regular oxidation activity and increased oxidative stress. (**c**) Antioxidant supplementation attempts to shift the biphasic response from adverse to beneficial phase to maintain nucleophilic tone. This mechanism is called parahormesis.

2.1. Endogenous Oxidative Stressors: Oxidative Enzymes and Reactive Species

Endogenous oxidative stressors are produced from cellular activities of cytosolic xanthine dehydrogenase (XDH), membrane-bound nicotinamide adenine dinucleotide phosphate (NADPH) oxidase, inflammatory lipoxygenase (LOX), and cyclooxygenase (COX), phagocytic myeloperoxidase (MPO) in respiratory burst, a second messenger nitrogen oxide (NO)-producing nitric oxide synthetase (NOS), mitochondrial and lysosomal electron transfer chain (ETC) enzymes, among others. Transition metals such as iron (Fe^{2+}) and copper (Cu^+) also play a crucial role in the formation of oxidative stressors via the Fenton reaction [41].

2.1.1. Oxidative Enzymes Generating Reactive Oxygen Species

Reactive oxygen species (ROS) include several free radicals, such as superoxide ($O_2^{-\bullet}$) and hydroxyl radical ($OH^\bullet$) and nonradical molecules such as hydrogen peroxide (H_2O_2) and organic hydroperoxide (ROOH) (Table 2). ROS are produced in endogenously in the cytosol, the plasma membrane, the membranes of mitochondria and endoplasmic reticulum, peroxisomes, and phagocytic cells [42,43] (Figure 2). ROS is difficult for direct measurement in biological tissues due to its highly reactivity and short life.

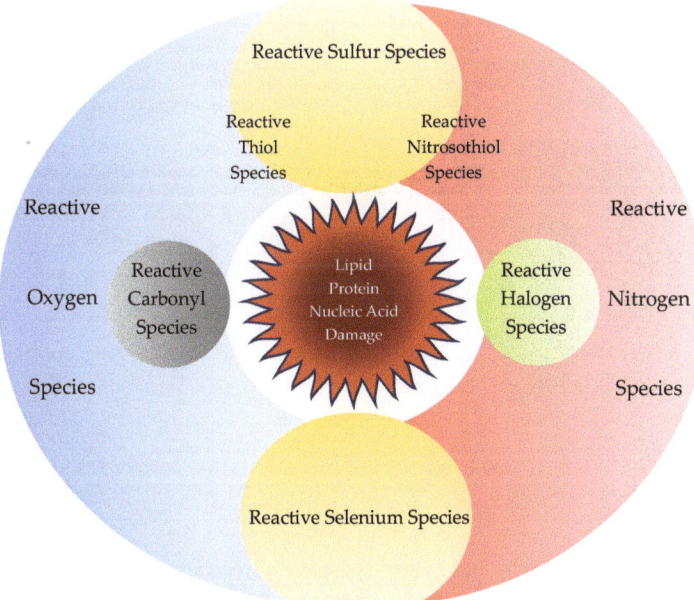

Figure 2. Reactive chemical species. Reactive chemical species comprise of not only reactive oxygen species and reactive nitrogen species, but also reactive sulfur, carbonyl, halogen, and selenium species. Sulfur reacts with oxygen or nitrogen to form reactive thiol or nitrosothiol species, respectively. All reactive chemical species react in concert during regular cellular activity but may cause oxidative stress to damage cellular components such as proteins, lipids, and nucleic acids.

Table 2. Reactive chemical species. During regular cellular activity living cells generate numerous reactive chemical species containing oxygen, nitrogen, sulfur, carbonyl, halogen, or selenium. Reactive sulfur species can contain thiols or nitrothiols. Free radicals possess at least one unpaired electron that makes highly reactive and short-lived. Nonradicals are oxidizing chemicals or easily converted to free radicals. Superoxide, reactive sulfur species, or reactive selenium species can be reducing agents as reactive nucleophilic species.

	Reactive Chemical Species
Reactive Oxygen Species (ROS)	Free Radicals Superoxide anion ($O_2^{-\bullet}$), Hydroxyl radical ($OH^\bullet$), Alkoxyl radical ($RO^\bullet$), Peroxyl radical ($ROO^\bullet$)
	Nonradicals Hydrogen peroxide (H_2O_2), Organic hydroperoxide (ROOH), Organic peroxide (ROOR), Singlet oxygen ($O_2{}^1\Delta_g$), Ozone (O_3)
Reactive Nitrogen Species (RNS)	Free Radicals Nitric oxide radical ($NO^\bullet$), Nitrogen dioxide radical ($NO_2{}^\bullet$)
	Nonradicals Nitrite (NO_2^-), Nitrate (NO_3^-), Nitroxyl anion (NO^-), Nitrosyl cation (NO^+), Peroxynitrite ($ONOO^-$), Peroxynitrate (O_2NOO^-), Nitrosoperoxycarbonate ($ONOOCO_2^-$), Dinitrogen trioxide (N_2O_3), Dinitrogen tetraoxide (N_2O_4), Nitryl chloride ($NClO_2$)
Reactive Sulfur Species (RSN)	Free Radicals Thiyl radical ($RS^\bullet$), Peroxysulphenyl radical ($RSOO^\bullet$)
	Nonradicals Hydrogen sulfide (H_2S), Thiolate anion (RS^-), Thiol (RSH), Hydropersulfide (RSSH), Disulfide (RSSR), Hydropolysulfide (RSS_nH), Dialkyl polysulfide (RSS_nR), Polysulfide (H_2Sx), Sulfenate (RSO^-), Sulfinate (RSO_2^-), Sulfonate (RSO_3^-), Thiosulmonate ($S_2O_3^{2-}$), Sulfite ($RS_2O_3^{2-}$), Sulfate (SO_4^{2-}), Thiosulfinate ($C_6H_{10}OS_2$), S-nitrosothiols (RSNOs), Nitrosopersulfide ($SSNO^-$), Dinitrosylated sulfite adduct (SULFI/NO)
Reactive Carbonyl Species (RCS)	Nonradicals Acetaldehyde (CH_3CHO), Acrolein (Proponel$^+$: C_3H_4O), Methylglyoxal 4-Hydroxy-nonenal ($C_9H_{16}O_2$), 3-Deoxyglucosone ($C_6H_{10}O_5$), Glyoxal ($C_2H_2O_2$), Methylglyoxal ($C_3H_4O_2$), Electronically excited triplet carbonyls ($^3L=O^*$)
Reactive Halogen Species (RHS)	Free Radicals Atomic chlorine ($Cl^\bullet$), Atomic bromine ($Br^\bullet$)
	Nonradicals Hypochlorite (OCl^-), Chloramines (RNHCl), Hypobromite (OBr^-), Hypoiodite (IO^-), Hypohalogenite (XO^-; X = F, Cl, Br, or I)
Reactive Selenium Species (RSeS)	Nonradicals Selenite (O_3Se^{-2}), Selenate (SeO_4^{2-}), Selenocysteine ($C_3H_7NO_2Se$), Selenomethionine ($C_5H_{11}NO_2Se$)
Reactive Nucleophilic Species	Free Radicals Superoxide anion ($O_2^{-\bullet}$)
	Nonradicals Hydrogen sulfide (H_2S), Thiolate (RS^-), Hydropersulfide (RSS^-), Disulfide (RSSR), Selenite (O_3Se^{-2}), Selenate (SeO_4^{2-}), Selenocysteine ($C_3H_7NO_2Se$), Selenomethionine ($C_5H_{11}NO_2Se$)

In the cytosol, ROS can be generated by soluble intercellular components, such as catecholamines, hydroquinones, flavins, and thiols (RSHs) that undergo reduction reactions [44]. The cytosolic enzyme XDH normally catalyzes xanthine, NAD^+, and water (H_2O) to urate, reduced form of NAD^+, NADH, and hydrogen ion (H^+). Reversible oxidation of cysteine residues or irreversible Ca^{2+}-stimulated proteolysis converts XDH to xanthine oxidase (XO) that transfers electrons to molecular oxygen (O_2), producing superoxide ($O_2^{-\bullet}$) during xanthine or hypoxanthine oxidation [45]. The serum levels of uric acid, a major endogenous antioxidant was measured in patients with PPMM, RRMM, and SPMM. The uric acid levels were significantly lower in active MS than inactive MS, and the uric acid levels were independently correlated with gender, disease activity and duration of the disease [46] (Table 3).

Table 3. Oxidative stress biomarkers of multiple sclerosis. The redox status can be monitored by the activities of oxidative and antioxidative enzymes and the presence of degradation products derived from cellular components. ↑: increase, ↓: decrease, -: unknown.

Classes		Types	Human Samples		Reference
			Blood	CSF	
Reactive Species		Reactive Nitrogen Species	↑	↑	[47]
Oxidative Enzymes		Xanthine Dehydrogenase (XDH)	↓	-	[46]
		Nicotinamide Adenine Dinucleotide Phosphate (NADPH) Oxidase	mixed	-	[48]
		Superoxide Dismutase (SOD)	↑	↓	[49–52]
		Inducible Nitric Oxide Synthase (iNOS)	↑	↑	[18,53–55]
		Myeloperoxidase (MPO)	mixed	-	[48]
Antioxidative Enzymes and Transcriptional Factors		Glutathione Peroxidase (GPx)	↑(relapse) ↓(remission)	↓	[56–61]
		Glutathione Reductase (GSR)	-	↑	[61,62]
		Catalase	↓	-	[61,62]
		Xanthine oxidase (XO)-Uric Acid	↓	-	[46]
		Nuclear Factor Erythroid 2-Related Factor (Nrf2)	↑	-	[52]
		Peroxisome proliferator-activated receptors (PPARs)	-	↑	[63]
		Peroxisome proliferator-activated receptor gamma coactivator 1-alpha (PGC-1α)	↓	-	[64]
Degradation Products and End Products	Protein	Protein carbonyls	↑	-	[65–71]
		3-nitrotyrosin (3-NO-Tyr)	↑	-	[68–70,72]
		Protein glutathionylation	-	↑	[73]
		Dityrosine	↑	-	[74]
		Advanced oxidation protein products (AOPPs)	↑	-	[49,74,75]
		Advanced glycation end products (AGEs)	↑	↑	[74,75]
	Amino acids	Asymmetric dimethylarginine (ADMA)	↓	-	[76]
	Lipid	F2-isoprostane (F2-isoP)	↑	↑	[77–81]
		Malondialdehyde (MDA)	mixed	↑	[61,82–85]
		4-hydroxynonenal (4-HNE)	-	↑	[86]
		Hydroxyoctadecadienoic acid (HODE)	↑	↑	[87]
		Oxysterol	mixed	↑	[88]
	DNA	8-dihydro-2′deoxyguanosine (8-oxodG)	↑	-	[56]

The plasma membrane is a network of phospholipid bilayer and integral proteins which protects the cellular organelles from the outer environment and is responsible for several cellular functions, such as cell adhesion, ion transport, cell signaling, and phagocytosis. The main ROS of the plasma membrane is a superoxide ($O_2^{-\bullet}$) produced by the membrane-bound enzyme nicotinamide adenine dinucleotide phosphate oxidase (NOX), which is composed of two membrane proteins, three cytosolic proteins, and a small GTP-binding protein [89,90]. The expression of NOX isoform NOX5 was significantly increased, but the expression NOX4 was significantly decreased in serum of RRMS patients, suggesting that differential NOX isoform expression contributes to OS-associated vascular changes in MS [48]. ROS is also produced by COX and LOX, which convert arachidonic acid to prostaglandins, thromboxanes, and leukotrienes. Phospholipase A_2 generates ROS during arachidonic acid oxidation [91]. In the presence of transition metal ions, such as Fe^{2+} and Cu^+, hydrogen peroxide (H_2O_2), organic hydroperoxide (ROOH), and organic peroxide (ROOR) produce hydroxyl ($OH^\bullet$), alkoxyl ($RO^\bullet$), and peroxyl radical ($ROO^\bullet$), respectively [92] (Table 3).

Superoxide dismutase (SOD) catalyzes the disproportionation of two superoxide ($O_2^{-\bullet}$) into molecular oxygen (O_2) and hydrogen peroxide (H_2O_2). These enzymes are present in almost all aerobic cells and in extracellular fluids. SODs contain metal ion cofactors that, depending on the isozyme, can be copper, zinc, manganese, or iron [93,94]. There are three isozymes in humans. Dimeric copper- and zinc-coordinated SOD1 is in the cytoplasm; tetrameric manganese-coordinated SOD2 is confined to the mitochondria; tetrameric copper- and zinc-coordinated SOD3 is extracellular [95]. The mitochondrial ROS production takes place at four protein complexes, ubiquinone, and cytochrome c of the ETC, embedded in the inner membrane of the mitochondria [96]. The Complexes I/III/IV utilize NADH as the substrate, while Complexes II/III/IV use succinic acid. The complex II is also glycerol 3-phosphate dependent. The primary mitochondrial ROS is superoxide ($O_2^{-\bullet}$) that is converted by mitochondrial SOD into hydrogen peroxide (H_2O_2), which can be turned into hydroxyl ($OH^\bullet$) via the Fenton reaction [97]. The Complex I and III release superoxide ($O_2^{-\bullet}$) into the mitochondrial matrix where it can damage the mitochondrial DNA, while the Complex III also releases superoxide ($O_2^{-\bullet}$) into the intermembrane space where it is accessible to the cytosol [98]. Reduced levels of antioxidant α-tocopherol was observed in the blood of patients with Leber's hereditary optic neuropathy, which is caused by mitochondrial mutation of the Complex I, suggesting that oxidative load was elevated and antioxidant capacity was compromised [99]. Other mitochondrial enzymes that contribute to hydrogen peroxide (H_2O_2) production are monoamine oxidases, dihydroorotate dehydrogenase, α-glycerophosphate dehydrogenase, and α-ketoglutarate dehydrogenase (α-KGDH) complex. Succinate dehydrogenase also generates ROS [100].

Significantly higher mean activity of SOD in erythrocyte lysates was reported in RRMS than controls. Interestingly, the SOD activity of CIS was higher than that of RRMS [101]. The erythrocyte SOD activity can be a diagnostic biomarker of CIS and RRMS. The SOD activity was significantly lower in the erythrocyte lysates of RRSM patients upon relapse than controls but increased following the intravenous administration of corticosteroid methylprednisolone and remained higher during remission period than controls. The SOD is a potent predictive and therapeutic biomarker. The serum/plasma samples also showed significantly higher mean SOD activity in RRMS compared to control groups [82]. However, platelet SOD1 and SOD2 activity was unchanged in MS patients [49]. Intriguingly, SOD activity was significantly low in CSF of CIS and RRMS patients, despite the significantly high activity of plasma SOD. Furthermore, there were negative correlations between the erythrocyte SOD activity and disease duration and expanded disability status scale (EDSS) in CIS and RRMS, between the erythrocyte SOD activity and Gd^+ enhancement lesion volume in CIS patients [50]. These findings suggest the SOD activity as a possible diagnostic and prognostic marker (Tables 3 and 4).

The peripheral blood mononuclear cells (PBMCs) SOD1 proteins and mRNA expression were significantly lower in RRMS patients than controls and became significantly more elevated following IFN-β1b treatment than the baseline [51]. These studies suggest SOD as a potential therapeutic biomarker (Table 4). However, the erythrocyte SOD activity remained unchanged following the treatment of natalizumab, a humanized monoclonal antibody against the cell adhesion molecule α4-integrin. But levels of carbonylated protein and oxidized guanosine were reduced [52].

In the inner membrane of mitochondria and the endoplasmic reticulum, a heme-containing monooxygenase cytochrome P450 (CYP) enzymes are responsible for oxidizing steroids, cholesterols, and fatty acids. The CYPs forms ROS superoxide ($O_2^{-\bullet}$) and hydrogen peroxide (ROOH) by substrate cycling [102]. Protonation of hydrogen peroxide (ROOH) forms hydrogen peroxide (H_2O_2) which, furthermore, cleaves into hydroxy radicals ($OH^\bullet$). The redox cycling produces free radical semiquinone from quinoid substrates [103]. In the mitochondrial transport chain, flavoprotein reductase forms ROS by direct reduction of O_2 and via the mediation of quinones. [104]. Superoxide ($O_2^{-\bullet}$) is produced by XO in the reperfusion phase of ischemia, LOX, COX, and NADPH-dependent oxidase [105]. In the endoplasmic reticulum NADH cytochrome b5 reductase can leak electrons to molecular oxygen (O_2) to generate superoxide ($O_2^{-\bullet}$) during the NADPH-dependent oxidation of xenobiotics [106].

Most enzymes in the peroxisomes produce ROS during the catalysis of fatty acid α- and β-oxidation, amino acid and glyoxylate metabolism, and synthesis of lipidic compounds. A large fraction of hydrogen peroxide (H_2O_2) generated inside peroxisomes was observed to penetrate the peroxisomal membrane and diffuse to the surrounding media [107]. The peroxide can diffuse through the channel formed by the peroxisomal membrane protein Pxmp2 and hydrogen peroxide (H_2O_2) generated by the peroxisomal urate oxidase can release through crystalloid core tubules into the cytosol [108]. Meanwhile, peroxisomes also possess protective mechanisms to counteract oxidative stress and maintain redox balance. Reduction in peroxisomal gene and protein expression was observed in MS gray matter [109].

Table 4. Possible redox biomarkers in multiple sclerosis. Reactive chemical species, oxidative enzymes, antioxidants, antioxidative enzymes, degradation products, and end products are potential biomarkers for multiple sclerosis (MS). Diagnostic biomarkers allow early detection and secondary prevention; prognostic biomarkers suggest the likely clinical course; predictive biomarkers predict the response of MS patients to a specific therapy; and therapeutic biomarkers indicate a target for therapy. CIS: clinically isolated syndrome, PPMS: primary progressive MS; RRMS: relapsing-remitting MS, SPMS: secondary progressive MS, mixedMM: mixed population of MS.

Class	Components	Biomarkers			
		Diagnostic	Prognostic	Predictive	Therapeutic
Reactive Chemical Species	Total nitrite (NO_2^-)/nitrite (NO_3^-) value (tNOx)	PPMS, RRMS, Relapse, SPMS	RRMS	-	-
	S-nitrosothiol	RRMS, SPMS	Spinal injury	-	-
Oxidative Enzymes	Superoxide dismutase (SOD)	CIS, RRMS	CIS, RRMS	RRMS	RRMS
	Myeloperoxidase (MPO)	RRMS	RRMS	-	-
	Inducible nitric oxide synthase (iNOS)	RRMS	-	-	-
Antioxidants and Antioxidative Enzymes	Xanthine oxidase (XO)-Uric acid	PPMM, RRMM, SPMM	-	-	-
	Selenium	RRMS	-	-	-
	Glutathione reductase (GSR)	mixedMM	MixedMM	-	-
	Catalase	CIS, RRMS	RRMS	-	-
	Thioredoxin-Peroxiredoxin (TRX-PRDX)	MS	-	-	-
	Nuclear factor erythroid 2-related factor (Nrf2)	RRMS	-	RRMS	-
	Peroxisome proliferator-activated receptors (PPARs)	RRMS	-	-	-
	Peroxisome proliferator-activated receptor gamma coactivator 1-alpha (PGC-1α)	PPMS, SPMS	-	-	-
Degradation Products and End Products	Protein carbonyls	RRMS, SPMS	RRMS, SPMS	RRMS	-
	3-nitrotyrosine (3-NO-Tyr)	RRMS, SPMS	-	RRMS	-
	Glutathionylation	Acute attack	-	-	-
	Dityrosine	RRSM	-	-	-
	Advanced oxidation protein products (AOPPs)	CIS, RRMS	RRMS	RRMS	-
	Advanced glycation end products (AGEs)	RRMS	-	-	-
	Asymmetric dimethylarginine (ADMA)	RRMS, SPMS	-	-	-
	F2-isoprostane (F2-isoP)	RRMS, SPMS	SPMS	-	-
	Malondialdehyde (MDA)	RRMS	RRMS	RRMS	-
	4-hydroxynonenal (4-HNE)	PPMS, RRMS, SPMS	-	-	-
	Hydroxyoctadecadienoic acid (HODE)	CIS, RRMS	-	-	-
	Oxocholesterols	MixedMS	SPMS	-	-
	Oxidized low-density lipoprotein (oxLDL)	RRMS, SPMS	-	-	-
	8-OH2dG	RRMS	-	-	-

The lysosomal ETC plays a central role to support the positive proton gradient to maintain an optimal pH of the acid hydrolases [110]. The ETC is made up of a flavin-adenine dinucleotide, a b-type cytochrome and ubiquinone with the donor NADH and ending to acceptor molecular oxygen (O_2), transferring three electrons. Superoxide ($O_2^{-•}$) is possibly produced in the acidic environment which favors dismutation of hydrogen peroxide (H_2O_2) into hydroxy radical ($OH^•$) by ferrous iron [111]. Furthermore, ozone (O_3) and ozone-like oxidants are generated from singlet oxygen ($O_2^1\Delta_g$) catalyzed by antibody or amino acid. Ozone (O_3) reacts with superoxide anion ($O_2^{-•}$) to form hydrogen peroxide (H_2O_2) in the presence of Fe^{+2} [112].

2.1.2. Oxidative Enzymes Generating Reactive Nitrogen Species

Reactive nitrogen species (RNS) are a group of nitrogen-congaing molecules including free radicals, nitric oxide (NO), and nitrogen dioxide (NO_2). Free radicals are nitric oxide ($NO^•$) and nitrogen dioxide ($NO_2^•$) radicals, while nonradicals are nitrite (NO_2^-) and nitrate (NO_3^-), among others (Table 2). RNS are derived from nitric oxide (NO) and superoxide anion ($O_2^{-•}$) produced by nitric oxide synthetase 2 (NOS2), NADPH oxidase, XO, LOX, and COX, among others [113,114]. At physiological concentrations, a gaseous molecule nitric oxide (NO) is a second messenger involved in blood pressure regulation, smooth muscle relaxation, defense mechanisms, immune regulation, and neurotransmission contributing the function of memory and learning [47].

Cross-sectional studies show that the levels of nitric oxide metabolites nitrite (NO_2^-) and nitrite (NO_3^-), measured as a total value (tNOx), are significantly higher in plasma or serum of patients with RRMS [83,115]. A longitudinal study revealed that higher serum tNOx is significantly correlated with relapsing rate, suggesting prognostic biomarker of NOS [116]. Many studies of CSF samples reported significantly higher levels of tNOx in RRMS and PPMS, compared to healthy controls [117,118]. A study observed significantly higher levels of CSF tNOx in RRMS than SPMS, suggesting an inflammatory role of RNS [119]. Significantly higher levels of CSF tNOx were reported in patients with acute relapsing phase of RRMS than those with stable remitting phase of RRMS [120,121] (Tables 3 and 4).

In cGMP-dependent pathways, nitric oxide radical ($NO^\bullet$) generated by endothelial NOS in endothelium, brain, and heart relaxes blood vessels and maintains normal blood pressure, while nitric oxide radicals ($NO^\bullet$) produced by neuronal NOS serve as a neurotransmitter to regulate blood pressure in the brain. Inducible NOS (iNOS) in macrophages and smooth muscle cells gives rise to nitric oxide radicals ($NO^\bullet$) as in reaction to bacterial lipopolysaccharides and/or cytokines [122].

Nitric oxide radical ($NO^\bullet$) is produced from the metabolism of L-arginine by NOS that converts L-arginine into L-citrulline and nitric oxide radical ($NO^\bullet$) by a 5-electron oxidation of a guanidine nitrogen of L-arginine [123]. In mitochondria nitric oxide radicals ($NO^\bullet$) react with respiratory Complex III to inhibit electron transfer and facilitate superoxide anion ($O_2^{\bullet-}$) production. The nitric oxide radicals ($NO^\bullet$) also compete with molecular oxygen (O_2) for the binding site at the binuclear center of cytochrome c oxidoreductase, inducing a reversible inhibition of cytochrome c oxidase. Nitric oxide (NO) neutralizes ROS [45]. However, RNS react with oxygen molecules (O_2) and ROS, giving rise to a variety of nitrogen oxides (NOs), such as nitrogen dioxide radical ($NO_2^\bullet$), nitrogen dioxide (NO_2), dinitrogen trioxide (N_2O_3), peroxynitrite ($ONOO^-$), nitrite (NO_2^-), and nitrate (NO_3^-). Higher concentrations of nitric oxide (NO) become toxic by forming nitrosothiols which oxidize tyrosine, cysteine, methionine, and GSH. In mitochondria, nitric oxide radicals ($NO^\bullet$) inhibit Complex I by S-nitrosation [124]. Together with other RNS, this contributes the damage of cell membranes, proteins, and lipid membrane leading to the degradation of mitochondria, lysosomes, and DNA. The chain of events culminates in the inhibition of immune response and production of carcinogenic nitrosamines [125]. Nitric oxide (NO) is also involved in metal homeostasis including Fe, Cu, and Zn [126].

Highly toxic peroxynitrite ($ONOO^-$) is formed by the reaction of nitric oxide (NO) and superoxide anions ($O_2^{-\bullet}$), leading to the production of more reactive compounds that oxidize methionine and tyrosine residues of proteins, lipids, and DNA. Reacting with superoxide anion ($O_2^{-\bullet}$), nitric oxide radicals ($NO^\bullet$) form peroxynitrite which causes reversible inhibition of cellular respiration in the mitochondria [127]. In peroxisomes nitric oxide radicals ($NO^\bullet$) react with superoxide anions ($O_2^{-\bullet}$) produced by XO to form peroxynitrite and hydrogen peroxides [111]. In addition, insulin resistance favors peroxintrite formation [128].

In response to bacterial lipopolysaccharides and inflammatory stimuli, iNOS generates nitric oxide (NO) that protects tissue hypoxia and serves as a neurotransmitter. However, overexpression iNOS, increase of nitric oxide (NO), and subsequent inflammation have been implicated in pathophysiology of neurodegenerative diseases including MS [47]. Calmodulin mediates the oxidative stress and inflammasome activation involving calmodulin-binding proteins, calcineurin, and calcium/calmodulin-dependent kinase II. Calmodulin inhibitors improved cognitive functions in an animal model of vascular dementia [129]. The iNOS activity is upregulated in acute MS plaques [19,53]. Increased activity and expression of iNOS in lymphocytes were found in active relapsing phase of RRMS [54]. CSF iNOS expression was shown in MS patients and mean CSF NOS activity was significantly higher, compared to controls [55] (Table 3).

2.1.3. Reactive Sulfur Species

Reactive sulfur species (RSS) are sulfur-based redox-active compounds able to oxidize or reduce biomolecules under physiological conditions, often formed by thiols (RSHs) and disulfides (RSSHs). RSS include cysteine and methionine, GSH, trypanothione, and mycothiol [130] (Table 2).

Thiyl radicals (RS$^\bullet$), very reactive oxidants produced in the active site of enzymes such as the ribonucleotide reductase can react with nitric oxide radicals (NO$^\bullet$) [131]. Thiolate ions (RS$^-$) are better nucleophiles than alkoxides because sulfur is more polarizable than oxygen [132]. Thiol (RSH) is a metal ligand [133]. Hydrogen sulfide (H$_2$S) is produced from from L-cysteine by cistationine-γ-lyase. Hydrogen sulfide (H$_2$S) increases the activity of N-methyl-D-aspartate receptor and β-adrenergic receptors through a cAMP-dependent protein kinase and activates NOS and the hemoxygenase favoring the formation of Nitric oxide (NO) and carbon monoxide (CO) from heme metabolism [134]. Hydrogen sulfide (H$_2$S) is a metal ligand that reacts with other biological electrophilic sulfur species such as hydropersulfide (RSSR) and sulfenic acid (RSOH) [135]. Cysteine residues in GSH were found to be readily oxidized by superoxide anions (O$_2^{-\bullet}$) to form singlet oxygen (O$_2{}^1\Delta_g$), glutathione disulfide (GSSG), and glutathione sulfonate (GSO$_3^-$) in a reaction involved with peroxysulphenyl radical (RSOO$^\bullet$). This mechanism may apply to cysteine residues in proteins [136]. Hydroxyl radicals (OH$^\bullet$) may also initiate the conversion of amino acids to peroxyl radicals [92]. Another reaction catalyzed by XO is the decomposition of S-nitrosothiols (RSNO), a RNS, to nitric oxide (NO), which reacts with a superoxide (O$_2^{-\bullet}$) anion to form peroxynitrite (ONOO$^-$) under aerobic conditions [137]. Hydropersulfide (RSSH) is a nucleophile, as well as electrophilic molecule that is readily reduced to extremely potent reductant thiol (RSH). Disulfide (RSSR) is electrophilic RSS that can be reduced to thiol (RSH). Hydropolysulfide (RSS$_n$H) and dialkyl polysulfide (RSS$_n$R) are like hydropersulfide (RSSH) [135]. RSS can interact with ROS, generating sulfur oxides such as peroxysulphenyl radical (RSOO$^\bullet$), sulfenate (RSO$^-$), sulfinate (RSO$_2^-$), sulfonate (RSO$_3^-$), thiosulmonate (S$_2$O$_3^{2-}$), and SO$_4^{2-}$ [138]. Sulfenate (RSO$^-$) reacts with other thiols to give disulfides, RSSR. RSS can also interact with RNS, leading to the formation of S-N hybrid molecules, such as thiazate (NSO$^-$), thionitrite (SNO$^-$) isomers, S-nitrosothiols (RSNOs), nitrosopersulfide (SSNO$^-$), and the dinitrosylated sulfite adduct, SULFI/NO. S-nitrosothiols (RSNOs) can be reduced to thiol (RSH) and nitroxyl (HNO) [139]. XO catalyzes S-nitrosothiols (RSNOs) to nitric oxide (NO), which reacts with a superoxide (O$_2^{-\bullet}$) anion to form peroxynitrite (ONOO$^-$) under aerobic conditions [123]. The properties of thiazate (NSO$^-$), thionitrite (SNO$^-$) isomers, nitrosopersulfide (SSNO$^-$) and polysulfides dinitrososulfites (Sulfi/NO), are to be determined and they appear to be a source of nitric oxide (NO) and nitroxyl (HNO) [140–142] (Table 2).

An antioxidant N-acetyl cysteine administration was reported to improve cognitive functions in patients in MS and N-acetyl cysteine supplement is under clinical trial for the treatment of fatigue in MS patients [143,144]. The levels of methionine reported mixed results. The plasma methionine levels were significantly reduced in RRMS and dietary methionine supplement was proposed for the treatment [145]. The level of methionine sulfoxide was elevated more than two-fold in CSF of MM patients and the reduction of dietary methionine was reported to slow the onset and progression of MM [146,147]. The levels of GSH in MS have not reached a consensus [147–149]. Trypanothione and mycothiol have not been investigated in MS. The serum S-nitrosothiol levels were increased in RRMS and SPMS, and selectively correlated with spinal cord injury and, thus, a high level of S-nitrosothiol is proposed to be a potential prognostic biomarker for spinal cord injury in MS [150] (Tables 3 and 4).

2.1.4. Reactive Carbonyl/Halogen/Selenium Species

Reactive carbonyl species (RCS) are metabolically generated highly reactive molecules with aldehydes and electronically excited (^{3}L=O*) triplet carbonyls, known for their harmful reactions to nucleic acids, proteins, and lipids [92]. In addition, RCS are considered to participate in electrophilic signaling of adaptive cell response and post-transcriptional protein modification [151]. RCS are classified into α,β-unsaturated aldehydes; keto-aldehyde and di-aldehydes. In the presence of catalase and bicarbonate, XO was found to produce the strong one-electron oxidant carbonate radical anion from oxidation with acetaldehyde. The carbonate radical was likely produced in one of the enzyme's redox centers with a peroxymonocarbonate intermediate [45]. Self-reaction of lipid peroxyl radical (LOO•) produced by the oxidation of polyunsaturated fatty acids (PUFAs) by hydroxyl radical (HO•) generates electronically excited triplet carbonyls (^{3}L=O*) yielding to singlet oxygen ($O_2{}^1\Delta_g$) [89] (Table 2). RCS react with amines and thiols leading to advanced glycation end products (AGEs), biomarkers of ageing and degenerative diseases [152].

MPO, a lysosomal heme-containing enzyme present in granulocytes and monocytes catalyzes the conversion of hydrogen peroxide (H_2O_2) and chloride anion (Cl^-) to hypochlorous acid (HClO) during the respiratory burst. An adipocyte producing hormone leptin stimulates the oxidative burst [153]. MPO also oxidizes tyrosine to tyrosyl radical [154]. MPO mediates protein nitrosylation, forming 3-chlorotyrosine (3-Cl-Tyr) and dityrosine crosslinks [155,156] (Table 2).

Studies on MPO activity reported mixed results. The mean MPO activity of peripheral leukocyte was observed reduced in a mixed population of MS patients, compared to controls [157]. Significantly higher serum MPO activity was measured in opticospinal phenotype (OSMS) of RRMS at relapse and remission and in conventional phenotype of RRMS at remission, compared to controls. A positive correlation was associated between Kurtzke's EDSS and MPO activity at remission of OSMS [158] (Table 4). The mean MPO activity of peripheral leukocytes was found higher, but statistically not significant in RRMS, compared to controls [56] (Table 3). No study regarding CSF MPO activity in MS was found. Selenium is an essential micronutrient with similar chemical and physical properties to sulfur, but more easily oxidized and kinetically more labile than sulfur. Selenium is a component of proteinogenic selenocysteine, naturally occurring selenomethionine and selenoproteins, such as glutathione peroxidase (GPx), thioredoxin reductase (TRXR), and selenoprotein P [57]. Reactive selenium species (RSeS) are selenium-containing inorganic and organic compounds including selenite (O_3Se^{-2}), selenocysteine ($C_3H_7NO_2Se$), and selenomethionine ($C_5H_{11}NO_2Se$) [58] (Table 2). Selenium have both beneficial and harmful actions. At low concentration it works as an antioxidant, inhibiting lipid peroxidation and detoxifying ROS as a component of GPx and TRXR, while at high concentration it becomes a toxic pro-oxidant, generating ROS, inducing lipid oxidation and forming cross linking in thioproteins [159] (Table 2). The serum selenium levels were measured significantly lower in MS patients, compared to controls, suggesting antioxidant capacity is impaired in MS [160] (Table 3).

2.1.5. Exogenous Oxidative Factors

Oxidative stressors are generated in reaction to exogenous stimuli such as pollutants, food and alcohol, cigarette smoke, heavy metals, chemotherapy, drug and xenobiotics, or radiation. Aging becomes more susceptible to their insults. Organic solvents, organic compounds such as quinone, pesticides and heavy metals including lead, arsenic, mercury, chromium, and cadmium are common sources of oxidative stressors [41]. Ultraviolet and infrared-B radiations generate oxygen radicals endogenously [161] (Figure 1a). The levels of serum arsenic, malondialdehyde (MDA), and lactate were elevated and ferric-reducing activity of plasma was reduced RRMS patients and the levels of serum lithium were significantly lower and the levels of nitric oxide (NO) were higher in RRMS patients, compared to healthy controls, suggesting environmental factors seem to play a role in pathogenesis of MS [162,163].

3. Reductive Stress

3.1. Reactive Nucleophilic Species

Endogenous reductive stressors include nucleophilic free radical, inorganic, and organic molecules and antioxidative enzyme. (Figure 1b). Superoxide ($O_2^{-\bullet}$) anion is one of the reactive nucleophilic species and a powerful reducing agent under physiological conditions, which initiates reaction cascades generating another ROS, such as hydrogen peroxide (H_2O_2) and sulfur dioxide (SO_2) derivatives. Hydrogen sulfide (H_2S), thiolate (RS^-), hydropersulfide (RSS^-), and disulfide (RSSR) are reactive nucleophilic species that can participate in nucleophilic substitution in vivo [133]. Selenium is more nucleophilic than sulfur due to its greater electron density. The selenol (RSeH) portion of selenocysteine ($C_3H_7NO_2Se$) is ionized at physiological pH, making it more nucleophilic against oxidative species [164,165] (Table 2).

3.2. Antioxidative Enzymes

Reductive stress is induced by excessive levels of reductive stressors that results from an elevation in GSH/GSSG ratio, NAD^+/NADH, $NADP^+$/NADPH and/or or overexpression of antioxidative enzymatic systems such as the GSH system, catalase, thioredoxin-peroxiredoxin (TRX-PRDX) system, α-ketoglutarate dehydrogenase (GPDH), and glycerol phosphate dehydrogenase [166,167]. The reductive stressors deplete reactive oxidative species and are harmful as oxidative stressors and implicated in pathological processes in AD, PD, and sporadic motor neuron disease, among others [168].

The GSH system consists of GSH, the enzymes for synthesis and recycling including gamma-glutamate cysteine ligase, glutathione synthetase, glutathione reductase (GSR), and gamma glutamyl transpeptidase, and the enzymes for metabolism and antioxidation including glutathione S-transferase and GPx [169]. The GPx is an enzyme containing four selenium-cofactors that catalyzes the reduction of hydrogen peroxide (H_2O_2) to water molecule (H_2O) and organic hydroperoxide (ROOH) to alcohol (ROH) by converting reduced monomeric GSH to GSSG. Glutathione s-transferases show high activity with lipid peroxides [170]. Eight isozymes are in the cytosol, membrane, and plasma, protecting the organisms from oxidative stress [171].

Most studies on peripheral blood GPx activity reported nonsignificant results in a mixed population of MS [56,59,172–174]. However, lower mean GPx activity of erythrocyte lysates in remission and higher mean GPx were reported in acute relapse of RRMS [60]. GPx activity in CSF was found lower in MS patients [61]. The GSR activity of lymphocyte and granulocyte lysates were not significantly different in MS, compared to controls. However, a significant correlation of GPx and GRx was observed in controls, but not in MS [62]. Mean GRx activity of CSF was found significantly higher in MS patients [61] (Tables 3 and 4).

Catalases a tetrameric heme- or manganese-containing dismutase that catalyzes the conversion of two hydrogen peroxide (H_2O_2) molecules to water (H_2O) in the presence of small amount of hydrogen peroxide. The cofactor is oxidized by one molecule of hydrogen peroxide and then regenerated by transferring the bound oxygen to a second molecule of substrate. The enzyme is located in the peroxisomes, the cytosol of erythrocytes, and the mitochondria, removing harmful hydrogen peroxides to prevent cellular and tissue damage [175].

Studies on the catalase activity of peripheral blood samples reported equivocal results in MS. The catalase activity of granulocyte lysates was found lower in MS patients, compared to controls [176]. The activities of CSF and plasma catalase were found increased in CIS and RRMS patients, compared to healthy controls, and MS patients with lower EDSS had higher plasma and CSF catalase activities [84] (Tables 3 and 4).

In TRX-PRDX system PRDXs catalyze the reduction of H_2O_2 to H_2O. H_2O_2 oxidizes the peroxidatic cysteine of PRDXs to protein sulfenic acid (PSOH), which can react with the thiol (SH) group of the resolving cysteine to yield the formation of an inter-(typical) or intramolecular (atypical) disulfide bond. TRX/TRXR system mediates the reduction of the PRDX disulfide bond. TRX reduced state is maintained by the flavoenzyme TRXR in the presence of NADPH. When H_2O_2 exceeds the normal levels, PRDXs are overoxidized from PSOH to protein sulfinic acids (PSO_2H). The latter can be reduced back to the native form of the enzyme by sulfiredoxin (SRX) in the presence of ATP. However, further oxidation of PRDXs to PSO_3H is irreversible [177].

Serum Trx1 was significantly increased in the newly diagnosed MS patients, compared to controls. *TRX1* and *APEX1* mRNA expressions were significantly higher in the newly diagnosed MS patients, patients under INF-β treatment, and patients who received immunosuppressant azathioprine or betamethasone, compared to healthy controls [178]. *PRDX2* mRNA is upregulated and PRDX2 expression is higher in MS lesions white matter of autopsy tissue of patients its expression level is positively correlated with the degree of inflammation and oxidative stress [179] (Tables 3 and 4).

α-KGDH is a mitochondrial enzyme in Krebs cycle, which catalyzes α-ketoglutarate, coenzyme A and NAD$^+$ to succinyl-CoA, NADH and CO_2, transferring an electron to the respiratory chain [180]. KGNH activity is sensitive to redox status. H_2O_2 reversibly inhibits KGNH by glutathionylation of lipoic acid cofactor, resulting reducing electron supply to the respiratory chain. A lipid peroxidation product 4-hydroxy-2-nonenal (4-HNE) reacts with lipoic acid cofactor, inhibiting α-KGDH activity [181]. The pyruvate tolerance test showed higher activity of α-KGDH in serum of MS patients [182]. However, reduced expression and activity of mitochondrial α-KGDH was observed in demyelinated axons that correlated with signs of axonal dysfunction (Table 3) [183].

α-GPDH catalyzes the reversible redox conversion of dihydroxyacetone phosphate to sn-glycerol 3-phosphate, linking carbohydrate and lipid metabolism. A loss of α-GPDH in oligodendrocytes were observed in chronic plaques of MS patients, suggesting the presence of antioxidant capacity impairment [63] (Table 3).

Nrf2 is a transcriptional factor of the antioxidative enzyme genes including catalase, GPx, GRx, glutathione S-transferase, and SOD. In response to oxidative stress, the Kelch-like ECH-associated protein 1 (KEAP1) inhibits the ubiquitin-proteasome system in the cytosol and facilitates the translocation of Nrf2 into the nucleus to bind to the *cis*-acting enhancer sequence of the promotor region, the antioxidant response elements [184,185]. Activation of the Nrf2-Keap1 pathway has been observed in various types of cancers, accompanied with reduced antioxidant capacity and elevated oxidative stress and inflammation [186]. The cytoplasmic and nucleic Nrf2 protein expression of PBMC was increased and correlated with clinical improvement in MS patients on 14-month course of natalizumab, an α4 integrin receptor blocker [110] (Tables 3 and 4).

Other transcriptional factors involved in energy metabolism have been investigated. Peroxisome proliferator-activated receptors (PPARs) are a transcriptional factor of the gene regulating energy metabolism including glucose metabolism, fatty acid oxidation, thermogenesis, lipid metabolism, and anti-inflammatory response [187]. PPARs have attracted growing attention as promising targets of many diseases such as diabetes and hyperlipidemia [188]. An isoform PPAR-gamma (PPAR-γ) was elevated in CSF samples of MS, compared to controls [64]. Peroxisome proliferator-activated receptor gamma coactivator 1-α (PGC-1α) 4 integrin receptor blocker is a transcriptional coactivator that regulates the genes involved in energy metabolism. Reduced PGC-1α expression was associated with mitochondria changes and correlated with neural loss in MS [189] (Tables 3 and 4).

3.3. Exogenous and Endogenous Antioxidants

A daily diet rich in naturally occurring polyphenolic antioxidants, such as flavonoids and phenolic acids are regularly recommended for disease prevention and antioxidant supplements, such as vitamin C, vitamin E, N-acetyl cysteine, L-carnitine and folic acid are frequently employed as a complementary therapy for various diseases [190,191]. Those preventive and therapeutic measures are based on the pathogenesis of diseases which are induced and developed under oxidative cellular environment. Furthermore, plant polyphenols were reported to alleviate oxidative stress and enhance neuroprotection [192]. Olive leaf-derived polyphenols are strong antioxidants and their therapeutic use are of particular interest against oxidant-induced diseases including cancer and neurodegenerative diseases [193–195]. The Mediterranean diet can present a biphasic dose-response curve toward hormetic stimuli, preventing low-grade inflammation and inflammageing [196,197]. There is a growing interest in supplementation of nonessential compounds that trigger the redox feedback loop activating the nucleophilic response, parahormesis (Figure 1c) [198].

N-Methyl-D-aspartic acid receptor antagonist memantine and memantine-ferulic acid conjugate improved oxidative stress in patients with AD [199]. A meta-analysis of randomized controlled trials showed that an exogenous antioxidant N-acetylcysteine supplement improved cognitive function in patients with schizophrenia [200]. Traditional Chinese medicine curcumin is an antioxidant and anti-inflammatory molecule that relieves pain and stress at least partly through the kynurenine metabolic pathway of tryptophan metabolism [201]. The kynurenine pathway produces endogenous oxidative and antioxidative metabolites. Single nucleotide polymorphism of the first rate-limiting enzyme indoleamine 2,3-dioxygenase 1 was associated with inflammation and depressive symptoms and influenced the age onset of neurodegenerative diseases [202]. The elevated levels of an oxidative metabolite 3-hydroxykynurenine and an antioxidative kynurenic acid were linked to depressive symptom of patients with stroke [203]. Meanwhile, administration of kynurenic acid induced antidepressant-like effects in animal model of depression [204].

However, unmonitored chronic antioxidant supplementation imposes reductive stress, the counterpart of oxidative stress. The reductive stress-induced inflammation is observed in hypertrophic cardiomyopathy, muscular dystrophy, pulmonary hypertension, rheumatoid arthritis, AD, and metabolic syndrome [168]. In adipose tissue a long-term antioxidant supplementation caused a paradoxical increase in oxidative stress which was associated with mitochondrial dysfunction [205]. Leptin secreted from adipose tissue serves as an inflammatory mediator and subsequent development of leptin resistance make obese individuals more susceptible to autoimmune disease including MS [206] (Figure 1c).

Vitamin supplements are recommended for the treatment of MS, as nutritional deficits are frequently observed in patients with MS [207]. MS induced by reductive stress has not been reported, but it deserves to monitor redox status in MS patients.

4. Degradation Products under Oxidative Stress

4.1. Proteins

Protein carbonyls are degradation products of reactions between reactive species and proteins, resulting in a loss of function or aggregation. Quantification with 2,4-Dinitrophenylhydrazine products showed increased carbonylation in plasma and serum of RRMS patients [65–67]. The plasma carbonyl levels were elevated in SPMS and correlated with the EDSS and the Beck Depression Inventory [208]. The levels of carbonyl groups were elevated in serum of patients with RRMS and lowered in the group of RRMS patients treated with INF-β [74]. The levels of CSF carbonyl proteins measured were elevated in RRMS and progressive MS [209,210] (Tables 3 and 4).

A highly active RNS reacts with tyrosine residues of proteins to form nitrotyrosines, leading to the alternation of protein conformation function. The main product of tyrosine oxidation is 3-nitrotyrosine (3-NO-Tyr), formed by the substitution of a hydrogen by a nitro group in the phenolic ring of the tyrosine residues. The content of 3-NO-Tyr is assessed by western blotting, high-performance liquid chromatography (HPLC), gas chromatography-mass spectrometry (GC/MS), and enzyme-linked immunosorbent assay (ELISA) [72]. Mean 3-NO-Tyr was observed significantly higher in plasma and serum of RRMS and SPMS patients and significantly higher 3-NO-Tyr was found in SPMS than RRMS [66,68,69]. Decreased mean 3-NO-Tyr was reported following a relapse and corticosteroid treatment [70]. In the serum of MS patients, 3-NO-Tyr was found significantly lower following INF-β1b treatment [71]. Following GA treatment, 3-NO-Tyr was found significantly reduced in peripheral leukocytes [69] (Tables 3 and 4).

Protein glutathionylation is a redox-dependent posttranslational modification that results in the formation of a mixed disulfide between GSH and the thiol group of a protein cysteine residue [211]. Protein glutathionylation is observed in response to oxidative or nitrosative stress and is redox-dependent, being readily reversible under reducing conditions. Extracellular SOD, α1-antitrypsin and phospholipid transfer protein were found glutathionylated at cysteine residues in CSF of MS Patients, witnessing the footprints of oxidative assault of MS [210].

Oxidative environments generate oxidized tyrosine orthologues such as o-tyrosine, m-tyrosine, nitrotyrosine, and dityrosine. Dityrosine was elevated in serum of RRMS patients [73,74]. Advanced oxidation protein products (AOPPs) are uremic toxins produced in reaction of plasma proteins with chlorinated oxidants such as chloramines and hypochlorous acid (HClO) [212]. The levels of AOPPs were significantly higher in plasma of MM patients [213]. The levels of AOPPs were significantly higher in plasma and CSF of CIS and RRMS patients than healthy controls, and the AOPPs levels were significantly higher CIS than RRMS. Furthermore, the levels of AOPPs were significantly higher in patients with higher EDSS scores than lower ones [50]. The AOPPs levels were decreased in serum of RRMS patients treated with IFN-β [74] (Tables 3 and 4).

AGEs are a group of glycotoxins produced in reaction of free amino groups of proteins, lipids, or nucleic acids and carbonyl groups of reducing sugars. The AGEs can accumulate in tissues and body fluids, resulting in protein malfunctions, reactive chemical production, and inflammation [214]. The levels of AGEs were significantly elevated in serum of RRMS patients, but no significant change was observed after IFN-β treatment [74]. The concentrations of AGEs were significantly higher in brain samples of MS patients, compared to nondemented counterparts. The levels of free AGEs were correlated in CSF and plasma samples of MS patients, but not protein-bound AGEs [75] (Tables 3 and 4).

4.2. Amino Acids

Asymmetric dimethylarginine (ADMA) is a L-arginine analogue produced in the cytoplasm in the process of protein modification. The formation of ADMA is dependent on oxidative stress status. ADMA is elevated by native or oxidized LDL and interferes with L-arginine in the production of nitric oxide (NO) [215]. Significantly higher ADMA concentrations were observed in serum and CSF of patients with RRMS and SPMS, while levels of arginine, L-homoarginine, nitrate, nitrite, ADMA did not differ between patients with MS and healthy controls [76] (Tables 3 and 4).

4.3. Lipid Membrane and Lipoproteins

Lipids in biological membrane are major target of OS. Peroxidation of lipid membrane is initiated by ROS, including superoxide anion ($O_2^{-\bullet}$), hydroxyl radical ($OH^{\bullet}$), hydrogen peroxide (H_2O_2), and singlet oxygen ($O_2{}^1\Delta_g$); and by RNS, including nitric oxide radical ($NO^{\bullet}$), peroxynitrite ($ONOO^-$), and nitrite (NO_2^-) stealing electron from PUFAs, such as arachidonic (20:4) and docosahexaenoic acid (22:6) [216]. The abstraction of *bis*-allylic hydrogen of PUFA leads to the formation of arachidonic acid hydroperoxyl radical ($ROO^{\bullet}$) and hydroperoxide (ROOH) in a chain reaction manner [45]. A portion of arachidonic acid peroxides and peroxy radicals generate endoperoxides rather than hydroperoxide (ROOH). The endoperoxides undergoes subsequent formation of a range of bioactive intermediates, such as F2-isoprostanes (F2-isoPs), MDA and 4-HNE. Hexanoyl-lysine (HEL) adduct is a lipid peroxidation by-product which is formed by the oxidation of omega-6 unsaturated fatty acid, such as linoleic acid [217]. Hydroxyoctadecadienoic acid (HODE) is derived from the oxidation of linoleates, the most abundant PUFAs in vivo [73,211]. Meanwhile, a cyclic sugar compound inositol is a major antioxidant component of the lipid membrane, which scavenges reactive species [54].

Studies on blood F2-isoPs levels reported increases in MS, especially in RRMS and SPMS subtypes compared to controls [77,78]. A study on CSF F2-isoPs levels presented three times higher in patients with MS than ones with other neurologic diseases [79]. The levels of F2-isoPs were moderately correlated with the degree of disability, suggesting a role as a prognostic marker [80]. MDA is highly reactive aldehyde generated by the reaction between reactive species and polyunsaturated lipids to form adducts with protein or DNA [81]. Studies on blood or serum MDA reported higher levels in MS patients [83,166]. The blood MDA levels were significantly higher in RRMS than controls or CIS, higher in RRMS than in remission, and higher in remission than controls. MDA levels were elevated at relapse, while lowered at day 5 of corticosteroid treatment [82,149]. Studies quantifying CSF MDA consistently reported higher levels in CIS and RRMS than controls [61,82,85,177]. There are positive correlations between MDA levels of plasma and CSF, and MDA levels in plasma/CSF and EDSS [84]. The levels of 4-HNE were elevated in the CSF of PPMS, RRMS, and SPMS patients, particularly in PPMS [86]. No study regarding HEL in MS was found in literature search. The serum 13-HODE was identified as a part of metabolomic signatures associated with more severe disease such as non-relapse-free MS or MS with higher EDSS [87]. The levels of 9-HODE and 13-HODE were significantly increased in CSF of CIS and RRMS patients, compared to healthy controls, but baseline levels of HODE did not differ between patients with signs of disease activity during up to four years of follow-up and patients without MS [218] (Tables 3 and 4).

Cholesterol oxidization products oxysterols were studied. Levels of plasma oxysterols increased in progressive MS patients and oxysterol levels were positively correlated with apolipoprotein C-II and apolipoprotein E. Furthermore, oxysterol and apolipoprotein changes were associated with conversion to SPMS [88]. Increased levels of oxidized low-density lipoprotein (oxLDL) in the serum and higher serum levels of autoantibodies against oxLDL were reported in MS patients [219,220]. Although studies on HDL levels in MS patients reported mixed results, lowered HDL antioxidant function in MS patients was observed, suggesting the involvement of lipoprotein function MS pathogenesis [219–222]. In mixed population of MS, decreased serum 24S-hydroxycholesterol and 27-hydroxycholesterol and increased CSF lathosterol, compared to healthy controls [223] (Tables 3 and 4).

4.4. Nucleic Acid

The biomarkers of oxidative damage of nucleic acids—8-Hydroxy-2'-deoxyguanosine (8-OH2dG) and 8-hydroxyguanosine (8-OHG)—can be assessed by ELISA, as well as by direct methods, such as HPLC and GC/MS [224,225]. Elevated levels of 8-OH2dG were reported in the blood of RRMS patients. DNA oxidation products were proposed as diagnostic biomarkers for MS [152] (Tables 3 and 4).

5. Conclusion and Future Perspectives

Redox biomarkers are classified by original cellular components and enzyme mechanisms of action in redox homeostasis. Redox status can be assessed by the measurement of reactive chemical species, oxidative or antioxidative enzyme activity, and degradation products derived from proteins, amino acids, lipid membrane, and nucleic acids. Measurement of reactive chemical species and oxidative enzyme activities assesses intensity of oxidative stress, while measurement of antioxidative activity analyses compensatory capacity. Fine measurement of the various redox components may reveal diagnostic, prognostic, or predicative value to differentiate the disease status and progression (Figure 3).

The levels of nitric oxide (NO) metabolites, S-nitrosothiol, and the activities of oxidative enzymes including SOD, MPO, and iNOS have been found significantly different to patients with MS, compared to healthy controls. The levels of antioxidants including uric acid and selenium, activities of antioxidative enzymes including GSR, catalase, and TRX-PRDX, and concentrations of transcriptional factors Nrf2, PPARs, and PGC-1α have been found significantly changed in MS patients. The protein degradation products including protein carbonyls, 3-NO-Tyr, glutathionylation, AOPPs, and AGEs, an amino acid by-product ADMA, the lipid and cholesterol degradation products including F2-isoP, MDA, 4-HNE, HODE, oxocholesterols, and oxLDL, and the nucleic acid degradation product 8-OH2dG significantly increased in samples of MS patients. Thus, the oxidative enzymes, antioxidative enzymes, and redox degradation products have been identified as promising biomarkers for the diagnosis of MS. Furthermore, SOD, 3-NO-Tyr, and MDA are sensitive to subtypes of MS, CIS and RRMS, RRMS and SPMS, RRMS and remission, respectively. tNOx, S-nitrosothiol, SOD, MPO, GSR, catalase, protein carbonyls, AOPPs, F2-isoP, MDA, and oxycholesterols were correlated with EDSS and thus they are potential prognostic biomarkers for MS. SOD, Nrf2, protein carbonyls, 3-NO-Tyr, AOPPs, and MDA were observed sensitive to the treatment of MS, being possible predictive biomarkers. Finally, SOD is a possible drug target of MS as a therapeutic marker (Table 3).

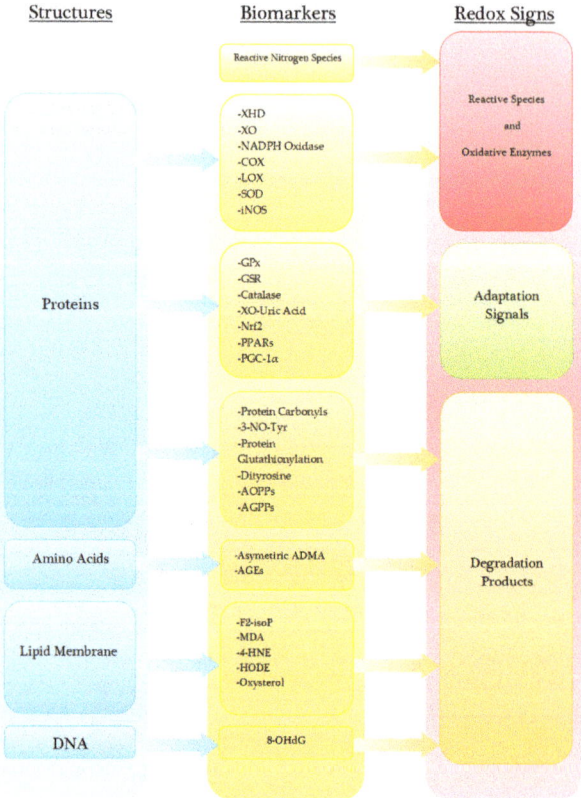

Figure 3. Classification of redox biomarkers according to cellular structures, biomarkers, and their modes of action in redox homeostasis.

In addition to biomarkers described above, the search for novel biomarkers has become a growing interest in neurodegenerative diseases. A micro RNA (miRNA) is a short non-coding RNA molecule consisting of approximately 22 nucleotides, which functions in posttranscriptional gene silencing. miRNAs have been linked to pathogenesis of various diseases including cancer, autoimmune diseases, and neurodegenerative disease such as PD [226]. Dysregulated interactions of miRNAs have been reported in mild cognitive impairment and AD. The associated genes were related to regulation of ageing and mitochondria [227]. Dysregulations of various miRNAs have been observed in AD, PD, Huntington's disease, and ALS and thus miRNAs were proposed to be potential diagnostic and therapeutic biomarkers of neurodegenerative diseases [228]. The link between environmental factors and miRNA dysregulations in MS was discussed [229]. Furthermore, miRNAs in blood and CSF samples of patients with MS as diagnostic and prognostic biomarkers have been reviewed recently [230].

Long Interspersed Nuclear Element-1 (LINE-1) is an autonomous non-long terminal repeat retrotransposon that creates genomic insertions through an RNA intermediate. The increased number of germline and somatic LINE-1s have been linked to the risk and progression of cancer as well as neurodegenerative and psychiatric diseases. An increased burden of highly active retrotranposition competent LINE-1s have been associated with the risk and progression of PD and LINE-1s were proposed as possible therapeutic biomarkers that can be targeted by reverse transcriptase [231]. Furthermore, LINE-1s was considered involved in irregular immune response and participate in pathogenesis of MS [232].

A search for demographic correlation between single nucleotide polymorphisms and MS has been under extensive study. Inflammation-mediating chemokine receptor V Δ32 deletion was not found correlated with MS [233]. Large-scale genome projects such as genome-wide association (GWA) studies generated polygenic risk scores for prediction of risk and progression of multifactorial neurodegenerative diseases. Large-scale pathway specific-genetic risk profiling expedited redox-related biological pathways to identify causal genes and potential therapeutic targets [234]. One of future challenges is a search for correlations with uncatalogued structural variants in MS.

Considering the dynamics of redox homeostasis, the amounts of reactive species, activities of oxidative and antioxidative enzymes, and concentrations of degradation products presumably differ during the progression of MS. The early phase presents an elevation of oxidative enzyme activity and a subsequent elevation of the activity of counteracting antioxidative enzymes with unchanged levels of degradation products. As the activity of antioxidative enzymes becomes compromised due to increasing oxidative stress, the amount of degradation products gradually increases, while the antioxidative enzyme activities slowly wane and fatigue. Eventually, the antioxidative response exhausts with elevated activities of oxidative enzymes and elevated levels of degradation products (Figure 4). Further studies and exploration into novel biomarkers are expected in search of a robust battery of biomarkers indicative to the redox status, in order to realize a fine calibration of major redox components that helps identify the disturbance of redox homeostasis, restore the nucleophilic tone and the most importantly build the best personalized treatment of MS for the sake of better quality of life [235].

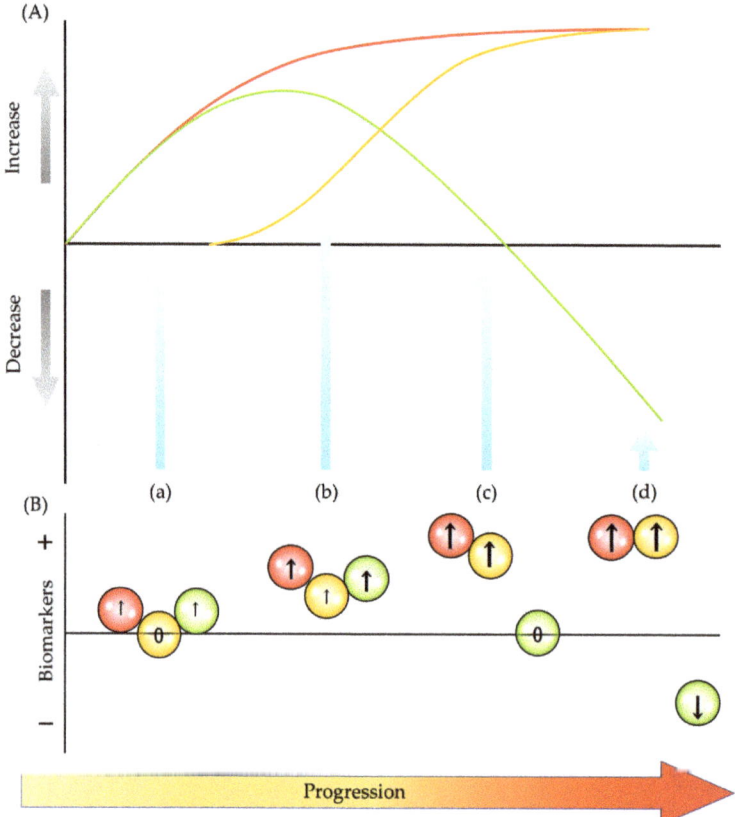

Figure 4. Dynamics of redox components in disease progression. (**A**) – (red line): reactive chemical species and activities of oxidative enzymes increase gradually. – (orange line): the degradation products increase accordingly upon exhaustion of antioxidative enzymes' activities. – (green line): antioxidative enzymes offset the effects of oxidative enzymes in the early phase, however; the antioxidative activities decline and, finally, fatigue in the later phase, resulting in the exacerbation of inflammation and cellular damage. (**B**) Biomarkers of three redox components may present different values. (a) The levels of oxidative enzyme slightly increase, but the degradation markers stay in a normal range. The antioxidative markers also slightly increase. (b) The oxidative markers further elevate, and the degradation markers start slightly increasing. The antioxidative markers also stay elevated. (c) The oxidative enzyme markers increase, but antioxidative markers return to normal range. The degradation product markers further elevate. (d) The oxidative markers greatly increase, but the antioxidative markers decline. The degradation products markers greatly elevate. ⬤: oxidative biomarkers; ⬤: degradation biomarkers; ⬤: antioxidative biomarkers; ↑: increase; ↓: decrease; and 0: unchanged.

Author Contributions: Conceptualization, M.T. and L.V.; writing—original draft preparation, M.T.; writing—review and editing, M.T., and L.V.; visualization, M.T.; project administration, M.T.; supervision, L.V.; funding acquisition, L.V. All authors have read and agreed to the published version of the manuscript.

Funding: The current work was supported by GINOP 2.3.2-15-2016-00034, Stay Alive GINOP 2.3.2-15-2016-00048, TUDFO/47138-1/2019-ITM University of Szeged Open Access Fund (FundRef), Grant number 4829.

Conflicts of Interest: The authors declare no conflict of interest.

Abbreviations

α	alpha
AD	Alzheimer's disease
ADMA	asymmetric dimethylarginine
AGEs	advanced glycation end products
ALS	amyotrophic lateral sclerosis
AOPPs	advanced oxidation protein products
β	beta
CIS	clinically isolated syndrome
CNS	central nervous system
COX	cyclooxygenase
CSF	cerebrospinal fluid
CYP	cytochrome P450
EDSS	expanded disability status scale
ELISA	enzyme-linked immunosorbent assay
ETC	electron transfer chain
F2-isoPs	F2-isoprostanes
GC/MS	gas chromatography-mass spectrometry
Gd^+	gadolinium
GPx	glutathione peroxidase
GSH	glutathione
GSSH	glutathione disulfide
GA	glatiramer
GPDH	ketoglutarat dehydrogenase
GSR	glutathione reductase
GWA	genome-wide association
HEL	hexanoyl-lysine
4-HNE	4-hydroxynonenal
HODE	hydroxyoctadecadienoic acid
HPLC	high-performance liquid chromatography
iNOS	inducible Nitric Oxide Synthase
IFN	Interferon
KEAP1	Kelch-like ECH-associated protein 1
KGDH	ketoglutarate dehydrogenase
LINE-1	Long Interspersed Nuclear Element-1
LOX	lipoxygenase
MDA	malondialdehyde
miRNA	micro RNA
MPO	myeloperoxidase
MRI	magnetic resonance imaging
MS	multiple sclerosis
NAD^+	nicotinamide adenine dinucleotide
NADPH	nicotinamide adenine dinucleotide phosphate
NOS	nitric oxide synthetase
3-NO-Tyr	3-nitrotyrosine
NOX	nicotinamide adenine dinucleotide phosphate oxidase

Nrf2	nuclear factor erythroid 2-related factor
8-OH2dG	8-Hydroxy-2′-deoxyguanosine
8-OHG	8-hydroxyguanosine
OSMS	opticospinal phenotype of relapsing-remitting multiple sclerosis
oxLDL	oxidized low-density lipoprotein
PD	Parkinson's disease
PGC-1	peroxisome proliferator-activated receptor gamma coactivator 1
PPARs	peroxisome proliferator-activated receptors
PUFAs	polyunsaturated fatty acids
RCS	reactive carbonyl species
redox	reduction-oxidation
RHS	reactive halogen species
RNS	reactive nitrogen species
ROS	reactive oxygen species
PPMS	primary progressive multiple sclerosis
PRMS	progressive-relapsing multiple sclerosis
RRMS	relapsing-remitting multiple sclerosis
RSS	reactive sulfur species
RSeS	reactive selenium species
SOD	superoxide dismutase
SPMS	secondary progressive multiple sclerosis
tNOx	total value nitric oxide
TRX-PRDX	thioredoxin-peroxiredoxin
TRXR	thioredoxin reductase
XDH	xanthine dehydrogenase
XO	xanthine oxidase

Appendix A

Assessment of the Methodological Quality

The methodological quality was assessed for each redox biomarker in multiple sclerosis.

Table A1. Classes and biomarkers, and risk of bias assessment included in this review.

Classes	Types	Risk of Bias
Reactive Species	Reactive Nitrogen Species	Unclear
Oxidative Enzymes	Xanthine Dehydrogenase (XDH)	Unclear
	Nicotinamide Adenine Dinucleotide Phosphate (NADPH) Oxidase	Unclear
	Superoxide Dismutase (SOD)	High risk
	Inducible Nitric Oxide Synthase (iNOS)	High risk
	Myeloperoxidase (MPO)	Unclear
Antioxidative Enzymes and Transcriptional Factors	Glutathione Peroxidase (GPx)	Low risk
	Glutathione Reductase (GSR)	High risk
	Catalase	High risk
	Xanthine oxidase (XO)-Uric Acid	Unclear
	Nuclear Factor Erythroid 2-Related Factor (Nrf2)	Unclear
	Peroxisome proliferator-activated receptors (PPARs)	Unclear
	Peroxisome proliferator-activated receptor gamma coactivator 1-alpha (PGC-1α)	Unclear

Table A1. Cont.

Classes		Types	Risk of Bias
Degradation Products and End Products	Protein	Protein carbonyls	Low risk
		3-nitrotyrosin (3-NO-Tyr)	High risk
		Protein glutathionylation	Unclear
		Dityrosine	Unclear
		Advanced oxidation protein products (AOPPs)	High risk
		Advanced glycation end products (AGEs)	High risk
	Amino acids	Asymmetric dimethylarginine (ADMA)	Unclear
	Lipid	F2-isoprostane (F2-isoP)	Low risk
		Malondialdehyde (MDA)	Low risk
		4-hydroxynonenal (4-HNE)	Unclear
		Hydroxyoctadecadienoic acid (HODE)	Unclear
		Oxysterol	Unclear
	DNA	8-dihydro-2'deoxyguanosine (8-oxodG)	Unclear

Table A2. Risk of bias was assessed according to the criteria of availability of meta-analysis or systematic review, study types, and with or without conflicting results, to judge evidence levels of high risk, low risk, or unclear.

Risk of Bias	Criteria
High risk	No meta-analysis or systematic review, fewer than five case–control and/or cohort studies, or presence of only expert review
Low risk	Presence of at least one meta-analysis or systematic review, without conflicting results
Unclear	Presence of only case–control study or cohort study, meta-analysis with conflicting results, or case–control studies with conflicting results

References

1. GBD 2016 Neurology Collaborators. Global, regional, and national burden of neurological disorders, 1990–2016: A systematic analysis for the Global Burden of Disease Study 2016. *Lancet Neurol.* **2019**, *18*, 459–480. [CrossRef]
2. Fricska-Nagy, Z.; Füvesi, J.; Rózsa, C.; Komoly, S.; Jakab, G.; Csépány, T.; Jobbágy, Z.; Lencsés, G.; Vécsei, L.; Bencsik, K. The effects of fatigue, depression and the level of disability on the health-related quality of life of glatiramer acetate-treated relapsing-remitting patients with multiple sclerosis in Hungary. *Mult. Scler. Relat. Disord.* **2016**, *7*, 26–32. [CrossRef] [PubMed]
3. Sandi, D.; Biernacki, T.; Szekeres, D.; Füvesi, J.; Kincses, Z.T.; Rózsa, C.; Mátyás, K.; Kása, K.; Matolcsi, J.; Zboznovits, D.; et al. Prevalence of cognitive impairment among Hungarian patients with relapsing-remitting multiple sclerosis and clinically isolated syndrome. *Mult. Scler. Relat. Disord.* **2017**, *17*, 57–62. [CrossRef] [PubMed]
4. Tanaka, M.; Toldi, J.; Vécsei, L. Exploring the Etiological Links behind Neurodegenerative Diseases: Inflammatory Cytokines and Bioactive Kynurenines. *Int. J. Mol. Sci.* **2020**, *21*, 2431. [CrossRef] [PubMed]
5. Boeschoten, R.E.; Braamse, A.M.J.; Beekman, A.T.F.; Cuijpers, P.; van Oppen, P.; Dekker, J.; Uitdehaag, B.M.J. Prevalence of Depression and Anxiety in Multiple Sclerosis: A Systematic Review and Meta-Analysis. *J. Neurol. Sci.* **2017**, *372*, 331–341. [CrossRef]

6. Hunt, C.; Macedo e Cordeiro, T.; Suchting, R.; de Dios, C.; Cuellar Leal, V.A.; Soares, J.C.; Dantzer, R.; Teixeira, A.L.; Selvaraj, S. Effect of immune activation on the kynurenine pathway and depression symptoms—A systematic review and meta-analysis. *Neurosci. Biobehav. Rev.* **2020**, *118*, 514. [CrossRef]
7. Jovanovic, F.; Candido, K.D.; Knezevic, N.N. The Role of the Kynurenine Signaling Pathway in Different Chronic Pain Conditions and Potential Use of Therapeutic Agents. *Int. J. Mol. Sci.* **2020**, *21*, 6045. [CrossRef]
8. Waubant, E.; Lucas, R.; Mowry, E.; Graves, J.; Olsson, T.; Alfredsson, L.; Langer-Gould, A. Environmental and genetic risk factors for MS: An integrated review. *Ann. Clin. Transl. Neurol.* **2019**, *6*, 1905–1922. [CrossRef]
9. Biernacki, T.; Sandi, D.; Kincses, Z.T.; Füvesi, J.; Rózsa, C.; Mátyás, K.; Vécsei, L.; Bencsik, K. Contributing factors to health-related quality of life in multiple sclerosis. *Brain Behav.* **2019**, *9*, e01466. [CrossRef]
10. Rajda, C.; Majláth, Z.; Pukoli, D.; Vécsei, L. Kynurenines and Multiple Sclerosis: The Dialogue between the Immune System and the Central Nervous System. *Int. J. Mol. Sci.* **2015**, *16*, 18270–18282. [CrossRef] [PubMed]
11. Chen, Y.Y.; Wang, M.C.; Wang, Y.N.; Hu, H.H.; Liu, Q.Q.; Liu, H.J.; Zhao, Y.Y. Redox signaling and Alzheimer's disease: From pathomechanism insights to biomarker discovery and therapy strategy. *Biomark. Res.* **2020**, *8*, 42. [CrossRef] [PubMed]
12. Filippi, M.; Bar-Or, A.; Piehl, F.; Preziosa, P.; Solari, A.; Vukusic, S.; Rocca, M.A. Multiple sclerosis. *Nat. Rev. Dis. Primers* **2018**, *4*, 43. [CrossRef] [PubMed]
13. Kincses, Z.T.; Tóth, E.; Bankó, N.; Veréb, D.; Szabó, N.; Csete, G.; Faragó, P.; Király, A.; Bencsik, K.; Vécsei, L. Grey matter atrophy in patients suffering from multiple sclerosis. *Ideggyogy Sz.* **2014**, *67*, 293–300. [PubMed]
14. Tóth, E.; Faragó, P.; Király, A.; Szabó, N.; Veréb, D.; Kocsis, K.; Kincses, B.; Sandi, D.; Bencsik, K.; Vécsei, L.; et al. The Contribution of Various MRI Parameters to Clinical and Cognitive Disability in Multiple Sclerosis. *Front. Neurol.* **2019**, *9*, 1172. [CrossRef]
15. Andravizou, A.; Dardiotis, E.; Artemiadis, A.; Sokratous, M.; Siokas, V.; Tsouris, Z.; Aloizou, A.M.; Nikolaidis, I.; Bakirtzis, C.; Tsivgoulis, G.; et al. Brain atrophy in multiple sclerosis: Mechanisms, clinical relevance and treatment options. *Autoimmun. Highlights* **2019**, *10*, 7. [CrossRef]
16. Hartung, H.P.; Graf, J.; Aktas, O.; Mares, J.; Barnett, M.H. Diagnosis of multiple sclerosis: Revisions of the McDonald criteria 2017—Continuity and change. *Curr. Opin. Neurol.* **2019**, *32*, 327–337. [CrossRef]
17. Iacobaeus, E.; Arrambide, G.; Pia Amato, M.; Derfuss, T.; Vukusic, S.; Hemmer, B.; Tintore, M.; Brundin, L.; 2018 ECTRIMS Focused Workshop Group. Aggressive multiple sclerosis (1): Towards a definition of the phenotype. *Mult. Scler.* **2020**, *26*, 1352458520925369. [CrossRef]
18. Correale, J.; Marrodan, M.; Ysrraelit, M.C. Mechanisms of Neurodegeneration and Axonal Dysfunction in Progressive Multiple Sclerosis. *Biomedicines* **2019**, *7*, 14. [CrossRef]
19. Melendez-Torres, G.J.; Armoiry, X.; Court, R.; Patterson, J.; Kan, A.; Auguste, P.; Madan, J.; Counsell, C.A.R.L.; Ciccarelli, O.; Clarke, A. Comparative effectiveness of beta-interferons and glatiramer acetate for relapsing-remitting multiple sclerosis: Systematic review and network meta-analysis of trials including recommended dosages. *BMC Neurol.* **2018**, *18*, 162. [CrossRef]
20. Goodman, A.D.; Anadani, N.; Gerwitz, L. Siponimod in the treatment of multiple sclerosis. *Expert Opin. Investig. Drugs* **2019**, *28*, 1051–1057. [CrossRef]
21. Robertson, D.; Moreo, N. Disease-Modifying Therapies in Multiple Sclerosis: Overview and Treatment Considerations. *Fed Pract.* **2016**, *33*, 28–34. [PubMed]
22. Jonasson, E.; Sejbaek, T. Diroximel fumarate in the treatment of multiple sclerosis. *Neurodegener. Dis. Manag.* **2020**, *10*, 267–276. [CrossRef]
23. Hauser, S.L.; Bar-Or, A.; Cohen, J.A.; Comi, G.; Correale, J.; Coyle, P.K.; Selmaj, K. Ofatumumab versus teriflunomide in multiple sclerosis. *N. Eng. J. Med.* **2020**, *383*, 546–557. [CrossRef] [PubMed]
24. Hojati, Z.; Kay, M.; Dehghanian, F. Mechanism of Action of Interferon Beta in Treatment of Multiple Sclerosis. In *Multiple Sclerosis, A Mechanistic View*, 1st ed.; Minagar, A., Ed.; Academic Press: Cambridge, MA, USA, 2016; pp. 365–392.
25. Ziemssen, T.; Schrempf, W. Glatiramer acetate: Mechanisms of action in multiple sclerosis. *Int. Rev. Neurobiol.* **2007**, *79*, 537–570.
26. De Angelis, F.; John, N.A.; Brownlee, W.J. Disease-modifying therapies for multiple sclerosis. *BMJ* **2018**, *363*, k4674. [CrossRef]
27. Rajda, C.; Bergquist, J.; Vécsei, L. Kynurenines, redox disturbances and neurodegeneration in multiple sclerosis. *J. Neural. Transm. Suppl.* **2007**, *72*, 323–329.

28. Rajda, C.; Pukoli, D.; Bende, Z.; Majláth, Z.; Vécsei, L. Excitotoxins, Mitochondrial and Redox Disturbances in Multiple Sclerosis. *Int. J. Mol. Sci.* **2017**, *18*, 353. [CrossRef]
29. Sas, K.; Szabó, E.; Vécsei, L. Mitochondria, Oxidative Stress and the Kynurenine System, with a Focus on Ageing and Neuroprotection. *Molecules* **2018**, *23*, 191. [CrossRef]
30. Fiorini, A.; Koudriavtseva, T.; Bucaj, E.; Coccia, R.; Foppoli, C.; Giorgi, A.; Schininà, M.E.; Di Domenico, F.; De Marco, F.; Perluigi, M. Involvement of oxidative stress in occurrence of relapses in multiple sclerosis: The spectrum of oxidatively modified serum proteins detected by proteomics and redox proteomics analysis. *PLoS ONE* **2013**, *8*, e65184. [CrossRef]
31. Choi, I.Y.; Lee, P.; Adany, P.; Hughes, A.J.; Belliston, S.; Denney, D.R.; Lynch, S.G. In vivo evidence of oxidative stress in brains of patients with progressive multiple sclerosis. *Mult. Scler.* **2018**, *24*, 1029–1038. [CrossRef]
32. Barcelos, I.P.; Troxell, R.M.; Graves, J.S. Mitochondrial Dysfunction and Multiple Sclerosis. *Biology* **2019**, *8*, 37. [CrossRef] [PubMed]
33. Cortese-Krott, M.M.; Koning, A.; Kuhnle, G.G.C.; Nagy, P.; Bianco, C.L.; Pasch, A.; Wink, D.A.; Fukuto, J.M.; Jackson, A.A.; van Goor, H.; et al. The Reactive Species Interactome: Evolutionary Emergence, Biological Significance, and Opportunities for Redox Metabolomics and Personalized Medicine. *Antioxid. Redox Signal* **2017**, *27*, 684–712. [CrossRef]
34. Santolini, J.; Wootton, S.A.; Jackson, A.A.; Feelisch, M. The Redox architecture of physiological function. *Curr. Opin. Physiol.* **2019**, *9*, 34–47. [CrossRef] [PubMed]
35. Sies, H. On the history of oxidative stress: Concept and some aspects of current development. *Curr. Opin. Toxicol.* **2018**, *7*, 122–126. [CrossRef]
36. Viña, J.; Lloret, A.; Vallés, S.L.; Borrás, C.; Badía, M.C.; Pallardó, F.V.; Sastre, J.; Alonso, M.D. Mitochondrial oxidant signalling in Alzheimer's disease. *J. Alzheimers Dis.* **2007**, *11*, 175–181. [CrossRef]
37. Pizzino, G.; Irrera, N.; Cucinotta, M.; Pallio, G.; Mannino, F.; Arcoraci, V.; Squadrito, F.; Altavilla, D.; Bitto, A. Oxidative Stress: Harms and Benefits for Human Health. *Oxid. Med. Cell Longev.* **2017**, *2017*, 8416763. [CrossRef]
38. Török, N.; Majláth, Z.; Fülöp, F.; Toldi, J.; Vécsei, L. Brain Aging and Disorders of the Central Nervous System: Kynurenines and Drug Metabolism. *Curr. Drug Metab.* **2016**, *17*, 412–429. [CrossRef]
39. Frijhoff, J.; Winyard, P.G.; Zarkovic, N.; Davies, S.S.; Stocker, R.; Cheng, D.; Knight, A.R.; Taylor, E.L.; Oettrich, J.; Ruskovska, T.; et al. Clinical Relevance of Biomarkers of Oxidative Stress. *Antioxid. Redox Signal* **2015**, *23*, 1144–1170. [CrossRef]
40. Tanaka, M.; Bohár, Z.; Vécsei, L. Are Kynurenines Accomplices or Principal Villains in Dementia? Maintenance of Kynurenine Metabolism. *Molecules* **2020**, *25*, 564. [CrossRef]
41. Bhattacharyya, A.; Chattopadhyay, R.; Mitra, S.; Crowe, S.E. Oxidative Stress: An Essential Factor in the Pathogenesis of Gastrointestinal Mucosal Diseases. *Physiol. Rev.* **2014**, *94*, 329–354. [CrossRef]
42. Aguilera, G.; Colín-González, A.L.; Rangel-López, E.; Chavarría, A.; Santamaría, A. Redox Signaling, Neuroinflammation, and Neurodegeneration. *Antioxid. Redox Signal.* **2018**, *28*, 1626–1651. [CrossRef] [PubMed]
43. Lushchak, V.I. Free radicals, reactive oxygen species, oxidative stress and its classification. *Chem. Biol. Interact.* **2014**, *224*, 164–175. [CrossRef] [PubMed]
44. Di Meo, S.; Reed, T.T.; Venditti, P.; Victor, V.M. Role of ROS and RNS Sources in Physiological and Pathological Conditions. *Oxid. Med. Cell Longev.* **2016**, *2016*, 1245049. [CrossRef] [PubMed]
45. Collin, F. Chemical Basis of Reactive Oxygen Species Reactivity and Involvement in Neurodegenerative Diseases. *Int. J. Mol. Sci.* **2019**, *20*, 2407. [CrossRef]
46. Drulovic, J.; Dujmovic, I.; Stojsavljevic, N.; Mesaros, S.; Andjelkovic, S.; Miljkovic, D.; Peric, V.; Dragutinovic, G.; Marinkovic, J.; Levic, Z.; et al. Uric acid levels in sera from patients with multiple sclerosis. *J. Neurol.* **2001**, *248*, 121–126. [CrossRef]
47. Nasyrova, R.F.; Moskaleva, P.V.; Vaiman, E.E.; Shnayder, N.A.; Blatt, N.L.; Rizvanov, A.A. Genetic Factors of Nitric Oxide's System in Psychoneurologic Disorders. *Int. J. Mol. Sci.* **2020**, *21*, 1604. [CrossRef]
48. Doğan, H.O.; Yildiz, Ö.K. Serum NADPH oxidase concentrations and the associations with iron metabolism in relapsing remitting multiple sclerosis. *J. Trace Elem. Med. Biol.* **2019**, *55*, 39–43. [CrossRef]
49. Inarrea, P.; Alarcia, R.; Alava, M.A.; Capablo, J.L.; Casanova, A.; Iñiguez, C.; Iturralde, M.; Larrodé, P.; Martín, J.; Mostacero, E.; et al. Mitochondrial complex enzyme activities and cytochrome C expression changes in multiple sclerosis. *Mol. Neurobiol.* **2014**, *49*, 1–9. [CrossRef]

50. Ljubisavljevic, S.; Stojanovic, I.; Vojinovic, S.; Stojanov, D.; Stojanovic, S.; Cvetkovic, T.; Savic, D.; Pavlovic, D. The patients with clinically isolated syndrome and relapsing remitting multiple sclerosis show different levels of advanced protein oxidation products and total thiol content in plasma and CSF. *Neurochem. Int.* **2013**, *62*, 988–997. [CrossRef]
51. Damiano, S.; Sasso, A.; De Felice, B.; Terrazzano, G.; Bresciamorra, V.; Carotenuto, A.; Orefice, N.S.; Orefice, G.; Vacca, G.; Belfiore, A.; et al. The IFN-beta 1b effect on Cu Zn superoxide dismutase (SOD1) in peripheral mononuclear blood cells of relapsing-remitting multiple sclerosis patients and in neuroblastoma SK-N-BE cells. *Brain Res. Bull.* **2015**, *118*, 1–6. [CrossRef]
52. Tasset, I.; Bahamonde, C.; Agüera, E.; Conde, C.; Cruz, A.H.; Pérez-Herrera, A.; Gascón, F.; Giraldo, A.I.; Ruiz, M.C.; Lillo, R.; et al. Effect of natalizumab on oxidative damage biomarkers in relapsing-remitting multiple sclerosis. *Pharmacol. Rep.* **2013**, *65*, 624–631. [CrossRef]
53. Gliozzi, M.; Scicchitano, M.; Bosco, F.; Musolino, V.; Carresi, C.; Scarano, F.; Maiuolo, J.; Nucera, S.; Maretta, A.; Paone, S.; et al. Modulation of Nitric Oxide Synthases by Oxidized LDLs: Role in Vascular Inflammation and Atherosclerosis Development. *Int. J. Mol. Sci.* **2019**, *20*, 3294. [CrossRef] [PubMed]
54. Lopez-Moratalla, N.; Gonzalez, A.; Aymerich, M.S.; López-Zabalza, M.J.; Pío, R.; de Castro, P.; Santiago, E. Monocyte inducible nitric oxide synthase in multiple sclerosis: Regulatory role of nitric oxide. *Nitric Oxide* **1997**, *1*, 95–104. [CrossRef] [PubMed]
55. Calabrese, V.; Scapagnini, G.; Ravagna, A.; Bella, R.; Foresti, R.; Bates, T.E.; Giuffrida Stella, A.M.; Pennisi, G. Nitric oxide synthase is present in the cerebrospinal fluid of patients with active multiple sclerosis and is associated with increases in cerebrospinal fluid protein nitrotyrosine and S-nitrosothiols and with changes in glutathione levels. *J. Neurosci. Res.* **2002**, *70*, 580–587. [CrossRef] [PubMed]
56. Tasset, I.; Aguera, E.; Sanchez-Lopez, F.; Feijóo, M.; Giraldo, A.I.; Cruz, A.H.; Gascón, F.; Túnez, I. Peripheral oxidative stress in relapsing remitting multiple sclerosis. *Clin. Biochem.* **2012**, *45*, 440–444. [CrossRef]
57. Cupp-Sutton, K.A.; Ashby, M.T. Biological Chemistry of Hydrogen Selenide. *Antioxidants* **2016**, *5*, 42. [CrossRef] [PubMed]
58. Misra, S.; Boylan, M.; Selvam, A.; Spallholz, J.E.; Björnstedt, M. Redox-Active Selenium Compounds—From Toxicity and Cell Death to Cancer Treatment. *Nutrients* **2015**, *7*, 3536–3556. [CrossRef]
59. Ljubisavljevic, S.; Stojanovic, I.; Cvetkovic, T.; Vojinovic, S.; Stojanov, D.; Stojanovic, D.; Bojanic, V.; Stokanovic, D.; Pavlovic, D. Glutathione homeostasis disruption of erythrocytes, but not glutathione peroxidase activity change, is closely accompanied with neurological and radiological scoring of acute CNS inflammation. *Neuroimmunomodulation* **2014**, *21*, 13–20. [CrossRef]
60. Zachara, B.; Gromadzinska, J.; Czernicki, J.; Maciejek, Z.; Chmielewski, H. Red blood cell glutathione peroxidase activity in multiple sclerosis. *Klin. Wochenschr.* **1984**, *62*, 179–182. [CrossRef]
61. Calabrese, V.; Raffaele, R.; Cosentino, E.; Rizza, V. Changes in cerebrospinal fluid levels of malondialdehyde and glutathione reductase activity in multiple sclerosis. *Int. J. Clin. Pharmacol. Res.* **1994**, *14*, 119–123.
62. Jensen, G.E.; Gissel-Nielsen, G.; Clausen, J. Leucocyte glutathione peroxidase activity and selenium level in multiple sclerosis. *J. Neurol. Sci.* **1980**, *48*, 61–67. [CrossRef]
63. Hirsch, H.E.; Blanco, C.E.; Parks, M.E. Glycerol phosphate dehydrogenase: Reduced activity in multiple sclerosis plaques confirms localization in oligodendrocytes. *J. Neurochem.* **1980**, *34*, 760–762. [CrossRef] [PubMed]
64. Ferret-Sena, V.; Capela, C.; Sena, A. Metabolic Dysfunction and Peroxisome Proliferator-Activated Receptors (PPAR) in Multiple Sclerosis. *Int. J. Mol. Sci.* **2018**, *19*, 1639. [CrossRef] [PubMed]
65. Oliveira, S.R.; Kallaur, A.P.; Simão, A.N.; Morimoto, H.K.; Lopes, J.; Panis, C.; Petenucci, D.L.; da Silva, E.; Cecchini, R.; Kaimen-Maciel, D.R.; et al. Oxidative stress in multiple sclerosis patients in clinical remission: Association with the expanded disability status scale. *J. Neurol. Sci.* **2012**, *321*, 49–53. [CrossRef] [PubMed]
66. Miller, E.; Walczak, A.; Saluk, J.; Ponczek, M.B.; Majsterek, I. Oxidative modification of patient's plasma proteins and its role in pathogenesis of multiple sclerosis. *Clin. Biochem.* **2012**, *45*, 26–30. [CrossRef] [PubMed]
67. Sadowska-Bartosz, I.; Adamczyk-Sowa, M.; Gajewska, A.; Bartosz, G. Oxidative modification of blood serum proteins in multiple sclerosis after interferon or mitoxantrone treatment. *J. Neuroimmunol.* **2014**, *266*, 7–74. [CrossRef] [PubMed]
68. Zabaleta, M.; Marino, R.; Borges, J.; Camargo, B.; Ordaz, P.; De Sanctis, J.B.; Bianco, N.E. Activity profile in multiple sclerosis: An integrative approach. A preliminary report. *Mult. Scler.* **2002**, *8*, 343–349. [CrossRef]

69. Iarlori, C.; Gambi, D.; Lugaresi, A.; Patruno, A.; Felaco, M.; Salvatore, M.; Speranza, L.; Reale, M. Reduction of free radicals in multiple sclerosis: Effect of glatiramer acetate (Copaxone). *Mult. Scler.* **2008**, *14*, 739–748. [CrossRef]
70. Seven, A.; Aslan, M.; Incir, S.; Altintas, A. Evaluation of oxidative and nitrosative stress in relapsing remitting multiple sclerosis: Effect of corticosteroid therapy. *Folia Neuropathol.* **2013**, *51*, 58–64. [CrossRef]
71. Stojanovic, I.; Vojinovic, S.; Ljubisavljevic, S.; Pavlovic, R.; Basic, J.; Pavlovic, D.; Ilic, A.; Cvetkovic, T.; Stukalov, M. INF-β1b therapy modulates L-arginine and nitric oxide metabolism in patients with relapse remittent multiple sclerosis. *J. Neurol. Sci.* **2012**, *323*, 187–192. [CrossRef]
72. Teixeira, D.; Fernandes, R.; Prudêncio, C.; Vieira, M. 3-Nitrotyrosine quantification methods: Current concepts and future challenges. *Biochimie* **2016**, *125*, 1–11. [CrossRef] [PubMed]
73. Srivastava, D.; Kukkuta Sarma, G.R.; Dsouza, D.S.; Muralidharan, M.; Srinivasan, K.; Mandal, A.K. Characterization of residue-specific glutathionylation of CSF proteins in multiple sclerosis—A MS-based approach. *Anal Biochem.* **2019**, *564-565*, 108–115. [CrossRef] [PubMed]
74. Adamczyk-Sowa, M.; Galiniak, S.; Żyracka, E.; Grzesik, M.; Naparło, K.; Sowa, P.; Bartosz, G.; Sadowska-Bartosz, I. Oxidative Modification of Blood Serum Proteins in Multiple Sclerosis after Interferon Beta and Melatonin Treatment. *Oxid. Med. Cell Longev.* **2017**, *2017*, 7905148. [CrossRef] [PubMed]
75. Wetzels, S.; Vanmierlo, T.; Scheijen, J.L.J.M.; van Horssen, J.; Amor, S.; Somers, V.; Schalkwijk, C.G.; Hendriks, J.J.A.; Wouters, K. Methylglyoxal-Derived Advanced Glycation Endproducts Accumulate in Multiple Sclerosis Lesions. *Front. Immunol.* **2019**, *10*, 855. [CrossRef] [PubMed]
76. Haghikia, A.; Kayacelebi, A.A.; Beckmann, B.; Hanff, E.; Gold, R.; Haghikia, A.; Tsikas, D. Serum and cerebrospinal fluid concentrations of homoarginine, arginine, asymmetric and symmetric dimethylarginine, nitrite and nitrate in patients with multiple sclerosis and neuromyelitis optica. *Amino Acids* **2015**, *47*, 1837–1845. [CrossRef]
77. Teunissen, C.E.; Sombekke, M.; van Winsen, L.; Killestein, J.; Barkhof, F.; Polman, C.H.; Dijkstra, C.D.; Blankenstein, M.A.; Pratico, D. Increased plasma 8,12-iso-iPF2alpha- VI levels in relapsing multiple sclerosis patients are not predictive of disease progression. *Mult. Scler.* **2012**, *18*, 1092–1098. [CrossRef] [PubMed]
78. Miller, E.; Mrowicka, M.; Saluk-Juszczak, J.; Ireneusz, M. The level of isoprostanes as a non-invasive marker for in vivo lipid peroxidation in secondary progressive multiple sclerosis. *Neurochem. Res.* **2011**, *36*, 1012–1016. [CrossRef]
79. Gonzalo, H.; Brieva, L.; Tatzber, F.; Jové, M.; Cacabelos, D.; Cassanyé, A.; Lanau-Angulo, L.; Boada, J.; Serrano, J.C.; González, C.; et al. Lipidome analysis in multiple sclerosis reveals protein lipoxidative damage as a potential pathogenic mechanism. *J. Neurochem.* **2012**, *123*, 622–634. [CrossRef]
80. Greco, A.; Minghetti, L.; Sette, G.; Fieschi, C.; Levi, G. Cerebrospinal fluid isoprostane shows oxidative stress in patients with multiple sclerosis. *Neurology* **1999**, *53*, 1876–1879. [CrossRef]
81. Pohl, E.E.; Jovanovic, O. The Role of Phosphatidylethanolamine Adducts in Modification of the Activity of Membrane Proteins under Oxidative Stress. *Molecules* **2019**, *24*, 4545. [CrossRef]
82. Mitosek-Szewczyk, K.; Gordon-Krajcer, W.; Walendzik, P.; Stelmasiak, Z. Free radical peroxidation products in cerebrospinal fluid and serum of patients with multiple sclerosis after glucocorticoid therapy. *Folia Neuropathol.* **2010**, *48*, 116–122. [PubMed]
83. Tavazzi, B.; Batocchi, A.P.; Amorini, A.M.; Nociti, V.; D'Urso, S.; Longo, S.; Gullotta, S.; Picardi, M.; Lazzarino, G. Serum Metabolic Profile in Multiple Sclerosis Patients. *Mult. Scler. Int.* **2011**, *2011*, 167156. [CrossRef] [PubMed]
84. Ljubisavljevic, S.; Stojanovic, I.; Vojinovic, S.; Stojanov, D.; Stojanovic, S.; Kocic, G.; Savic, D.; Cvetkovic, T.; Pavlovic, D. Cerebrospinal fluid and plasma oxidative stress biomarkers in different clinical phenotypes of neuroinflammatory acute attacks. Conceptual accession: From fundamental to clinic. *Cell Mol. Neurobiol.* **2013**, *33*, 767–777. [CrossRef] [PubMed]
85. Ghabaee, M.; Jabedari, B.; Al-E-Eshagh, N.; Ghaffarpour, M.; Asadi, F. Serum and cerebrospinal fluid antioxidant activity and lipid peroxidation in Guillain-Barre syndrome and multiple sclerosis patients. *Int. J. Neurosci.* **2010**, *120*, 301–304. [CrossRef] [PubMed]
86. Pawlowski, J.; Shukla, P.; Bielekova, B. Identifying CSF Biomarkers of Oxidative Stress in Patients with Multiple Sclerosis. 2011. Available online: https://www.researchgate.net/publication/290998239_Identifying_CSF_Biomarkers_of_Oxidative_Stress_in_Patients_with_Multiple_Sclerosis (accessed on 28 August 2020).

87. Villoslada, P.; Alonso, C.; Agirrezabal, I.; Kotelnikova, E.; Zubizarreta, I.; Pulido-Valdeolivas, I.; Saiz, A.; Comabella, M.; Montalban, X.; Villar, L.; et al. Metabolomic signatures associated with disease severity in multiple sclerosis. *Neurol. Neuroimmunol. Neuroinflamm.* **2017**, *4*, e321. [CrossRef] [PubMed]
88. Fellows Maxwell, K.; Bhattacharya, S.; Bodziak, M.L.; Jakimovski, D.; Hagemeier, J.; Browne, R.W.; Weinstock-Guttman, B.; Zivadinov, R.; Ramanathan, M. Oxysterols and apolipoproteins in multiple sclerosis: A 5 year follow-up study. *J. Lipid Res.* **2019**, *60*, 1190–1198. [CrossRef] [PubMed]
89. Prasad, A.; Balukova, A.; Pospíšil, P. Triplet Excited Carbonyls and Singlet Oxygen Formation during Oxidative Radical Reaction in Skin. *Front. Physiol.* **2018**, *9*, 1109. [CrossRef]
90. Nordzieke, D.E.; Medraño-Fernandez, I. The Plasma Membrane: A Platform for Intra- and Intercellular Redox Signaling. *Antioxidants* **2018**, *7*, 168. [CrossRef]
91. Yahfoufi, N.; Alsadi, N.; Jambi, M.; Matar, C. The Immunomodulatory and Anti-Inflammatory Role of Polyphenols. *Nutrients* **2018**, *10*, 1618. [CrossRef]
92. Azadmanesh, J.; Borgstahl, G.E.O. A Review of the Catalytic Mechanism of Human Manganese Superoxide Dismutase. *Antioxidants* **2018**, *7*, 25. [CrossRef]
93. Pospíšil, P.; Prasad, A.; Rác, M. Mechanism of the Formation of Electronically Excited Species by Oxidative Metabolic Processes: Role of Reactive Oxygen Species. *Biomolecules* **2019**, *9*, 258. [CrossRef] [PubMed]
94. Di Marzo, N.; Chisci, E.; Giovannoni, R. The Role of Hydrogen Peroxide in Redox-Dependent Signaling: Homeostatic and Pathological Responses in Mammalian Cells. *Cells* **2018**, *7*, 156. [CrossRef] [PubMed]
95. Case, A.J. On the Origin of Superoxide Dismutase: An Evolutionary Perspective of Superoxide-Mediated Redox Signaling. *Antioxidants* **2017**, *6*, 82. [CrossRef]
96. Tang, J.X.; Thompson, K.; Taylor, R.W.; Oláhová, M. Mitochondrial OXPHOS Biogenesis: Co-Regulation of Protein Synthesis, Import, and Assembly Pathways. *Int. J. Mol. Sci.* **2020**, *21*, 3820. [CrossRef] [PubMed]
97. Weidinger, A.; Kozlov, A.V. Biological Activities of Reactive Oxygen and Nitrogen Species: Oxidative Stress *versus* Signal Transduction. *Biomolecules* **2015**, *5*, 472–484. [CrossRef]
98. Ježek, J.; Cooper, K.F.; Strich, R. Reactive Oxygen Species and Mitochondrial Dynamics: The Yin and Yang of Mitochondrial Dysfunction and Cancer Progression. *Antioxidants* **2018**, *7*, 13. [CrossRef]
99. Klivenyi, P.; Karg, E.; Rozsa, C.; Horvath, R.; Komoly, S.; Nemeth, I.; Turi, S.; Vecsei, L. alpha-Tocopherol/lipid ratio in blood is decreased in patients with Leber's hereditary optic neuropathy and asymptomatic carriers of the 11,778 mtDNA mutation. *J. Neurol. Neurosurg. Psychiatry* **2001**, *70*, 359–362. [CrossRef]
100. Ahmad, W.; Ijaz, B.; Shabbiri, K.; Ahmed, F.; Rehman, S. Oxidative toxicity in diabetes and Alzheimer's disease: Mechanisms behind ROS/RNS generation. *J. Biomed. Sci.* **2017**, *24*, 76. [CrossRef]
101. Ljubisavljevic, S.; Stojanovic, I.; Cvetkovic, T.; Vojinovic, S.; Stojanov, D.; Stojanovic, D.; Stefanovic, N.; Pavlovic, D. Erythrocytes' antioxidative capacity as a potential marker of oxidative stress intensity in neuroinflammation. *J. Neurol. Sci.* **2014**, *337*, 8–13. [CrossRef]
102. Spinello, A.; Ritacco, I.; Magistrato, A. The Catalytic Mechanism of Steroidogenic Cytochromes P450 from All-Atom Simulations: Entwinement with Membrane Environment, Redox Partners, and Post-Transcriptional Regulation. *Catalysts* **2019**, *9*, 81. [CrossRef]
103. Irazabal, M.V.; Torres, V.E. Reactive Oxygen Species and Redox Signaling in Chronic Kidney Disease. *Cells* **2020**, *9*, 1342. [CrossRef] [PubMed]
104. Onukwufor, J.O.; Berry, B.J.; Wojtovich, A.P. Physiologic Implications of Reactive Oxygen Species Production by Mitochondrial Complex I Reverse Electron Transport. *Antioxidants* **2019**, *8*, 285. [CrossRef] [PubMed]
105. Aggarwal, V.; Tuli, H.S.; Varol, A.; Thakral, F.; Yerer, M.B.; Sak, K.; Varol, M.; Jain, A.; Khan, M.A.; Sethi, G. Role of Reactive Oxygen Species in Cancer Progression: Molecular Mechanisms and Recent Advancements. *Biomolecules* **2019**, *9*, 735. [CrossRef] [PubMed]
106. Siendones, E.; Ballesteros, M.; Navas, P. Cellular and Molecular Mechanisms of Recessive Hereditary Methaemoglobinaemia Type II. *J. Clin. Med.* **2018**, *7*, 341. [CrossRef]
107. Lismont, C.; Revenco, I.; Fransen, M. Peroxisomal Hydrogen Peroxide Metabolism and Signaling in Health and Disease. *Int. J. Mol. Sci.* **2019**, *20*, 3673. [CrossRef]
108. Chu, R.; Lin, Y.; Reddy, K.C.; Pan, J.; Rao, M.S.; Reddy, J.K.; Yeldandi, A.V. Transformation of epithelial cells stably transfected with H_2O_2-generating peroxisomal urate oxidase. *Cancer Res.* **1996**, *56*, 4846–4852.
109. Gray, E.; Rice, C.; Hares, K.; Redondo, J.; Kemp, K.; Williams, M.; Brown, A.; Scolding, N.; Wilkins, A. Reductions in neuronal peroxisomes in multiple sclerosis grey matter. *Mult. Scler.* **2014**, *20*, 651–659. [CrossRef]

110. Lin, K.-J.; Lin, K.-L.; Chen, S.-D.; Liou, C.-W.; Chuang, Y.-C.; Lin, H.-Y.; Lin, T.-K. The Overcrowded Crossroads: Mitochondria, Alpha-Synuclein, and the Endo-Lysosomal System Interaction in Parkinson's Disease. *Int. J. Mol. Sci.* **2019**, *20*, 5312. [CrossRef]
111. Chobot, V.; Hadacek, F.; Kubicova, L. Effects of Selected Dietary Secondary Metabolites on Reactive Oxygen Species Production Caused by Iron(II) Autoxidation. *Molecules* **2014**, *19*, 20023–20033. [CrossRef]
112. Onyango, A.N. Endogenous Generation of Singlet Oxygen and Ozone in Human and Animal Tissues: Mechanisms, Biological Significance, and Influence of Dietary Components. *Oxid. Med. Cell Longev.* **2016**, *2016*, 2398573. [CrossRef]
113. Adams, L.; Franco, M.C.; Estevez, A.G. Reactive nitrogen species in cellular signaling. *Exp. Biol. Med.* **2015**, *240*, 711–717. [CrossRef] [PubMed]
114. Marrocco, I.; Altieri, F.; Peluso, I. Measurement and Clinical Significance of Biomarkers of Oxidative Stress in Humans. *Oxid. Med. Cell Longev.* **2017**, *2017*, 6501046. [CrossRef] [PubMed]
115. Rejdak, K.; Petzold, A.; Stelmasiak, Z.; Giovannoni, G. Cerebrospinal fluid brain specific proteins in relation to nitric oxide metabolites during relapse of multiple sclerosis. *Mult. Scler.* **2008**, *14*, 59–66. [CrossRef] [PubMed]
116. Giovannoni, G.; Miller, D.H.; Losseff, N.A.; Sailer, M.; Lewellyn-Smith, N.; Thompson, A.J.; Thompson, E.J. Serum inflammatory markers and clinical/MRI markers of disease progression in multiple sclerosis. *J. Neurol.* **2001**, *248*, 487–495. [CrossRef] [PubMed]
117. Peltola, J.; Ukkonen, M.; Moilanen, E.; Elovaara, I. Increased nitric oxide products in CSF in primary progressive MS may reflect brain atrophy. *Neurology* **2001**, *57*, 895–896. [CrossRef]
118. Acar, G.; Idiman, F.; Idiman, E.; Kirkali, G.; Cakmakci, H.; Ozakbas, S. Nitric oxide as an activity marker in multiple sclerosis. *J. Neurol.* **2003**, *250*, 588–592. [CrossRef]
119. Danilov, A.I.; Andersson, M.; Bavand, N.; Wiklund, N.P.; Olsson, T.; Brundin, L. Nitric oxide metabolite determinations reveal continuous inflammation in multiple sclerosis. *J. Neuroimmunol.* **2003**, *136*, 112–118. [CrossRef]
120. Svenningsson, A.; Petersson, A.S.; Andersen, O.; Hansson, G.K. Nitric oxide metabolites in CSF of patients with MS are related to clinical disease course. *Neurology* **1999**, *53*, 1880–1882. [CrossRef]
121. Brundin, L.; Morcos, E.; Olsson, T.; Wiklund, N.P.; Andersson, M. Increased intrathecal nitric oxide formation in multiple sclerosis; cerebrospinal fluid nitrite as activity marker. *Eur. J. Neurol.* **1999**, *6*, 585–590. [CrossRef]
122. Xue, Q.; Yan, Y.; Zhang, R.; Xiong, H. Regulation of iNOS on Immune Cells and Its Role in Diseases. *Int. J. Mol. Sci.* **2018**, *19*, 3805. [CrossRef]
123. Fernando, V.; Zheng, X.; Walia, Y.; Sharma, V.; Letson, J.; Furuta, S. S-Nitrosylation: An Emerging Paradigm of Redox Signaling. *Antioxidants* **2019**, *8*, 404. [CrossRef] [PubMed]
124. Pérez-Torres, I.; Manzano-Pech, L.; Rubio-Ruíz, M.E.; Soto, M.E.; Guarner-Lans, V. Nitrosative Stress and Its Association with Cardiometabolic Disorders. *Molecules* **2020**, *25*, 2555. [CrossRef] [PubMed]
125. Bryll, A.; Skrzypek, J.; Krzyściak, W.; Szelągowska, M.; Śmierciak, N.; Kozicz, T.; Popiela, T. Oxidative-Antioxidant Imbalance and Impaired Glucose Metabolism in Schizophrenia. *Biomolecules* **2020**, *10*, 384. [CrossRef] [PubMed]
126. Zhang, X.; Zhang, D.; Sun, W.; Wang, T. The Adaptive Mechanism of Plants to Iron Deficiency via Iron Uptake, Transport, and Homeostasis. *Int. J. Mol. Sci.* **2019**, *20*, 2424. [CrossRef] [PubMed]
127. Venditti, P.; Di Meo, S. The Role of Reactive Oxygen Species in the Life Cycle of the Mitochondrion. *Int. J. Mol. Sci.* **2020**, *21*, 2173. [CrossRef]
128. López-Gambero, A.J.; Sanjuan, C.; Serrano-Castro, P.J.; Suárez, J.; Rodríguez de Fonseca, F. The Biomedical Uses of Inositols: A Nutraceutical Approach to Metabolic Dysfunction in Aging and Neurodegenerative Diseases. *Biomedicines* **2020**, *8*, 295. [CrossRef]
129. O'Day, D.H. Calmodulin Binding Proteins and Alzheimer's Disease: Biomarkers, Regulatory Enzymes and Receptors That Are Regulated by Calmodulin. *Int. J. Mol. Sci.* **2020**, *21*, 7344. [CrossRef]
130. Giles, G.I.; Nasim, M.J.; Ali, W.; Jacob, C. The Reactive Sulfur Species Concept: 15 Years On. *Antioxidants* **2017**, *6*, 38. [CrossRef]
131. Schöneich, C. Thiyl Radical Reactions in the Chemical Degradation of Pharmaceutical Proteins. *Molecules* **2019**, *24*, 4357. [CrossRef]

132. Ramírez, R.E.; García-Martínez, C.; Méndez, F. Understanding the Nucleophilic Character and Stability of the Carbanions and Alkoxides of 1-(9-Anthryl)ethanol and Derivatives. *Molecules* **2013**, *18*, 10254–10265. [CrossRef]
133. Bjørklund, G.; Crisponi, G.; Nurchi, V.M.; Cappai, R.; Buha Djordjevic, A.; Aaseth, J. A Review on Coordination Properties of Thiol-Containing Chelating Agents towards Mercury, Cadmium, and Lead. *Molecules* **2019**, *24*, 3247. [CrossRef] [PubMed]
134. Głowacka, U.; Brzozowski, T.; Magierowski, M. Synergisms, Discrepancies and Interactions between Hydrogen Sulfide and Carbon Monoxide in the Gastrointestinal and Digestive System Physiology, Pathophysiology and Pharmacology. *Biomolecules* **2020**, *10*, 445. [CrossRef]
135. Benchoam, D.; Cuevasanta, E.; Möller, M.N.; Alvarez, B. Hydrogen Sulfide and Persulfides Oxidation by Biologically Relevant Oxidizing Species. *Antioxidants* **2019**, *8*, 48. [CrossRef] [PubMed]
136. McBean, G.J. Cysteine, Glutathione, and Thiol Redox Balance in Astrocytes. *Antioxidants* **2017**, *6*, 62. [CrossRef] [PubMed]
137. Marozkina, N.; Gaston, B. An Update on Thiol Signaling: S-Nitrosothiols, Hydrogen Sulfide and a Putative Role for Thionitrous Acid. *Antioxidants* **2020**, *9*, 225. [CrossRef]
138. McNeil, N.M.R.; McDonnell, C.; Hambrook, M.; Back, T.G. Oxidation of Disulfides to Thiolsulfinates with Hydrogen Peroxide and a Cyclic Seleninate Ester Catalyst. *Molecules* **2015**, *20*, 10748–10762. [CrossRef]
139. Grman, M.; Nasim, M.J.; Leontiev, R.; Misak, A.; Jakusova, V.; Ondrias, K.; Jacob, C. Inorganic Reactive Sulfur-Nitrogen Species: Intricate Release Mechanisms or Cacophony in Yellow, Blue and Red? *Antioxidants* **2017**, *6*, 14. [CrossRef]
140. Nagahara, N.; Wróbel, M. H_2S, Polysulfides, and Enzymes: Physiological and Pathological Aspects. *Biomolecules* **2020**, *10*, 640. [CrossRef]
141. Kolluru, G.K.; Shen, X.; Kevil, C.G. Reactive Sulfur Species: A New Redox Player in Cardiovascular Pathophysiology. *Arterioscler. Thromb. Vasc. Biol.* **2020**, *40*, 874–884. [CrossRef]
142. Bild, W.; Ciobica, A.; Padurariu, M.; Bild, V. The interdependence of the reactive species of oxygen, nitrogen, and carbon. *J. Physiol. Biochem.* **2013**, *69*, 147–154. [CrossRef]
143. Monti, D.A.; Zabrecky, G.; Leist, T.P.; Wintering, N.; Bazzan, A.J.; Zhan, T.; Newberg, A.B. N-acetyl Cysteine Administration Is Associated with Increased Cerebral Glucose Metabolism in Patients With Multiple Sclerosis: An Exploratory Study. *Front. Neurol.* **2020**, *11*, 88. [CrossRef] [PubMed]
144. Krysko, K.; Bischof, A.; Nourbakhsh, B.; Henry, R.; Revirajan, N.; Manguinao, M.; Li, Y.; Waubant, E. N-acetyl cysteine for fatigue in progressive multiple sclerosis: A pilot randomized double-blind placebo-controlled trial (P5.2-093). *Neurology* **2019**, *92* (Suppl. 15), P5.2-093.
145. Singhal, N.K.; Freeman, E.; Arning, E.; Wasek, B.; Clements, R.; Sheppard, C.; Blake, P.; Bottiglieri, T.; McDonough, J. Dysregulation of methionine metabolism in multiple sclerosis. *Neurochem. Int.* **2018**, *112*, 1–4. [CrossRef] [PubMed]
146. Methionine Metabolism Disrupted in MS. Available online: https://www.medpagetoday.com/meetingcoverage/sfn/69274 (accessed on 24 June 2020).
147. Roy, D.; Chen, J.; Mamane, V. Methionine Metabolism Shapes T Helper Cell Responses through Regulation of Epigenetic Reprogramming. *Cell Metab.* **2020**, *31*, 250–266. [CrossRef] [PubMed]
148. Ferreira, B.; Mendes, F.; Osório, N.; Caseiro, A.; Gabriel, A.; Valado, A. Glutathione in multiple sclerosis. *Br. J. Biomed. Sci.* **2013**, *70*, 75–79. [CrossRef]
149. Karg, E.; Klivényi, P.; Németh, I.; Bencsik, K.; Pintér, S.; Vécsei, L. Nonenzymatic antioxidants of blood in multiple sclerosis. *J. Neurol.* **1999**, *246*, 533–539. [CrossRef]
150. Fominykh, V.; Onufriev, M.V.; Vorobyeva, A.; Brylev, L.; Yakovlev, A.A.; Zakharova, M.N.; Gulyaeva, N.V. Increased S-nitrosothiols are associated with spinal cord injury in multiple sclerosis. *J. Clin. Neurosci.* **2016**, *28*, 38–42. [CrossRef]
151. Antognelli, C.; Perrelli, A.; Armeni, T.; Nicola Talesa, V.; Retta, S.F. Dicarbonyl Stress and S-Glutathionylation in Cerebrovascular Diseases: A Focus on Cerebral Cavernous Malformations. *Antioxidants* **2020**, *9*, 124. [CrossRef]
152. Hwang, S.W.; Lee, Y.-M.; Aldini, G.; Yeum, K.-J. Targeting Reactive Carbonyl Species with Natural Sequestering Agents. *Molecules* **2016**, *21*, 280. [CrossRef]
153. Pérez-Pérez, A.; Sánchez-Jiménez, F.; Vilariño-García, T.; Sánchez-Margalet, V. Role of Leptin in Inflammation and Vice Versa. *Int. J. Mol. Sci.* **2020**, *21*, 5887. [CrossRef]

154. Khan, A.A.; Alsahli, M.A.; Rahmani, A.H. Myeloperoxidase as an Active Disease Biomarker: Recent Biochemical and Pathological Perspectives. *Med. Sci.* **2018**, *6*, 33. [CrossRef]
155. Mannino, M.H.; Patel, R.S.; Eccardt, A.M.; Janowiak, B.E.; Wood, D.C.; He, F.; Fisher, J.S. Reversible Oxidative Modifications in Myoglobin and Functional Implications. *Antioxidants* **2020**, *9*, 549. [CrossRef] [PubMed]
156. Gonos, E.S.; Kapetanou, M.; Sereikaite, J.; Bartosz, G.; Naparło, K.; Grzesik, M.; Sadowska-Bartosz, I. Origin and pathophysiology of protein carbonylation, nitration and chlorination in age-related brain diseases and aging. *Aging (Albany NY)* **2018**, *10*, 868–901. [CrossRef] [PubMed]
157. Mostert, J.P.; Ramsaransing, G.S.; Heersema, D.J.; Heerings, M.; Wilczak, N.; De Keyser, J. Serum uric acid levels and leukocyte nitric oxide production in multiple sclerosis patients outside relapses. *J. Neurol. Sci.* **2005**, *231*, 41–44. [CrossRef] [PubMed]
158. Minohara, M.; Matsuoka, T.; Li, W.; Osoegawa, M.; Ishizu, T.; Ohyagi, Y.; Kira, J. Upregulation of myeloperoxidase in patients with opticospinal multiple sclerosis: Positive correlation with disease severity. *J. Neuroimmunol.* **2006**, *178*, 156–160. [CrossRef] [PubMed]
159. Zoidis, E.; Seremelis, I.; Kontopoulos, N.; Danezis, G.P. Selenium-Dependent Antioxidant Enzymes: Actions and Properties of Selenoproteins. *Antioxidants* **2018**, *7*, 66. [CrossRef]
160. Socha, K.; Kochanowicz, J.; Karpińska, E.; Soroczyńska, J.; Jakoniuk, M.; Mariak, Z.; Borawska, M.H. Dietary habits and selenium, glutathione peroxidase and total antioxidant status in the serum of patients with relapsing-remitting multiple sclerosis. *Nutr. J.* **2014**, *13*, 62. [CrossRef]
161. Grandi, C.; D'Ovidio, M.C. Balance between Health Risks and Benefits for Outdoor Workers Exposed to Solar Radiation: An Overview on the Role of Near Infrared Radiation Alone and in Combination with Other Solar Spectral Bands. *Int. J. Environ. Res. Public Health* **2020**, *17*, 1357. [CrossRef]
162. Karimi, A.; Bahrampour, K.; Momeni Moghaddam, M.A.; Asadikaram, G.; Ebrahimi, G.; Torkzadeh-Mahani, M.; Esmaeili Tarzi, M.; Nematollahi, M.H. Evaluation of lithium serum level in multiple sclerosis patients: A neuroprotective element. *Mult. Scler. Relat. Disord.* **2017**, *17*, 244–248. [CrossRef]
163. Juybari, K.B.; Ebrahimi, G.; Momeni Moghaddam, M.A.; Asadikaram, G.; Torkzadeh-Mahani, M.; Akbari, M.; Mirzamohammadi, S.; Karimi, A.; Nematollahi, M.H. Evaluation of serum arsenic and its effects on antioxidant alterations in relapsing-remitting multiple sclerosis patients. *Mult. Scler. Relat. Disord.* **2018**, *19*, 79–84. [CrossRef]
164. Carroll, L.D.; Davies, M.J. Reaction of Selenium Compounds with Oxygen Species and the Control of Oxidative Stress. In *Organoselenium Compounds in Biology and Medicine: Synthesis, Biological and Therapeutic Treatments*; Jain, V.K., Priyadarsini, K.I., Eds.; Royal Society of Chemistry: London, UK, 2018; pp. 254–275.
165. Xiao, W.; Loscalzo, J. Metabolic Responses to Reductive Stress. *Antioxid. Redox Signal* **2020**, *32*, 1330–1347. [CrossRef] [PubMed]
166. Korge, P.; Calmettes, G.; Weiss, J.N. Increased reactive oxygen species production during reductive stress: The roles of mitochondrial glutathione and thioredoxin reductases. *Biochim. Biophys. Acta* **2015**, *1847*, 514–525. [CrossRef] [PubMed]
167. Bradshaw, P.C. Cytoplasmic and Mitochondrial NADPH-Coupled Redox Systems in the Regulation of Aging. *Nutrients* **2019**, *11*, 504. [CrossRef] [PubMed]
168. Pérez-Torres, I.; Guarner-Lans, V.; Rubio-Ruiz, M.E. Reductive Stress in Inflammation-Associated Diseases and the Pro-Oxidant Effect of Antioxidant Agents. *Int. J. Mol. Sci.* **2017**, *18*, 2098. [CrossRef] [PubMed]
169. Jozefczak, M.; Remans, T.; Vangronsveld, J.; Cuypers, A. Glutathione Is a Key Player in Metal-Induced Oxidative Stress Defenses. *Int. J. Mol. Sci.* **2012**, *13*, 3145–3175. [CrossRef] [PubMed]
170. Singhal, S.S.; Singh, S.P.; Singhal, P.; Horne, D.; Singhal, J.; Awasthi, S. Antioxidant Role of Glutathione S-Transferases: 4-Hydroxynonenal, a Key Molecule in Stress-Mediated Signaling. *Toxicol. Appl. Pharmacol.* **2015**, *289*, 361–370. [CrossRef]
171. Bocedi, A.; Noce, A.; Marrone, G.; Noce, G.; Cattani, G.; Gambardella, G.; Di Lauro, M.; Di Daniele, N.; Ricci, G. Glutathione Transferase P1-1 an Enzyme Useful in Biomedicine and as Biomarker in Clinical Practice and in Environmental Pollution. *Nutrients* **2019**, *11*, 1741. [CrossRef]
172. Shukla, V.K.; Jensen, G.E.; Clausen, J. Erythrocyte glutathione peroxidase deficiency in multiple sclerosis. *Acta Neurol. Scand.* **1977**, *56*, 542–550. [CrossRef]
173. Szeinberg, A.; Golan, R.; Ben Ezzer, J.; Sarova-Pinhas, I.; Sadeh, M.; Braham, J. Decreased erythrocyte glutathione peroxidase activity in multiple sclerosis. *Acta Neurol. Scand.* **1979**, *60*, 265–271. [CrossRef]

174. Szeinberg, A.; Golan, R.; Ben-Ezzer, J.; Sarova-Pinhas, I.; Kindler, D. Glutathione peroxidase activity in various types of blood cells in multiple sclerosis. *Acta Neurol. Scand.* **1981**, *63*, 67–75. [CrossRef]
175. Reiter, R.J.; Tan, D.X.; Rosales-Corral, S.; Galano, A.; Zhou, X.J.; Xu, B. Mitochondria: Central Organelles for Melatonin's Antioxidant and Anti-Aging Actions. *Molecules* **2018**, *23*, 509. [CrossRef] [PubMed]
176. Jensen, G.E.; Clausen, J. Glutathione peroxidase and reductase, glucose-6-phosphate dehydrogenase and catalase activities in multiple sclerosis. *J. Neurol. Sci.* **1984**, *63*, 45–53. [CrossRef]
177. Belcastro, E.; Gaucher, C.; Corti, A.; Leroy, P.; Lartaud, I.; Pompella, A. Regulation of Protein Function by S-nitrosation and S-glutathionylation: Processes and Targets in Cardiovascular Pathophysiology. *Biol. Chem.* **2017**, *398*, 1267–1293. [CrossRef] [PubMed]
178. Mahmoudian, E.; Khalilnezhad, A.; Gharagozli, K.; Amani, D. Thioredoxin-1, redox factor-1 and thioredoxin-interacting protein, mRNAs are differentially expressed in Multiple Sclerosis patients exposed and non-exposed to interferon and immunosuppressive treatments. *Gene* **2017**, *634*, 29–36. [CrossRef] [PubMed]
179. Voigt, D.; Scheidt, U.; Derfuss, T.; Brück, W.; Junker, A. Expression of the Antioxidative Enzyme Peroxiredoxin 2 in Multiple Sclerosis Lesions in Relation to Inflammation. *Int. J. Mol. Sci.* **2017**, *18*, 760. [CrossRef]
180. Todisco, S.; Convertini, P.; Iacobazzi, V.; Infantino, V. TCA Cycle Rewiring as Emerging Metabolic Signature of Hepatocellular Carcinoma. *Cancers* **2020**, *12*, 68. [CrossRef]
181. Schaur, R.J.; Siems, W.; Bresgen, N.; Eckl, P.M. 4-Hydroxy-nonenal—A Bioactive Lipid Peroxidation Product. *Biomolecules* **2015**, *5*, 2247–2337. [CrossRef]
182. McArdle, B.; Mackenzie, I.C.; Webster, G.R. STUDIES ON INTERMEDIATE CARBOHYDRATE METABOLISM IN MULTIPLE SCLEROSIS. *J. Neurol. Neurosurg. Psychiatry* **1960**, *23*, 127–132. [CrossRef]
183. Nijland, P.G.; Molenaar, R.J.; van der Pol, S.M.; van der Valk, P.; van Noorden, C.J.; de Vries, H.E.; van Horssen, J. Differential expression of glucose-metabolizing enzymes in multiple sclerosis lesions. *Acta Neuropathol. Commun.* **2015**, *3*, 79. [CrossRef]
184. Cores, Á.; Piquero, M.; Villacampa, M.; León, R.; Menéndez, J.C. NRF2 Regulation Processes as a Source of Potential Drug Targets against Neurodegenerative Diseases. *Biomolecules* **2020**, *10*, 904. [CrossRef]
185. Orrù, C.; Perra, A.; Kowalik, M.A.; Rizzolio, S.; Puliga, E.; Cabras, L.; Giordano, S.; Columbano, A. Distinct Mechanisms Are Responsible for Nrf2-Keap1 Pathway Activation at Different Stages of Rat Hepatocarcinogenesis. *Cancers* **2020**, *12*, 2305. [CrossRef] [PubMed]
186. Lamichane, S.; Dahal Lamichane, B.; Kwon, S.-M. Pivotal Roles of Peroxisome Proliferator-Activated Receptors (PPARs) and Their Signal Cascade for Cellular and Whole-Body Energy Homeostasis. *Int. J. Mol. Sci.* **2018**, *19*, 949. [CrossRef] [PubMed]
187. Xi, Y.; Zhang, Y.; Zhu, S.; Luo, Y.; Xu, P.; Huang, Z. PPAR-Mediated Toxicology and Applied Pharmacology. *Cells* **2020**, *9*, 352. [CrossRef] [PubMed]
188. Vargas-Mendoza, N.; Morales-González, Á.; Madrigal-Santillán, E.O.; Madrigal-Bujaidar, E.; Álvarez-González, I.; García-Melo, L.F.; Anguiano-Robledo, L.; Fregoso-Aguilar, T.; Morales-Gonzalez, J.A. Antioxidant and Adaptative Response Mediated by Nrf2 during Physical Exercise. *Antioxidants* **2019**, *8*, 196. [CrossRef] [PubMed]
189. Witte, M.E.; Nijland, P.G.; Drexhage, J.A.; Gerritsen, W.; Geerts, D.; van Het Hof, B.; Reijerkerk, A.; de Vries, H.E.; van der Valk, P.; van Horssen, J. Reduced expression of PGC-1α partly underlies mitochondrial changes and correlates with neuronal loss in multiple sclerosis cortex. *Acta Neuropathol.* **2013**, *125*, 231–243. [CrossRef] [PubMed]
190. Del Bo', C.; Bernardi, S.; Marino, M.; Porrini, M.; Tucci, M.; Guglielmetti, S.; Cherubini, A.; Carrieri, B.; Kirkup, B.; Kroon, P.; et al. Systematic Review on Polyphenol Intake and Health Outcomes: Is there Sufficient Evidence to Define a Health-Promoting Polyphenol-Rich Dietary Pattern? *Nutrients* **2019**, *11*, 1355.
191. Shenkin, A. Micronutrients in health and disease. *Postgrad. Med. J.* **2006**, *82*, 559–567. [CrossRef]
192. Leri, M.; Scuto, M.; Ontario, M.L.; Calabrese, V.; Calabrese, E.J.; Bucciantini, M.; Stefani, M. Healthy Effects of Plant Polyphenols: Molecular Mechanisms. *Int. J. Mol. Sci.* **2020**, *21*, 1250. [CrossRef]
193. Brunetti, G.; Di Rosa, G.; Scuto, M.; Leri, M.; Stefani, M.; Schmitz-Linneweber, C.; Calabrese, V.; Saul, N. Healthspan Maintenance and Prevention of Parkinson's-like Phenotypes with Hydroxytyrosol and Oleuropein Aglycone in *C. elegans*. *Int. J. Mol. Sci.* **2020**, *21*, 2588. [CrossRef]

194. Di Rosa, G.; Brunetti, G.; Scuto, M.; Trovato Salinaro, A.; Calabrese, E.J.; Crea, R.; Schmitz-Linneweber, C.; Calabrese, V.; Saul, N. Healthspan Enhancement by Olive Polyphenols in *C. elegans* Wild Type and Parkinson's Models. *Int. J. Mol. Sci.* **2020**, *21*, 3893. [CrossRef]
195. Siracusa, R.; Scuto, M.; Fusco, R.; Trovato, A.; Ontario, M.L.; Crea, R.; Di Paola, R.; Cuzzocrea, S.; Calabrese, V. Anti-inflammatory and Anti-oxidant Activity of Hidrox® in Rotenone-Induced Parkinson's Disease in Mice. *Antioxidants* **2020**, *9*, 824. [CrossRef] [PubMed]
196. Scuto, M.; Di Mauro, P.; Ontario, M.L.; Amato, C.; Modafferi, S.; Ciavardelli, D.; Trovato Salinaro, A.; Maiolino, L.; Calabrese, V. Nutritional Mushroom Treatment in Meniere's Disease with *Coriolus versicolor*: A Rationale for Therapeutic Intervention in Neuroinflammation and Antineurodegeneration. *Int. J. Mol. Sci.* **2020**, *21*, 284. [CrossRef] [PubMed]
197. Miquel, S.; Champ, C.; Day, J.; Aarts, E.; Bahr, B.A.; Bakker, M.; Bánáti, D.; Calabrese, V.; Cederholm, T.; Cryan, J.; et al. Poor cognitive ageing: Vulnerabilities, mechanisms and the impact of nutritional interventions. *Ageing Res. Rev.* **2018**, *42*, 40–55. [CrossRef] [PubMed]
198. Calabrese, E.J. Preconditioning is hormesis part II: How the conditioning dose mediates protection: Dose optimization within temporal and mechanistic frameworks. *Pharmacol. Res.* **2016**, *110*, 265–275. [CrossRef] [PubMed]
199. Koola, M.M. Galantamine-Memantine combination in the treatment of Alzheimer's disease and beyond. *Psychiatry Res.* **2020**, *293*, 113409. [CrossRef] [PubMed]
200. Koola, M.M.; Jafarnejad, S.; Looney, S.; Praharaj, S.; Pillai, A.; Ahmed, A.; Slifstein, M. Meta-Analyses of Randomized Controlled Trials and Potential Novel Combination Treatments in Schizophrenia. *Biol. Psychiatry* **2020**, *87*, S306. [CrossRef]
201. Zhang, Y.; Li, L.; Zhang, J. Curcumin in antidepressant treatments: An overview of potential mechanisms, pre-clinical/clinical trials and ongoing challenges. *Basic Clin. Pharmacol. Toxicol.* **2020**, *127*, 243–253. [CrossRef]
202. Török, N.; Maszlag-Török, R.; Molnár, K.; Szolnoki, Z.; Somogyvári, F.; Boda, K.; Tanaka, M.; Klivényi, P.; Vécsei, L. Single Nucleotide Polymorphisms of Indoleamine 2,3-Dioxygenase 1 Influenced the Age Onset of Parkinson's Disease. *Preprints* **2020**, 2020090470. [CrossRef]
203. Carrillo-Mora, P.; Pérez-De la Cruz, V.; Estrada-Cortés, B.; Toussaint-González, P.; Martínez-Cortéz, J.A.; Rodríguez-Barragán, M.; Quinzaños-Fresnedo, J.; Rangel-Caballero, F.; Gamboa-Coria, G.; Sánchez-Vázquez, I.; et al. Serum Kynurenines Correlate With Depressive Symptoms and Disability in Poststroke Patients: A Cross-sectional Study. *Neurorehabil. Neural Repair* **2020**, 154596832095367. [CrossRef]
204. Tanaka, M.; Bohár, Z.; Martos, D.; Telegdy, G.; Vécsei, L. Antidepressant-like effects of kynurenic acid in a modified forced swim test. *Pharmacol. Rep.* **2020**, *72*, 449–455. [CrossRef]
205. Peris, E.; Micallef, P.; Paul, A.; Palsdottir, V.; Enejder, A.; Bauzá-Thorbrügge, M.; Olofsson, C.S.; Asterholm, W.I. Antioxidant treatment induces reductive stress associated with mitochondrial dysfunction in adipocyte. *J. Biol. Chem.* **2019**, *294*, 2340–2352. [CrossRef] [PubMed]
206. Becerril, S.; Rodríguez, A.; Catalán, V.; Ramírez, B.; Unamuno, X.; Portincasa, P.; Gómez-Ambrosi, J.; Frühbeck, G. Functional Relationship between Leptin and Nitric Oxide in Metabolism. *Nutrients* **2019**, *11*, 2129. [CrossRef] [PubMed]
207. Feige, J.; Moser, T.; Bieler, L.; Schwenker, K.; Hauer, L.; Sellner, J. Vitamin D Supplementation in Multiple Sclerosis: A Critical Analysis of Potentials and Threats. *Nutrients* **2020**, *12*, 783. [CrossRef] [PubMed]
208. Morel, A.; Bijak, M.; Niwald, M.; Miller, E.; Saluk, J. Markers of oxidative/nitrative damage of plasma proteins correlated with EDSS and BDI scores in patients with secondary progressive multiple sclerosis. *Redox Rep.* **2017**, *22*, 547–555. [CrossRef] [PubMed]
209. Rommer, P.S.; Greilberger, J.; Salhofer-Polanyi, S.; Auff, E.; Leutmezer, F.; Herwig, R. Elevated levels of carbonyl proteins in cerebrospinal fluid of patients with neurodegenerative diseases. *Tohoku J. Exp. Med.* **2014**, *234*, 313–317. [CrossRef] [PubMed]
210. Irani, D.N. Cerebrospinal fluid protein carbonylation identifies oxidative damage in autoimmune demyelination. *Ann. Clin. Transl. Neurol.* **2016**, *4*, 145–150. [CrossRef]
211. Poerschke, R.L.; Fritz, K.S.; Franklin, C.C. Methods to detect protein glutathionylation. *Curr. Protoc. Toxicol.* **2013**, *57*, 6.17.1–6.17.18. [CrossRef]

212. Garibaldi, S.; Barisione, C.; Marengo, B.; Ameri, P.; Brunelli, C.; Balbi, M.; Ghigliotti, G. Advanced Oxidation Protein Products-Modified Albumin Induces Differentiation of RAW264.7 Macrophages into Dendritic-Like Cells Which Is Modulated by Cell Surface Thiols. *Toxins* **2017**, *9*, 27. [CrossRef]
213. Hányšová, S.; Čierny, D.; Petráš, M.; Lehotský, J. Elevated plasma levels of advanced oxidation protein products in Slovak multiple sclerosis patients: Possible association with different disability states. *Act Nerv. Super Rediviva.* **2017**, *59*, 45–50.
214. Gill, V.; Kumar, V.; Singh, K.; Kumar, A.; Kim, J.-J. Advanced Glycation End Products (AGEs) May Be a Striking Link Between Modern Diet and Health. *Biomolecules* **2019**, *9*, 888. [CrossRef]
215. Tain, Y.; Hsu, C. Toxic Dimethylarginines: Asymmetric Dimethylarginine (ADMA) and Symmetric Dimethylarginine (SDMA). *Toxins* **2017**, *9*, 92. [CrossRef] [PubMed]
216. Zarkovic, N. Antioxidants and Second Messengers of Free Radicals. *Antioxidants* **2018**, *7*, 158. [CrossRef]
217. Ito, F.; Sono, Y.; Ito, T. Measurement and Clinical Significance of Lipid Peroxidation as a Biomarker of Oxidative Stress: Oxidative Stress in Diabetes, Atherosclerosis, and Chronic Inflammation. *Antioxidants* **2019**, *8*, 72. [CrossRef] [PubMed]
218. Håkansson, I.; Gouveia-Figueira, S.; Ernerudh, J.; Vrethem, M.; Ghafouri, N.; Ghafouri, B.; Nording, M. Oxylipins in cerebrospinal fluid in clinically isolated syndrome and relapsing remitting multiple sclerosis. *Prostaglandins Other Lipid Mediat.* **2018**, *138*, 41–47. [CrossRef] [PubMed]
219. Palavra, F.; Marado, D.; Mascarenhas-Melo, F.; Sereno, J.; Teixeira-Lemos, E.; Nunes, C.C.; Gonçalves, G.; Teixeira, F.; Reis, F. New markers of early cardiovascular risk in multiple sclerosis patients: Oxidized-LDL correlates with clinical staging. *Dis. Mark.* **2013**, *34*, 341–348. [CrossRef]
220. Besler, H.T.; Comoğlu, S. Lipoprotein oxidation, plasma total antioxidant capacity and homocysteine level in patients with multiple sclerosis. *Nutr. Neurosci.* **2003**, *6*, 189–196. [CrossRef] [PubMed]
221. Salemi, G.; Gueli, M.C.; Vitale, F.; Battaglieri, F.; Guglielmini, E.; Ragonese, P.; Trentacosti, A.; Massenti, M.F.; Savettieri, G.; Bono, A. Blood lipids, homocysteine, stress factors, and vitamins in clinically stable multiple sclerosis patients. *Lipids Health Dis.* **2010**, *9*, 19. [CrossRef] [PubMed]
222. Meyers, L.; Groover, C.J.; Douglas, J.; Lee, S.; Brand, D.; Levin, M.C.; Gardner, L.A. A role for Apolipoprotein A-I in the pathogenesis of multiple sclerosis. *J. Neuroimmunol.* **2014**, *277*, 176–185. [CrossRef] [PubMed]
223. van de Kraats, C.; Killestein, J.; Popescu, V.; Rijkers, E.; Vrenken, H.; Lütjohann, D.; Barkhof, F.; Polman, C.H.; Teunissen, C.E. Oxysterols and cholesterol precursors correlate to magnetic resonance imaging measures of neurodegeneration in multiple sclerosis. *Mult. Scler.* **2014**, *20*, 412–417. [CrossRef]
224. Graille, M.; Wild, P.; Sauvain, J.-J.; Hemmendinger, M.; Guseva Canu, I.; Hopf, N.B. Urinary 8-OHdG as a Biomarker for Oxidative Stress: A Systematic Literature Review and Meta-Analysis. *Int. J. Mol. Sci.* **2020**, *21*, 3743. [CrossRef]
225. Ibitoye, R.; Kemp, K.C.; Rice, C.M.; Hares, K.M.; Scolding, N.J.; Wilkins, A. Oxidative stress-related biomarkers in multiple sclerosis: A review. *Biomark. Med.* **2016**, *10*, 889–902. [CrossRef] [PubMed]
226. Taguchi, Y.-H.; Wang, H. Exploring MicroRNA Biomarkers for Parkinson's Disease from mRNA Expression Profiles. *Cells* **2018**, *7*, 245. [CrossRef] [PubMed]
227. Brito, L.M.; Ribeiro-dos-Santos, Â.; Vidal, A.F.; de Araújo, G.S.; on behalf of the Alzheimer's Disease Neuroimaging Initiative. Differential Expression and miRNA–Gene Interactions in Early and Late Mild Cognitive Impairment. *Biology* **2020**, *9*, 251. [CrossRef]
228. Catanesi, M.; d'Angelo, M.; Tupone, M.G.; Benedetti, E.; Giordano, A.; Castelli, V.; Cimini, A. MicroRNAs Dysregulation and Mitochondrial Dysfunction in Neurodegenerative Diseases. *Int. J. Mol. Sci.* **2020**, *21*, 5986. [CrossRef]
229. Mohammed, E.M.A. Environmental Influencers, MicroRNA, and Multiple Sclerosis. *J. Cent. Nerv. Syst. Dis.* **2020**, *12*, 1179573519894955. [CrossRef] [PubMed]
230. Martinez, B.; Peplow, P.V. MicroRNAs in blood and cerebrospinal fluid as diagnostic biomarkers of multiple sclerosis and to monitor disease progression. *Neural. Regen. Res.* **2020**, *15*, 606–619.
231. Pfaff, A.L.; Bubb, V.J.; Quinn, J.P.; Koks, S. An increased burden of highly active 3 retrotransposition competent L1s is associated with 4 Parkinson's disease risk and progression in the PPMI 5 cohort. *Int. J. Mol. Sci.* **2020**, *21*, 6562. [CrossRef]
232. Geis, F.K.; Goff, S.P. Silencing and Transcriptional Regulation of Endogenous Retroviruses: An Overview. *Viruses* **2020**, *12*, 884. [CrossRef]

233. Török, N.; Molnár, K.; Füvesi, J.; Karácsony, M.; Zsiros, V.; Fejes-Szabó, A.; Fiatal, S.; Ádány, R.; Somogyvári, F.; Stojiljković, O.; et al. Chemokine receptor V Δ32 deletion in multiple sclerosis patients in Csongrád County in Hungary and the North-Bácska region in Serbia. *Hum Immunol.* **2015**, *76*, 59–64. [CrossRef]
234. Hall, A.; Bandres-Ciga, S.; Diez-Fairen, M.; Billingsley, K.J. Genetic risk profiling in Parkinson's disease and utilizing genetics to gain insight into disease-related biological pathways. *Int. J. Mol. Sci.* **2020**, *19*, 7332. [CrossRef]
235. Dhama, K.; Latheef, S.K.; Dadar, M.; Samad, H.A.; Munjal, A.; Khandia, R.; Karthik, K.; Tiwari, R.; Yatoo, M.I.; Bhatt, P.; et al. Biomarkers in Stress Related Diseases/Disorders: Diagnostic, Prognostic, and Therapeutic Values. *Front. Mol. Biosci.* **2019**, *6*, 91. [CrossRef] [PubMed]

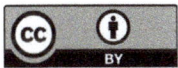

© 2020 by the authors. Licensee MDPI, Basel, Switzerland. This article is an open access article distributed under the terms and conditions of the Creative Commons Attribution (CC BY) license (http://creativecommons.org/licenses/by/4.0/).

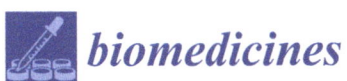

Article

An Exploratory Pilot Study with Plasma Protein Signatures Associated with Response of Patients with Depression to Antidepressant Treatment for 10 Weeks

Eun Young Kim [1,2,†], Hee-Sung Ahn [3,†], Min Young Lee [4], Jiyoung Yu [3], Jeonghun Yeom [5], Hwangkyo Jeong [6], Hophil Min [7], Hyun Jeong Lee [8,9], Kyunggon Kim [3,5,10,11,*] and Yong Min Ahn [12,13,*]

1. Mental Health Center, Seoul National University Health Care Center, 1 Gwanak-ro, Gwanak-gu, Seoul 08826, Korea; ey00@snu.ac.kr
2. Department of Human Systems Medicine, Seoul National University College of Medicine, 101 Daehak-ro, Jongno-gu, Seoul 03080, Korea
3. Asan Institute for Life Sciences, Asan Medical Center, Seoul 05505, Korea; zaulim3@gmail.com (H.-S.A.); yujiyoung202@gmail.com (J.Y.)
4. Institute for Systems Biology, Seattle, Washington, DC 98109, USA; minyoung.lee@gmail.com
5. Convergence Medicine Research Center, Asan Institute for Life Sciences, Asan Medical Center, Seoul 05505, Korea; nature8309@gmail.com
6. Department of Biomedical Sciences, University of Ulsan College of Medicine, Seoul 05505, Korea; hkyo723@naver.com
7. Doping Control Center, Korea Institute of Science and Technology, Hwarang-ro 14-gil 5, Seongbuk-gu, Seoul 02792, Korea; mhophil@kist.re.kr
8. Department of Psychiatry & Behavioral Science, National Cancer Center, Ilsandong-gu, Goyang-si, Gyeonggi-do 10408, Korea; hjlee.np@gmail.com
9. Division of Cancer Control & Policy, National Cancer Control Institute, National Cancer Center, Ilsandong-gu, Goyang-si, Gyeonggi-do 10408, Korea
10. Clinical Proteomics Core Laboratory, Convergence Medicine Research Center, Asan Medical Center, Seoul 05505, Korea
11. Bio-Medical Institute of Technology, Asan Medical Center, Seoul 05505, Korea
12. Department of Neuropsychiatry, Seoul National University Hospital, 101 Daehak-ro, Jongno-gu, Seoul 03080, Korea
13. Department of Psychiatry and Behavioral Science, Institute of Human Behavioral Medicine, Seoul National University College of Medicine, 101 Daehak-ro, Jongno-gu, Seoul 03080, Korea

* Correspondence: kkkon1@amc.seoul.kr (K.K.); aym@snu.ac.kr (Y.M.A.); Tel.: +82-2-1688-7575 (K.K.); +82-2-2072-0710 (Y.M.A.)
† These authors contributed equally to this work.

Received: 21 October 2020; Accepted: 26 October 2020; Published: 28 October 2020

Abstract: Major depressive disorder (MDD) is a leading cause of global disability with a chronic and recurrent course. Recognition of biological markers that could predict and monitor response to drug treatment could personalize clinical decision-making, minimize unnecessary drug exposure, and achieve better outcomes. Four longitudinal plasma samples were collected from each of ten patients with MDD treated with antidepressants for 10 weeks. Plasma proteins were analyzed qualitatively and quantitatively with a nanoflow LC–MS/MS technique. Of 1153 proteins identified in the 40 longitudinal plasma samples, 37 proteins were significantly associated with response/time and clustered into six according to time and response by the linear mixed model. Among them, three early-drug response markers (PHOX2B, SH3BGRL3, and YWHAE) detectable within one week were verified by liquid chromatography-multiple reaction monitoring/mass spectrometry (LC-MRM/MS) in the well-controlled 24 patients. In addition, 11 proteins correlated significantly with two or more psychiatric measurement indices. This pilot study might be useful in finding protein marker candidates that can monitor response to antidepressant treatment during follow-up visits within 10 weeks after the baseline visit.

Keywords: major depressive disorder; longitudinal study; LC-MS/MS; plasma protein biomarker; drug response monitoring; multiple reaction monitoring

---

1. Introduction

Major depressive disorder (MDD) is one of the leading causes of disability worldwide [1], with a high prevalence among individuals of all ages and races [2]. MDD is a chronic condition with a high recurrence rate with a full recovery rate of only 20% and 80% of recovered patients experiencing at least one relapse in their entire life [3]. Antidepressants have long been used in the acute and long-term treatment of MDD, with selective serotonin reuptake inhibitors (SSRIs) being the first-line antidepressants. The process of selecting an antidepressant agent is primarily prescribed based on trial and error. Patients with poor efficacy of the initial course of medication for at least 4–6 weeks require alternative therapeutic strategies, containing changing within and between classes of antidepressants. Unfortunately, the treatment outcomes from antidepressants are discouraging. About 50% of patients enrolled in the Sequenced Treatment Alternative to Relieve Depression (STAR*D) study failed to respond to standard SSRI treatment, and only about 30% experienced complete remission in response to the first antidepressant used [4]. After unsuccessful treatment for MDD patients with a SSRI, the choice of a second drug is important for remission [5]. Biomarkers for response to antidepressant treatment can reduce the time to symptom relief and costs, minimize unnecessary drug exposure, and improve patient outcomes.

Proteomics, the quantitative analysis of all proteins expressed in samples, is a powerful tool for identifying novel molecular biomarkers and enables the detection of molecular signatures reflecting multiple biological pathways involved in response to treatment in patients with MDD [6]. Proteomic analysis of peripheral body fluids, such as blood plasma and serum, may not only enable prediction of response to treatment in clinical practice, but also assist in monitoring drug activity during early stages of clinical trials. To date, however, there have been few proteomic analyses of peripheral blood samples that can predict response to antidepressant treatment [7,8]. A previous liquid chromatography tandem mass spectrometry (LC-MS/MS) analysis found that several plasma proteins might be potential biomarkers for the prediction of antidepressant response over a 6-week treatment period [7]. A multiplex immunoassay testing of up to 258 blood-based markers related to immune, endocrine, and metabolic mechanisms identified 9 markers as potential pre-treatment biomarkers associated with antidepressants treatment response [8].

Longitudinal data are commonly used in biomedical studies [9,10]. In statistical analyses, mixed-effect models (MEMs) [11] and generalized estimating equations (GEEs) [12] are widely applied. To further elaborate, MEM is a subject-level approach that could employ random effects to acquire a between-subjects variable by considering the correlations with observations from the same subject based on the full-likelihood method. Conversely, GEE is a population-level model that relies on a partial-likelihood function. In this study, repeated drug efficacy measurements (baseline and follow-up visits after treatment) were performed on the surrogate plasma protein over time for each patient, with the subject of interest being some of the time-varying changes. In proteomic studies, the MEM method is more popularly used than the GEE method [13–15]. This is because after fixing the desired effect, it is possible to estimate by measuring a random effect of the technical or biological repeated measurement with actual MS [16,17]. In addition, it is technically easier to reflect the variance of any effect on repeated measurements of the same sample after more than two times of MS. Conversely, GEE is robust to the misspecification of correlation structure using quasi likelihood, and many modified variance estimation methods for small samples have been developed [18]. We identified biological implications primarily with the results of the analysis with linear mixed model (LMM) and compared the results after performing with the same data with GEE.

In this preliminary study, LC–MS/MS profiling was performed to identify candidate blood-based protein biomarkers that could monitor early (0–1 week), mid (1–4 week), or late (4–10 week) response to antidepressants, before and after their administration. This study also assessed whether changes in plasma protein concentrations after antidepressant treatment were associated with changes in the severity of depressive symptoms. Blood samples were collected at four time points during the 10-week treatment of ten depressed patients, five responders, and five non-responders, who were taking escitalopram. Plasma proteins were profiled, as were differences in protein abundance between the two groups. Unlike biomarker studies that don't take into account the time of disease occurrence [19–22], this study attempted to identify more reliable candidate biomarkers by time-dependent longitudinal changes in the plasma proteome of these patients. Furthermore, the identified biomarkers predicting early-drug response were validated in 19 responders and five non-responders by the liquid chromatography-multiple reaction monitoring/mass spectrometry (LC-MRM/MS) technique. In addition, significant markers were identified assessing the correlation between protein concentrations, as determined by molecular diagnostic techniques, and psychological parameters.

2. Materials and Methods

2.1. Study Subjects

Since MADRS score is regarded as the criterion for determining response to drug administration, plasma samples were collected from ten patients with MDD who participated in a clinical trial testing the efficacy and safety of escitalopram dose escalation at Seoul National University Hospital, Seoul, Republic of Korea, from February 2013 to February 2016 [23]. All the participants are Korean patients. The trial included two phases: open-label treatment for 4 weeks with a standard dose (10–20 mg/day) of escitalopram, followed by randomized, double-blinded treatment for 6 weeks with 20 mg/day or 30 mg/day escitalopram. Patients aged 18–65 years with a primary diagnosis of MDD, as defined by the Diagnostic and Statistical Manual of Mental Disorders, 4th edition (text revision), were included. All patients had a total MADRS score ≥ 18 at initial screening and baseline visits. Subjects were excluded if they experienced hypersensitivity to escitalopram, had received any psychoactive medications such as antipsychotics, mood stabilizers, or selective monoamine oxidase inhibitors, had symptoms of depression and were deemed resistant to two or more antidepressant treatments, had psychiatric disorders other than MDD or a prior history of psychiatric disorders, such as manic or hypomanic episodes, schizophrenia, schizoaffective disorder, or substance abuse disorder, were at significant risk of suicide, as evaluated by an investigator or with score of ≥ 5 on item 10 of MADRS, or had a history of neurologic disorders or medically unstable conditions (e.g., renal or hepatic impairment, or cardiovascular, pulmonary, or gastrointestinal disorders). Of the patients who entered the clinical trial, five responders (1 male and 4 females) and five non-responders (1 male and 4 females) were selected, from each of whom plasma samples were obtained at four time points: baseline, week 1, week 4 (randomization), and week 10 (6 weeks after randomization) for proteomic analysis. An additional 24 patients were selected, 19 responders and five non-responders, from each of whom plasma samples were obtained at baseline and at week 1. The primary efficacy outcome was a change in total MADRS score. Response was defined as ≥50% reduction in baseline MADRS score after 4 and 10 weeks of treatment. None of these patients were taking medication that could alter the blood levels of relevant factors, such as nonsteroidal anti-inflammatory agents or steroids, and none had any acute or chronic diseases, such as cardiovascular disease, pulmonary disease, hypertension, endocrine abnormalities, rheumatic diseases, or cerebrovascular disease. The study protocol was approved by the Institutional Review Board of Seoul National University Hospital (Number: 1008-116-329, approved on 2 December 2010). The study was performed in accordance with the ethical principles stated in the Declaration of Helsinki and the International Conference on Harmonization Good Clinical Practice guidelines. All patients provided written informed consent and were free to discontinue the study at any time.

2.2. Blood Collection and Plasma Preparation

Plasma was prepared as suggested by the Human Proteome Organization Plasma Proteome Project. Blood samples (3 mL) were collected into ethylenediaminetetraacetic acid-containing tubes at baseline, week 1, week 4 (randomization), and week 10 (post-randomization week 6), and the blood samples were obtained from subjects after an overnight fast (at least 12 h) from 9:30 to 11:30 AM. Blood samples centrifuged at 2000× g for 15 min at room temperature (RT) immediately after sample collection. Plasma was transferred to 0.5 mL tubes and frozen within 20 min after centrifugation. Then, the samples were placed on ice and transported to the laboratory and immediately frozen at −80 °C until assayed.

2.3. Plasma Manipulation and Digestion

Plasma samples were sequentially subjected to high abundant plasma protein depletion and trypsin/Lys-C digestion. To remove the 14 most abundant plasma proteins (albumin, IgA, IgG, IgM, α1-antitrypsin, α1-acid glycoprotein, apolipoprotein A1, apolipoprotein A2, complement C3, transferrin, α2-macroglobulin, transthyretin, haptoglobin, and fibrinogen), a 40 µL aliquot of plasma diluted 4-fold with a proprietary "Buffer A" was injected into a MARS14 depletion column (Agilent Technology, Palo Alto, CA, USA) on a binary HPLC system (20A Prominence, Shimadzu, Tokyo, Japan). The unbound fraction was buffer-exchanged into 8 M urea in 50 mM Tris (pH 8), concentrated to approximately 50 µL by ultrafiltration using a Vivaspin 500 3 kDa cutoff filter (Sartorius, Goettingen, Germany), and then transferred to a new filter unit (Nanosep, 30 kDa; Pall Corporation, NY, USA). A 200 µL aliquot of 8 M urea in 50 mM Tris (pH 8.5) was added, and the mixture was centrifuged at 14,000× g for 15 min, with the procedure repeated twice. The flow-through from the collection tube was discarded, 100 µL of 0.05 M iodoacetamide solution was added, and the preparation was mixed at 600 rpm in a thermo-mixer for 1 min and incubated without mixing for 20 min. The filter units were centrifuged at 14,000× g for 10 min; 100 µL of 8 M urea in 50 mM Tris (pH 8.5) was added, and the filter units were again centrifuged at 14,000× g for 15 min, with this step repeated twice. A 100 µL aliquot of 0.05 M ammonium bicarbonate was added to the filter unit, and the unit was centrifuged at 14,000× g for 10 min, with this step also repeated twice. A 40 µL aliquot of 0.05 M ammonium bicarbonate containing 2.5 µg Lys-C/trypsin was added, and the preparation was mixed at 600 rpm in a thermo-mixer for 1 min. The units were incubated in a wet chamber at 37 °C for 12 h and transferred to new collection tubes. The filter units were centrifuged at 14,000× g for 10 min, 40 µL of 0.5 M NaCl was added, and the filter units were again centrifuged at 14,000× g for 10 min. The digestion reaction was stopped by the addition of formic acid to a final concentration of 0.3%. The peptide mixture was desalted with a Sep Pak C-18 cartridge (Waters, Milford, MA, USA), lyophilized with a cold trap (CentriVap Cold Traps, Labconco, Kansas City, MO, USA), and stored at −80 °C until used.

2.4. Nano-LC-ESI-MS/MS Analysis

Peptides were separated using a Dionex UltiMate 3000 RSLCnano system (Thermo Fisher Scientific, Waltham, MA, USA). Tryptic peptides from a bead column were reconstituted in 0.1% formic acid and separated on a 50 cm Easy-Spray column with a 75 µm inner diameter packed with 2 µm C18 resin (Thermo Fisher Scientific) over 200 min (250 nL/min). The column was developed using a 0–45% acetonitrile gradient in 0.1% formic acid and 5% DMSO at 50 °C. The LC was coupled to a Q Exactive mass spectrometer with a nano-ESI source. Mass spectra were acquired in a data-dependent mode with an automatic switch between a full scan and 20 data-dependent MS/MS scans. The target value for the full scan MS spectra was 3,000,000, with a maximum injection time of 120 ms and a resolution of 70,000 at m/z 400. Repeated peptides were dynamically excluded for 20 s. All MS data have been deposited in the PRIDE archive (www.ebi.ac.uk/pride/archive/projects/PXD017211) under Project PXD017211 [24].

2.5. Database Searching and Label-free Quantification

The acquired MS/MS spectra were searched using the SequestHT on Proteome discoverer (version 2.2, Thermo Fisher Scientific) against the SwissProt human database (May 2017). The search parameters were set as default including cysteine carbamidomethylation as a fixed modification, and N-terminal acetylation and methionine oxidation as variable modifications with two miscleavages. Peptides were identified based on a search with an initial mass deviation of the precursor ion of up to 10 ppm, with the allowed fragment mass deviation set to 20 ppm. When assigning proteins to peptides, both unique and razor peptides were used. Label-free quantitation (LFQ) was performed using peak intensity for unique peptides of each protein [25].

2.6. Analysis of Public Microarray Data

We downloaded the gene expression profile data (series accession number: GSE146446 [26] and GSE45468 [27]) in the Gene Expression Omnibus database for using Biobase and GEOquery package in R. Both data used the GPL570 platform (Affymetrix Human Genome U133 Plus 2.0 Array; Agilent Technologies, Palo Alto, CA, USA). We found the Affymetrix probe IDs by searching for the gene name. Then, subsequent statistical analysis was performed using the gene expression level value of each gene.

2.7. Batch Mean-Centering Correction, Missing Data Imputation, and Normalization

Three batches were prepared, with batch 1 consisting of S15 (non-responders) and S29 (responders); batch 2 of S54 (non-responders) and S52 (responders); and batch 3 of S6 (non-responders), S11 (non-responders), S32 (responders), S34 (non-responders), S38 (responders), and S46 (responders), based on sample preparation date [28]. Mean-centering correction per protein was applied to raw data from 104 LC-MS/MS analyses to avoid the batch effect [29,30].

Then, missing data imputation was performed. Of 316 quantified proteins measured at one time in each individual sample, 180 were completely quantified, whereas missing data for the remaining 136 proteins were determined by a local least-squares imputation method [31]. Using this method, the 180 completely quantified proteins were clustered into 15 groups by Pearson's correlation analysis, and missing values were estimated by a linear optimal combination of the 15 selected clusters.

These data were normalized relative to endogenous normalizing proteins without spike-in standards [32]. From the complete data, six of 210 proteins were finally selected as suitable for LFQ normalization based on the following criteria: (1) their plasma concentrations remained nearly constant in all samples, as determined by their NormFinder stability value [33]; (2) their plasma concentrations did not differ significantly in the five responders and five non-responders, as shown by LMM analysis (p-value > 0.05); and (3) there were no reports of depression. The raw abundance of the six selected normalizing proteins, BTD, C8B, C1S, ITIH2, IGFALS, and SERPINA3, in each sample was divided by the geometric mean of six raw abundances in all samples. The median of these six ratios in a sample was defined as the normalization scaling factor (NSF) for that sample. The NSF for sample s can be calculated using the following equation:

$$NSF_s = geomean\left(\frac{N_{1,s}}{\hat{N}_1}, \frac{N_{2,s}}{\hat{N}_2}, \ldots, \frac{N_{6,s}}{\hat{N}_6}\right)$$

where $N_{i,s}$ is the raw protein abundance of a normalization protein i in sample s, and $\hat{N}_i$ is the median abundance of protein i in all the samples. The normalized abundance of the intensity of each biomarker candidate in a sample was calculated by dividing its raw peak intensity by the NSF:

$$P\check{A}_{j,s} = \frac{PA_{j,s}}{NSF_s}$$

where $P\check{A}_{j,s}$ is the normalized abundance of the j-th biomarker candidate in sample s, and $PA_{j,s}$ is the raw abundance of the corresponding protein.

2.8. LC-ESI-MRM/MS Analysis

Liquid chromatography (LC) was performed on an Agilent 1290 Infinity UHPLC System with a reverse-phase ultra-high-performance LC (UHPLC) column (Agilent ZORBAX Eclipse Plus C18 Column, 95 Å, 2.1 mm i.d. × 100 mm, packed with 1.8 μm C18 resin) at a temperature of 50 °C. The mobile phases used in this study were 0.1% formic acid in water (solvent A) and 0.1% formic acid in acetonitrile (solvent B). The column was developed using a gradient of 0–2% solvent B for 5 min, 2–3% solvent B for 5 min, 3–50% solvent B for 10 min, 50–50% solvent B for 4 min, 50–0% solvent B for 1 min, and 0–0% solvent B for 9 min at a flow rate of 0.3 mL/min. The injected sample consisted of a mixture of digested plasma peptides (initial plasma volume: 40 μL) and isotope-labeled internal standard peptides. The UHPLC system was coupled to a triple quadrupole mass spectrometer (Agilent 6495 QQQ) by a standard-flow Jet Stream electrospray source operated in positive ion mode. Additional parameters included capillary voltage, 3.5 kV; nozzle voltage, 1 kV; gas temperature, 290 °C; drying gas flow rate, 11 L/min at 350 °C; nebulizer gas pressure, 40 PSI at 350 °C; and unit resolution for Q1 and Q3. MRM transitions were selected, and their collision energies optimized by Skyline (64-bit, version 19.1.0.193) software (Supplementary Table S4). The cell accelerator voltage was set to 5 V. Quantification experiments were performed using dynamic MRM (delta retention time: 3 min), with a total cycle time of approximately 1.5 s. The mass spectrometer was operated with MassHunter software (version B.08.00, Agilent), which generated MRM/MS data (*.d). MRM results from extracted ion chromatograms were analyzed by Skyline and quantified relative to the corresponding stable isotope-labeled peptides (SpikeTides™; JPT Peptdie Technologies Berlin, Germany).

2.9. Statistical Analysis

Data were analyzed using RStudio (version 1.1.456) including R (version 3.6.0). Longitudinal plasma protein abundance was assessed by LMM analysis (lme4 package), with drug response (non-response or response), sampling time (baseline, 1 week, 4 weeks, and 10 weeks), and response/time interaction and technical replications as fixed variables, and individual patients nesting for fixed variables and individuals as random variables. In the GEE analysis (geesmv package), we merged plasma abundance as the median of two or three technical replicates and then analyzed drug response, sampling time, and drug/sampling time. The working correlation structure was set independently, and Gaussian estimation was performed.

Clustering analysis was based on median protein concentrations in each group (responders and non-responders) at the four time points, and t-stochastic neighbor embedding (t-SNE) [34] (perplexity = 2, theta = 0, and dims = 2) and affinity propagation (method = correlation symmetry matrix and Spearman) were computed using Rtsne and apcluster [35] packages, respectably. Other software packages included ggline for scatter plots and psygenet2r for mapping proteins on the psychiatric disorders gene association network (PsyGeNet) at database = "ALL" [36]. To control type I error by multiple comparisons, we applied the Bayesian sequential goodness of fit metatest (SGoF) method of default option (alpha = 0.05, gamma = 0.05, P0 = 0.5, a0 = 1, b0 = 1) in the SGoF R package [37] for p-values of response/time interaction by LMM analysis and Benjamini–Hochberg procedure [38] for p-values of MRM paired analysis, and then, we calculated permutated p-values for correlation analysis [39].

2.10. Literature Search

We performed a literature search on PubTabor central [40] using the keywords "protein name" AND "major depressive disorder" and identified 48 plasma proteins (37 proteins showing significance for response/interaction term in LMM and 11 proteins that significantly correlate with two or more psychiatric indexes). As used here, PubTator Central (PTC) is an online-based web page that automatically annotates the association between genes and diseases in PubMed abstracts and PMC full-text articles.

3. Results

3.1. Demographic and Clinical Characteristics of Study Subjects

The baseline characteristics of the ten study subjects, five responders, and five non-responders, are summarized in Table 1. Mean (standard deviation (SD)) subject age was similar in responders (44.2 (14.2) years) and non-responders (42.8 (16.4) years). There were no significant differences between the two groups in affective symptoms and disease severity, including their scores on the Montgomery and Asberg Depression Rating Scale (MADRS), the Clinical Global Impression-Severity (CGI-S), Beck's Depression Inventory (BDI), the Hamilton Rating Scale for Depression (HAM-D), the Clinically Useful Depression Outcome Scale (CUDOS), and the World Health Organization Quality of Life abbreviated version scores including physical, psychological, social, and environmental quality of life (Supplementary Table S1).

Table 1. Demographic and clinical variables of study subjects.

Variable	Responders (N = 5)	Non-Responders (N = 5)	p-Value
Age (SD)	44.2 (14.2)	42.8 (16.4)	0.841
Male (%)	1 (20)	1 (20)	1.000
Age at onset (SD)	41.8 (11.9)	33.4 (9.8)	0.093
Body mass index (kg/m^2) (SD)	23.1 (3.7)	24.7 (4.6)	0.309
Clinical characteristics at baseline			
Montgomery and Asberg Depression Rating Scale (SD)	31.0 (4.6)	28.8 (2.5)	0.599
Clinical Global Impression-Severity (SD)	5.0 (0.7)	4.2 (1.3)	0.344
Beck's Depression Inventory (SD)	32.6 (7.3)	26.8 (3.6)	0.206
Hamilton Rating Scale for Depression (SD)	21.6 (3.4)	21.0 (2.9)	1.000
Clinically Useful Depression Outcome Scale (SD)	38.4 (12.8)	40.4 (3.0)	0.917
World Health Organization Quality of Life abbreviated version			
Physical quality of life (SD)	8.8 (1.7)	8.5 (0.9)	0.831
Psychological quality of life (SD)	8.0 (0.8)	8.3 (1.7)	0.827
Social quality of life (SD)	10.1 (1.5)	11.7 (2.4)	0.193
Environmental quality of life (SD)	10.1 (1.7)	10.1 (1.1)	0.914

p-values appropriately calculated using the Mann–Whitney U test or Fisher's exact test.

3.2. Plasma Sample Preparations and Development of LC-MS/MS

Four plasma samples were obtained from each of the ten patients, for a total of 40 samples, and their proteins profiled by LC-MS/MS, with each sample assayed in duplicate or triplicate. A total of 1159 proteins were identified, with 684 proteins quantified by more than half and 206 proteins completely quantified in 104 of the LC-MS/MS measurements (Supplementary Table S2). Before comparing plasma protein abundance by the label-free quantification (LFQ) method, six relatively stable and abundant endogenous proteins (BTD, C8B, C1S, ITIH2, IGFALS, and SERPINA3) were chosen for data normalization of the abundance of other proteins, as described in the Materials and Methods section [41,42]. Following normalization of protein abundances in all experiments, sample-to-sample variations were corrected (Supplementary Figure S1A–C). Normalized abundances showed statistically significant correlations with the concentrations of plasma proteins (ng/mL) in the plasma proteome database [43], with a Pearson's correlation coefficient of 0.677 (adjusted p-value < 0.001; Supplementary Figure S1D). Assuming technical variations were exceedingly small, only 346 detected proteins measured at one time in each individual sample were considered, followed by the elimination of 24 proteins associated with plasma depletion, including 14 plasma depletion target proteins and ten immunoglobulin-related proteins, and six normalization factors. A total of 316 proteins were analyzed in the next step, with missing values determined by a least-squares regression approach (Supplementary Table S3) [31,44].

3.3. Time-Dependent Changes in Plasma Proteins in Responders and Non-Responders

Statistical comparisons of paired plasma protein abundances at baseline and after 1, 4, and 10 weeks of treatment showed that seven, four, and six proteins, respectively, were upregulated in responders and 16, 17, and 10 proteins, respectively, were upregulated in non-responders using the Mann–Whitney test without correction (p-value < 0.05; Figure 1A). The Venn diagram of the three time points, T_1, T_4, and T_{10} is shown in Figure 1B. Proteins upregulated in non-responders were associated with responses to wounding and stimuli, responses to wounding, and tube morphogenesis in the gene ontology (GO) biological process (Figure 1C). These findings may reflect the greater number of active inflammatory pathways with neural circuits of the brain in non-responders [45]. Proteins that fit the GO terms extracellular structure organization, regulation of complement activation, and triglyceride-rich lipoprotein particle remodeling were enriched in both groups.

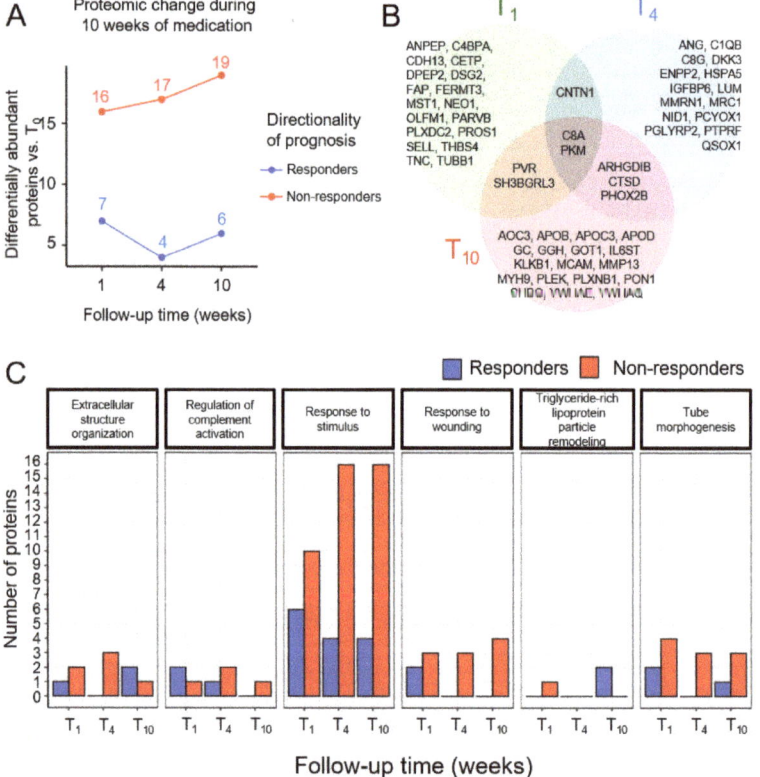

Figure 1. Plasma proteomic analyses and functional annotations identifying changes in differentially abundant proteins over the first week of drug administration. (**A**) Time-dependent up- and downregulation of differentially abundant proteins compared with the start of drug administration; T_0. The number of proteins altered at each time point is shown above each time point. (**B**) Venn diagram of proteins differentially abundant at T_1, T_4, and T_{10} vs. T_0. (**C**) Gene ontology terms of proteins differentially up- and downregulated at T_1, T_4, and T_{10} vs. T_0.

LMM is appropriate for identifying differentially abundant plasma proteins based on longitudinal proteome data. The response/time interaction term is important in measuring inter-group differences in time-dependent responsiveness to SSRIs. Through the LMM multiple comparison analysis, we identified 37 significant proteins which were corrected by a SGoF method [37] (adjusted p-value < 0.05; response/time interaction term). These proteins over time, as well as the between-group differences, are shown as lowest adjusted p-values in Table 2.

Table 2. 37 differentially abundant proteins corresponding to response/time interaction.

UNIPROT Accession	Adjusted p-Value	Gene Name	Protein Name	Cluster No.	COR [a]
P04278	2.70×10^{-3}	SHBG	Sex hormone-binding globulin	5	0.12
P05090	2.95×10^{-3}	APOD	Apolipoprotein D	6	−0.34 [b]
Q06033	4.01×10^{-3}	ITIH3	Inter-alpha-trypsin inhibitor heavy chain H3	5	−0.21
P08567	4.36×10^{-3}	PLEK	Pleckstrin	4	0.04
P04275	4.69×10^{-3}	VWF	von Willebrand factor	6	−0.19
P52566	5.11×10^{-3}	ARHGDIB	Rho GDP-dissociation inhibitor 2	1	−0.15
P02656	6.89×10^{-3}	APOC3	Apolipoprotein C-III	6	−0.06
P06276	7.13×10^{-3}	BCHE	Cholinesterase	6	−0.11
P27169	8.89×10^{-3}	PON1	Serum paraoxonase/arylesterase 1	5	−0.08
P22105-4	9.85×10^{-3}	TNXB	Tenascin-X	6	−0.25
P02774-3	1.09×10^{-2}	GC	Vitamin D-binding protein	5	0.04
P0C0L5	1.10×10^{-2}	C4B	Complement C4-B	5	−0.21
P02649	1.15×10^{-2}	APOE	Apolipoprotein E	6	−0.04
P07339	1.45×10^{-2}	CTSD	Cathepsin D	4	0.02
Q92820	1.50×10^{-2}	GGH	Gamma-glutamyl hydrolase	5	−0.01
P09172	1.69×10^{-2}	DBH	Dopamine beta-hydroxylase	2	0.03
P40189	1.75×10^{-2}	IL6ST	Interleukin-6 receptor subunit beta	4	0.15
Q8NBP7	1.81×10^{-2}	PCSK9	Proprotein convertase subtilisin/kexin type 9	3	−0.14
Q16610	1.83×10^{-2}	ECM1	Extracellular matrix protein 1	2	0.02
P62258	1.83×10^{-2}	YWHAE	14-3-3 protein epsilon	6	0.18
P80188	1.83×10^{-2}	LCN2	Neutrophil gelatinase-associated lipocalin	6	−0.11
Q9H299	1.99×10^{-2}	SH3BGRL3	SH3 domain-binding glutamic acid-rich-like protein 3	1	0.13
P27918	2.05×10^{-2}	CFP	Properdin	6	0.08
P08571	2.12×10^{-2}	CD14	Monocyte differentiation antigen CD14	2	0.24
P08697	2.33×10^{-2}	SERPINF2	Alpha-2-antiplasmin	5	0.22
P36980	2.34×10^{-2}	CFHR2	Complement factor H-related protein 2	4	0.16
P08253	2.57×10^{-2}	MMP2	72 kDa type IV collagenase	6	0.13
P13671	2.65×10^{-2}	C6	Complement component C6	5	0.13
O43852-3	2.80×10^{-2}	CALU	Calumenin	3	0.10
P14543	2.93×10^{-2}	NID1	Nidogen-1	4	−0.05
P35579	2.95×10^{-2}	MYH9	Myosin-9	1	0.05
P05160	3.70×10^{-2}	F13B	Coagulation factor XIII B chain	6	−0.17
P02765	3.75×10^{-2}	AHSG	Alpha-2-HS-glycoprotein	2	0.20
Q99453	3.85×10^{-2}	PHOX2B	Paired mesoderm homeobox protein 2B	2	−0.12
O43157	4.01×10^{-2}	PLXNB1	Plexin-B1	5	−0.01
P06396	4.26×10^{-2}	GSN	Gelsolin	6	0.04
O43866	4.41×10^{-2}	CD5L	CD5 antigen-like	3	−0.27

[a] Spearman's correlation coefficient of protein abundance and Montgomery and Asberg Depression Rating Scale (MADRS) for each protein. [b] Adjusted p-values < 0.05 on a permutated correlation test based on Spearman's coefficient analysis.

To better understand the abundance patterns and to cluster proteins with similar patterns, protein abundance at three different times (T_1, T_4, and T_{10}) was subtracted from that at baseline (T_0), followed by t-SNE and affinity propagation (Figure 2A). Six clusters of unique patterns were obtained (Figure 2B). The three and five proteins in clusters 1 and 4, respectively, decreased over time in responders and increased over time in non-responders. Cluster 2, which included five proteins, showed little change over time in responders but decreased over time in non-responders. In cluster 3, three proteins showed increase from week 1 and appeared flat week 4 onward in responders; conversely, the proteins showed a sharp decrease at week 4 and then flattened at week 10 in non-responders. In cluster 5, 10 proteins showed little change over time in responders but increased over time in non-responders. In cluster 6, 11 proteins showed decreases at 4 weeks and increases at 10 weeks in responders but little change over time in non-responders. The individual abundance profiles of the 37 proteins are shown in Supplementary Figure S2.

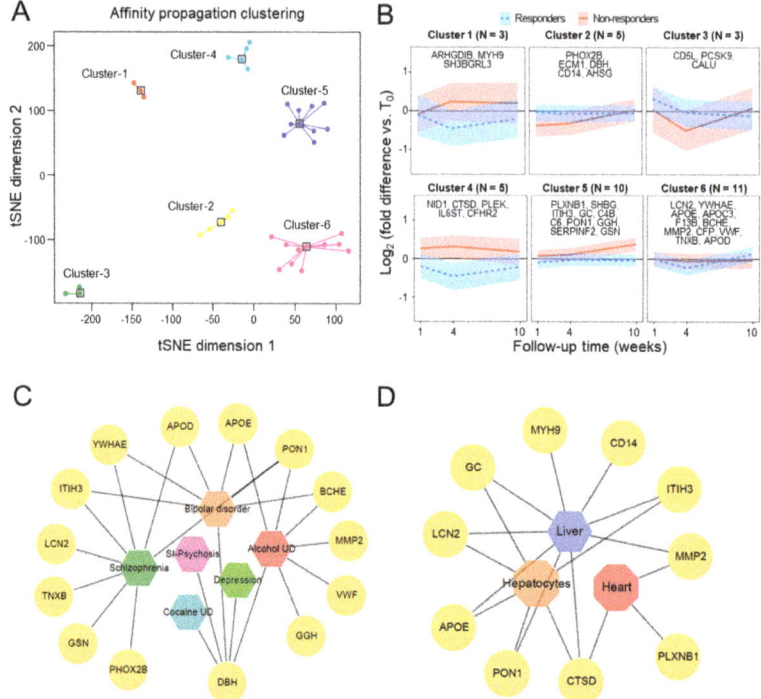

Figure 2. Affinity propagation clustering, profile analysis, and public database search of the 37 proteins found to differ significantly in the response/time interaction of linear mixed model (LMM). (**A**) Identification of seven protein clusters by t-SNE-based affinity propagation clustering. (**B**) Change over time in protein amount in responders and non-responders. (**C**) Association of 14 proteins found on PsyGeNet with psychiatric diseases. (**D**) Association of ten proteins found in the DrugMatrix category of Enrichr with responses of rat tissues and cells to selective serotonin reuptake inhibitors (SSRIs).

To assess whether the functional roles of these proteins were associated with antidepressant response and psychiatric disorders, we searched for the 37 proteins in the PsyGeNet (Figure 2C) [36]. APOD, APOE, BCHE, DBH, GGH, GSN, ITIH3, LCN2, MMP2, PHOX2B, PON1, TNXB, VWF, YWHAE, 14 of these proteins were found to be associated with psychiatric symptoms, such as schizophrenia, bipolar disorder, cocaine use disorders, substance-induced psychosis, alcohol use disorders, and depression. In addition, we assessed whether these 37 proteins were associated with citalopram, an analog of escitalopram, by searching responses of rat tissues and cells to SSRIs in the DrugMatrix category of Enrichr [46], a web-based gene enrichment analysis tool. We found that expression of nine proteins, ITIH3, PON1, MMP2, MYH9, APOE, GC, CD14, LCN2, and CTSD, differed significantly in SSRI-treated and control, corn oil-treated rat liver; the expression of seven proteins, ITIH3, PON1, LCN2, APOE, GC, CLU, and CTSD, differed significantly in SSRI- and corn oil-treated rat hepatocytes; and three proteins, PLXNB1, MMP2, and CTSD, differed significantly in SSRI- and corn oil-treated rat hearts (Figure 2D). It indicated that the drug reaction of these proteins causes quantitative changes not only in the blood but also in the organs of the liver and heart.

3.4. External Validation in Public Studies of mRNA Expression

Because we could not find a benchmark study on blood protein-based drug responsiveness to antidepressants, we examined the expression patterns of LMM-significant 37 proteins described in the results of large-scale studies at the blood circulating cell-free mRNA level from two publicly available GEO datasets—(GSE146446 [26] and GSE45468 [27]). Unlike the proteomic study above, the two GEO studies contained results on the effects of patients receiving a placebo. In the first GSE146446 dataset, mRNA expression in the blood of 171 depressed patients was studied, and patients' responses to an antidepressant vs. the placebo were monitored. The antidepressant used was duloxetine. These data contain quantitative mRNA expressions in patients before and after 8 weeks of taking the antidepressant and placebo. There were 96 patients who received the drug, including 75 responders and 21 non-responders; and 107 patients received the placebo, including 44 responders and 63 non-responders. The 37 plasma proteins that were significant in time and response were all found in the dataset, and these were analyzed by LMM. Among them, *MYH9* represented significance for the treatment/response/time interaction term, *PCSK9* showed significance for the treatment/response interaction term (p-value < 0.05), and *PLEK* showed significance for treatment/response and treatment/time/response interaction terms (p-value < 0.05; Figure 3A). The second GSE45468 dataset reflected blood mRNA expression in 52 patients. These data included mRNA expression in patients before and after 6 h, 24 h, and 2 weeks of infusion of infliximab and a placebo. There were 23 patients who received the drug, including 12 responders and 11 non-responders, and there were 15 responders and 14 non-responders among 29 patients who received the placebo. In this dataset, only 13 out of 37 proteins were found and subjected to LMM analysis. Among them, *CALU* represented significance for the treatment/time/response interaction term (p-value < 0.05), and *CTSD* and *SH3BGRL3* represented significance for the treatment/response interaction term (p-value < 0.05; Figure 3B).

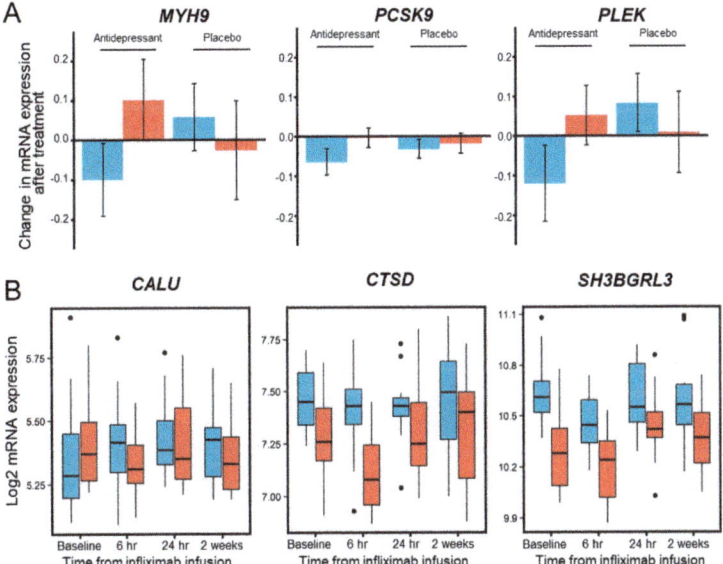

Figure 3. External validation of LMM-significant 37 proteins in two public GEO datasets (GSE146446 and GSE45468). (**A**) In the GSE146446 dataset, the quantitative mRNA expression changes in three genes, *MYH9*, *PCSK9*, and *PLEK*, before and after 8 weeks of taking the antidepressant and placebo in responders (blue color) and non-responders (red color). Error bars represent standard error of the mean. (**B**) In the GSE45468 dataset, the mRNA expression level of patients for three genes, *CALU*, *CTSD* and *SH3BGRL3*, before infliximab infusion and after 6 h, 24 h, and 2 weeks is shown in box plots. Responders are shown in blue color and non-responders are shown in red color.

3.5. LC-MRM/MS Validation of Candidate Plasma Proteins Predictive of Early Response

The differentially abundant ten proteins that were commonly significant between two groups at baseline, early treatment phase (from baseline to 1 week; Mann–Whitney U test: p-value < 0.05) and on the response/time interaction in LMM were selected (Figure 4A) and validated by serial isotope dilute-MRM/MS [47]. Among them, surrogate peptides were chosen by criteria except for CFHR2, which had no reliable peptide [48,49].

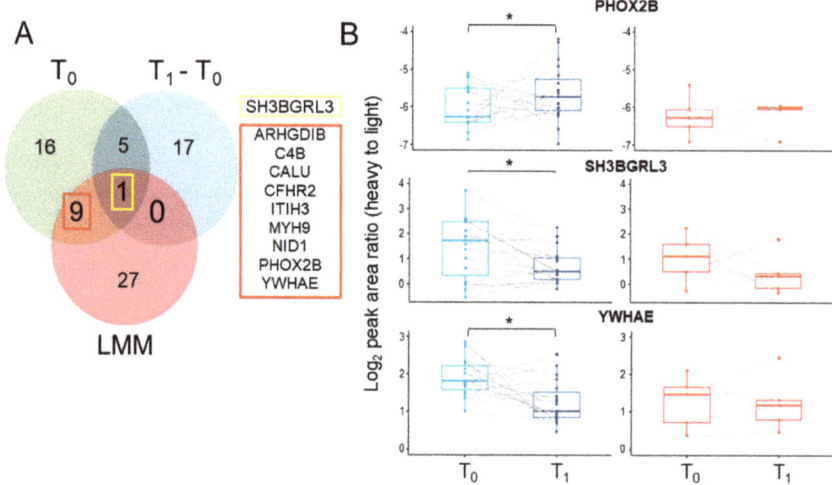

Figure 4. Liquid chromatography-multiple reaction monitoring/mass spectrometry (LC-MRM/MS) validation of ten candidate predictive biomarkers of early-drug response. (**A**) Venn diagram for detection of candidate biomarkers by three statistical analyses (T_0 vs. T_1 and T_1–T_0 between two groups, and response/time terms in LMM). (**B**) Boxplot of abundance of PHOX2B, SH3BGRL3, and YWHAE at T_1 vs. T_0, as determined by LC-MRM/MS, in responders (blue color) and non-responders (red color). * The asterisk identifies the adjusted p-values that are significant at the 0.05 level.

Based on reverse standard calibration curves (Supplementary Figure S3), 15 surrogate peptides representing nine proteins were selected for protein quantification, and a representative peptide with a strong signal for each protein was selected based on the LC-MRM/MS results (Supplementary Table S4). In the validation MRM result, comparing 19 responders and five non-responders, the MYH9 could not be quantified because the heavy-light ratio was below the limit of quantitation. Of the remaining eight proteins, the three proteins, PHOX2B, SH3BGRL3, and YWHAE, showed significant differences on baseline and week 1 in responders (Wilcoxon signed-rank test: FDR-adjusted p-value < 0.05) but not in non-responders (Wilcoxon signed-rank test: FDR-adjusted p-value > 0.05; Figure 4B). After 1 week, PHOX2B protein levels increased significantly, whereas SH3BGRL3 and YWHAE protein levels decreased significantly in responders; conversely, the three proteins did not show any significant changes in non-responders. By contrast, the level of the other five proteins did not differ significantly in the two groups (Supplementary Figure S4).

3.6. Relationship between Plasma Proteins and Psychiatric Morbidity Survey Scores

Because MADRS score is the standard criterion for determining response to drug administration, plasma proteins with high positive or negative correlation with MADRS scores indirectly reflect the efficacy of the drug. Using Spearman's correlation analysis of 316 quantified proteins, we determined the significant correlation relationship between the abundance of the 64 identified plasma proteins and at least one other psychiatric index, such as CGI-S, BDI, HAM-D, CUDOS, and psychological quality of life (PsychoQOL) scores by permutation-based analysis (Supplementary Table S5). Each of these 11 proteins, EXT1, PROC, NUCB1, PROS1, LYVE1, F9, ATRN, HRG, FUCA1, CD109 and ANGPTL6, significantly correlated with two or more of the psychiatric indices (adjusted p-value < 0.05; Figure 5).

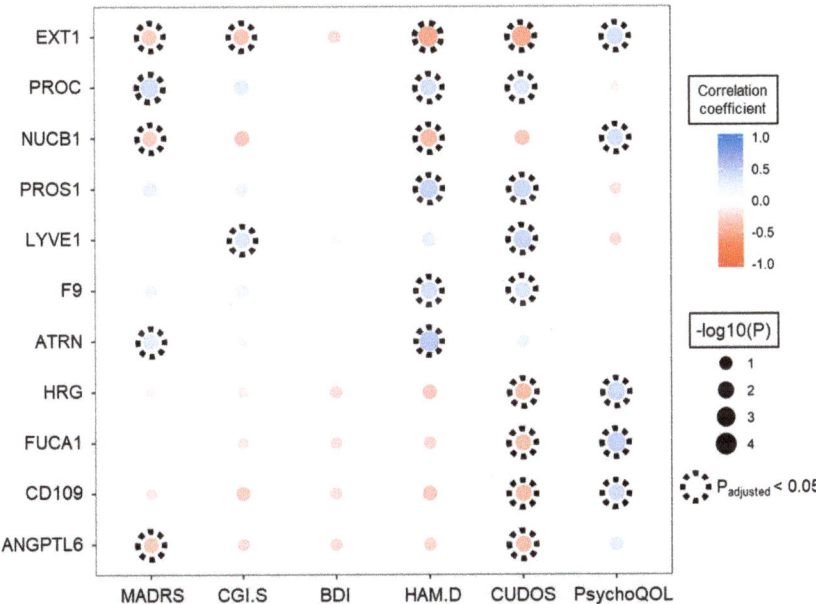

Figure 5. Plots showing correlations between the abundance of 11 plasma proteins and psychological indices; these 11 proteins correlated significantly with two or more of the six indices. Positive and negative correlation coefficients are colored blue and red, respectively, with the size of the bubble indicating the minus log10 adjusted p-value, and the dotted circles indicating significant correlation relationships (adjusted p-value < 0.05).

4. Discussion

In this pilot study, longitudinal analysis with a small sample size (N = 10) may estimate biased variation and cause inflation of type I error. Statistical techniques using a small sample number have been developed in psychiatry for circumstances wherein sample collection is not easy [50]. To discuss this part, we built a GEE model in addition to the LMM model. Compared to LMM, GEE showed greater statistical validity with a devised variance estimate even in a small number of samples [18]. We applied one of them, the Wang and Long method [51], modified bias-correction and efficiency improvement. Consequently, we found seven significant proteins for the time/response interaction term (adjusted p-value < 0.05; Wald test and corrected by SGoF; Supplementary Table S6), overlapping with five (AHSG, IL6ST, APOD, PHOX2B, and SHBG) of 37 significant proteins found in LMM. Unlike a GEE, which is a population level-based model and relatively easy to compute, LMM can consider random effects with technical or biological variation obtained from the whole data, and thus, we considered the LMM technique more suitable than GEEs [15,50,52].

Regarding protein biomarker candidates, we identified 37 plasma proteins significantly associated with MDD by the LMM analysis, and these protein biomarkers could be biologically or physiologically divided into four functional categories through the literature search on PubTabor central [40]. First, six plasma markers, GC, LCN2, ITIH3, VWF, PHOX2B and YWHAE, were previously reported to be associated with SSRI efficacy, with the abundances of GC, LCN2, and ITIH3 in plasma samples associated with response to SSRIs [21,53–55]. Among them, PHOX2B and YWHAE were validated by

LC-MRM/MS analysis in this study. SSRI stress in human brain cells was reported to be associated with a PHOX2B transcription factor [56]. The YWHAE genes have been reported to play a significant role in MDD in the Han Chinese population, with alterations in their protein–protein interactions [57]. The second category is that sex hormones, neurotransmitters, and related proteins have been strongly associated with depression [58]. In this study, plasma SHBG, which has been previously linked to depression [59–61], showed the sharpest difference over time between responders and non-responders (adjusted p-value = 2.70×10^{-3}), decreasing gradually with time in responders and increasing gradually with time in non-responders. We also found that plasma dopamine beta-hydroxylase (DBH) concentrations increased in responders from 4 to 10 weeks, consistent with low plasma DBH levels associated with low activity of the noradrenaline system in patients with depression [62–66]. Third, we found that the plasma proteins GSN and C4B were biomarkers of depression, similar to findings in previous studies using the same LC-MS platform [67–69]. The level of C4B was significantly higher in responders than in non-responders and showed a significant change over time. Subsequently, APOD, PON1, BCHE, and IL6ST were reported to be related to depression, a finding consistent with our results [21,70–74]. Finally, APOE, CSTD and MMP2 that varied genetically and in mRNA level of abundance were reported to be associated with depression. We found that the levels of abundance of two of these proteins, APOE and CSTD, with single nucleotide polymorphisms (SNPs) differed significantly in responders and non-responders [75–78]. The expression of the MMP2 gene in the brain was associated with recurrence of depression [55].

Moreover, 11 plasma proteins that strongly correlated with two or more psychiatric indexes were related with neurological mechanisms and SSRI response. EXT1 was involved in the biosynthesis of heparan sulfate, which played an important role in the development of the nervous systems in the brain, and its deletion caused autism-like behavior in mice [79,80]. NUCB1 is known as a Golgi-resident marker of neurons [81] and interrupts amyloid fibrillation in the brain [82]. PROS1 turned out to be a novel Aβ-responsive protein based on proteome profiling of the hippocampus in the 5XFAD mouse model [83]. LYVE1 was the upregulated gene expressed in SSRI responders to non-responders [84], and differential LYVE1 and MHC II expression was used to identify CNS border-associated macrophages in single cell experiments [85]. ATRN, a neuroprotectant [86], was high in the SSRI responder in blood proteins. CD109 was higher in the disease group in the plasma proteome comparison between the psychotic disorder and the normal group [87].

This preliminary retrospective study had several limitations, including its small sample size, the lack of racial diversity among the study subjects, and the collection of plasma samples at a single center. Proteomics studies using small specimens are frequent. Typically, 10–50 samples are used during the preclinical discovery and validation phase, given the analysis of large data sets and limited timelines [88]. Thus, our results should be considered preliminary findings. All participants were Korean population, and our results may not be generalizable to other ethnic groups. In addition, plasma protein abundance may be affected by the plasma preparation method [89,90], but plasma was rapidly prepared from blood and stored frozen at −80 °C to avoid any pre-analytical effect [91–93]. Moreover, alterations in plasma protein abundance may be dependent on the SSRI type and dosage. In this study, we used samples treated with the same antidepressant (escitalopram) in a relatively certain range of doses, and this may be a limitation in using the results of this study to predict treatment responses with other antidepressants. However, this can be considered the strength of this study. As it is clinically difficult to collect plasma samples using the same type and dose of antidepressants for patients with major depressive disorders in a prospective design, so far, most studies on protein biomarkers for antidepressant treatment response have not been able to control the types or doses of antidepressants [69]. In the view of personalized treatment, predicting whether an individual with depression will benefit from a particular antidepressant is critical in choosing the right antidepressant; furthermore, how different types of antidepressants affect plasma proteins should be considered. In this study, the use of samples treated with the same antidepressant (escitalopram) in a relatively certain range of doses is considered a strength of this study. A controlled prospective study with a large sample size is necessary to establish a clear differential influence of several types of antidepressants on plasma proteins. Therefore, prospective studies in larger patient cohorts are needed to validate our findings.

5. Conclusions

To monitor the association between the efficacy of SSRIs and biomarker abundance, plasma samples were collected for 10 weeks during treatment of patients with MDD. Biomarkers have been identified through longitudinal measurements of protein concentrations, with some showing significant correlation with mental disease variables. These findings suggest that the liquid biopsy technique may solve unmet clinical problems.

Supplementary Materials: The following are available online at http://www.mdpi.com/2227-9059/8/11/455/s1: Figure S1. Box plots for protein abundances in each LC-MS/MS run. Protein abundances (a) before and (b) after endogenous protein-based normalization. (c) Two-dimensional global t-SNE map comparing the responders (blue) and non-responders (red) at each sampling time (1, 4, and 10 weeks) and 3 t-SNE parameters of perplexity. (d) Plasma protein log2 abundances (ng/mL) in the Plasma Proteome Database (bottom) and normalized protein abundance (right). Figure S2. Changes in responders over time to the amounts of 37 significant proteins belonging to six clusters, as determined by response/time interaction. Clusters 1 through 6 included 3, 5, 3, 5, 10 and 11 proteins, respectively. Figure S3. Calibration curves of 15 surrogate peptides relative to nine proteins based on heavy-to-light extracted ion chromatogram ratio. Figure S4. MRM results of five proteins at T_0 vs. T_1. Boxplot of five quantified proteins paired at T_0 and T_1 in responders and non-responders. Table S1. Demographic and clinical characteristics of the ten depressed patients at each of the four hospital visits. Table S2. The 1,159 plasma proteins identified in 104 LC-MS/MS measurements. The notation system is (sample name)_(response)_(time)_(experiment number). Table S3. Log2 transformed normalized protein abundance of 316 proteins in 104 LC-MS/MS measurements. Table S4. MRM parameters optimized for 14 target peptides of nine proteins. Table S5. Spearman's rank correlation coefficients and adjusted *p*-values for the relationships between 316 protein abundance and six psychiatric symptom indices. Table S6. Estimation results in generalized estimation equation.

Author Contributions: Conceptualization, E.Y.K., M.Y.L., H.J.L., K.K. and Y.M.A.; methodology, H.M., J.Y. (Jiyoung Yu), J.Y. (Jeonghum Yeom), M.Y.L., and H.-S.A.; validation, H.-S.A.; formal analysis, H.J.; resources, E.Y.K., H.J.L., and Y.M.A.; data curation, H.-S.A.; writing—original draft preparation, H.-S.A., E.Y.K. and K.K.; writing—review and editing, H.-S.A., E.Y.K., M.Y.L., and K.K.; visualization, H.-S.A.; supervision, K.K.; funding acquisition, E.Y.K., K.K., and Y.M.A. All authors have read and agreed to the published version of the manuscript.

Funding: This research was supported by the Basic Science Research Program through the National Research Foundation of Korea (NRF) funded by the Ministry of Education (NRF-2017R1D1A1B03028787) and the Korean government (MSIT) (NRF-2019M3E5D3073106 and NRF-2019M3E5D30733690).

Acknowledgments: The authors gratefully acknowledge the participation of all patients and investigators involved in this trial.

Conflicts of Interest: Yong Min Ahn has received research support from or served as a speaker for Janssen Korea, Ltd., Lundbeck Korea Co., Ltd., and Korea Otsuka Pharmaceutical. Janssen Korea, Ltd., Lundbeck Korea Co., Ltd., and Korea Otsuka Pharmaceutical and the funder had no role in the design of the study; in the collection, analyses, or interpretation of data; in the writing of the manuscript, or in the decision to publish the results.

Abbreviations

MDD	Major depressive disorder
SSRIs	Selective serotonin reuptake inhibitors
STAR*D	Sequenced Treatment Alternative to Relieve Depression
LC-MS/MS	Liquid chromatography tandem mass spectrometry
MEM	mixed-effect model
GEE	generalized estimating equation
LMM	Linear mixed model
LC-MRM/MS	Liquid chromatography-multiple reaction monitoring/mass spectrometry
LFQ	Label-free quantification
SD	Standard deviation

MADRS	Montgomery and Asberg Depression Rating Scale
CGI-S	Clinical Global Impression-Severity
BDI	Beck's Depression Inventory
HAM-D	Hamilton Rating Scale for Depression
CUDOS	Clinically Useful Depression Outcome Scale
GO	Gene ontology
SGoF	Sequential goodness of fit metatest
t-SNE	t-stochastic neighbor embedding
PsyGeNet	Psychiatric disorders gene association network
PsychoQOL	Psychological quality of life
DBH	Dopamine beta-hydroxylase
NSF	Normalization scaling factor

References

1. Vos, T.; Flaxman, A.D.; Naghavi, M.; Lozano, R.; Michaud, C.; Ezzati, M.; Shibuya, K.; Salomon, J.A.; Abdalla, S.; Aboyans, V.; et al. Years lived with disability (YLDs) for 1160 sequelae of 289 diseases and injuries 1990–2010: A systematic analysis for the Global Burden of Disease Study 2010. *Lancet* **2012**, *380*, 2163–2196. [CrossRef]
2. Fava, M.; Kendler, K.S. Major depressive disorder. *Neuron* **2000**, *28*, 335–341. [CrossRef]
3. Burcusa, S.L.; Iacono, W.G. Risk for recurrence in depression. *Clin. Psychol. Rev.* **2007**, *27*, 959–985. [CrossRef] [PubMed]
4. Cain, R.A. Navigating the Sequenced Treatment Alternatives to Relieve Depression (STAR*D) study: Practical outcomes and implications for depression treatment in primary care. *Prim. Care* **2007**, *34*, 505–519. [CrossRef] [PubMed]
5. Rush, A.J.; Trivedi, M.H.; Wisniewski, S.R.; Stewart, J.W.; Nierenberg, A.A.; Thase, M.E.; Ritz, L.; Biggs, M.M.; Warden, D.; Luther, J.F.; et al. Bupropion-SR, sertraline, or venlafaxine-XR after failure of SSRIs for depression. *N. Engl. J. Med.* **2006**, *354*, 1231–1242. [CrossRef]
6. Martins-de-Souza, D.; Harris, L.W.; Guest, P.C.; Turck, C.W.; Bahn, S. The role of proteomics in depression research. *Eur. Arch. Psychiatry Clin. Neurosci.* **2010**, *260*, 499–506. [CrossRef]
7. Turck, C.W.; Guest, P.C.; Maccarrone, G.; Ising, M.; Kloiber, S.; Lucae, S.; Holsboer, F.; Martins-de-Souza, D. Proteomic Differences in Blood Plasma Associated with Antidepressant Treatment Response. *Front. Mol. Neurosci.* **2017**, *10*, 272. [CrossRef]
8. Chan, M.K.; Cooper, J.D.; Bot, M.; Birkenhager, T.K.; Bergink, V.; Drexhage, H.A.; Steiner, J.; Rothermundt, M.; Penninx, B.W.; Bahn, S. Blood-based immune-endocrine biomarkers of treatment response in depression. *J. Psychiatr. Res.* **2016**, *83*, 249–259. [CrossRef]
9. Feng, Z.; Diehr, P.; Peterson, A.; McLerran, D. Selected statistical issues in group randomized trials. *Annu. Rev. Public Health* **2001**, *22*, 167–187. [CrossRef]
10. Gibbons, R.D.; Hedeker, D.; DuToit, S. Advances in analysis of longitudinal data. *Annu. Rev. Clin. Psychol.* **2010**, *6*, 79–107. [CrossRef]
11. Laird, N.M.; Ware, J.H. Random-effects models for longitudinal data. *Biometrics* **1982**, *38*, 963–974. [CrossRef] [PubMed]
12. Liang, K.Y.; Zeger, S.L. Longitudinal Data-Analysis Using Generalized Linear-Models. *Biometrika* **1986**, *73*, 13–22. [CrossRef]
13. Pedroza, C.; Truong, V.T.T. Estimating relative risks in multicenter studies with a small number of centers—Which methods to use? A simulation study. *Trials* **2017**, *18*, 512. [CrossRef] [PubMed]
14. Aktas Samur, A.; Coskunfirat, N.; Saka, O. Comparison of predictor approaches for longitudinal binary outcomes: Application to anesthesiology data. *PeerJ* **2014**, *2*, e648. [CrossRef] [PubMed]
15. McNeish, D.M.; Harring, J.R. Clustered data with small sample sizes: Comparing the performance of model-based and design-based approaches. *Commun. Stat-Simul. C* **2017**, *46*, 855–869. [CrossRef]
16. Zhou, C.; Simpson, K.L.; Lancashire, L.J.; Walker, M.J.; Dawson, M.J.; Unwin, R.D.; Rembielak, A.; Price, P.; West, C.; Dive, C.; et al. Statistical considerations of optimal study design for human plasma proteomics and biomarker discovery. *J. Proteome Res.* **2012**, *11*, 2103–2113. [CrossRef]

17. Cairns, D.A.; Barrett, J.H.; Billingham, L.J.; Stanley, A.J.; Xinarianos, G.; Field, J.K.; Johnson, P.J.; Selby, P.J.; Banks, R.E. Sample size determination in clinical proteomic profiling experiments using mass spectrometry for class comparison. *Proteomics* **2009**, *9*, 74–86. [CrossRef]
18. Wang, M.; Kong, L.; Li, Z.; Zhang, L. Covariance estimators for generalized estimating equations (GEE) in longitudinal analysis with small samples. *Stat. Med.* **2016**, *35*, 1706–1721. [CrossRef]
19. Ren, J.; Zhao, G.; Sun, X.; Liu, H.; Jiang, P.; Chen, J.; Wu, Z.; Peng, D.; Fang, Y.; Zhang, C. Identification of plasma biomarkers for distinguishing bipolar depression from major depressive disorder by iTRAQ-coupled LC-MS/MS and bioinformatics analysis. *Psychoneuroendocrinology* **2017**, *86*, 17–24. [CrossRef]
20. Park, D.I.; Stambuk, J.; Razdorov, G.; Pucic-Bakovic, M.; Martins-de-Souza, D.; Lauc, G.; Turck, C.W. Blood plasma/IgG N-glycome biosignatures associated with major depressive disorder symptom severity and the antidepressant response. *Sci. Rep.* **2018**, *8*, 179. [CrossRef]
21. Lee, M.Y.; Kim, E.Y.; Kim, S.H.; Cho, K.C.; Ha, K.; Kim, K.P.; Ahn, Y.M. Discovery of serum protein biomarkers in drug-free patients with major depressive disorder. *Prog. Neuropsychopharmacol. Biol. Psychiatry* **2016**, *69*, 60–68. [CrossRef] [PubMed]
22. Zheng, P.; Fang, Z.; Xu, X.J.; Liu, M.L.; Du, X.; Zhang, X.; Wang, H.; Zhou, J.; Xie, P. Metabolite signature for diagnosing major depressive disorder in peripheral blood mononuclear cells. *J. Affect Disord.* **2016**, *195*, 75–81. [CrossRef] [PubMed]
23. Kim, E.Y.; Kim, S.H.; Lee, H.J.; Lee, N.Y.; Kim, H.Y.; Park, C.H.K.; Ahn, Y.M. A randomized, double-blind, 6-week prospective pilot study on the efficacy and safety of dose escalation in non-remitters in comparison to those of the standard dose of escitalopram for major depressive disorder. *J. Affect. Disord.* **2019**, *259*, 91–97. [CrossRef] [PubMed]
24. Deutsch, E.W.; Bandeira, N.; Sharma, V.; Perez-Riverol, Y.; Carver, J.J.; Kundu, D.J.; Garcia-Seisdedos, D.; Jarnuczak, A.F.; Hewapathirana, S.; Pullman, B.S.; et al. The ProteomeXchange consortium in 2020: Enabling 'big data' approaches in proteomics. *Nucleic Acids Res.* **2020**, *48*, D1145–D1152. [CrossRef]
25. Ahn, H.S.; Kim, J.H.; Jeong, H.; Yu, J.; Yeom, J.; Song, S.H.; Kim, S.S.; Kim, I.J.; Kim, K. Differential Urinary Proteome Analysis for Predicting Prognosis in Type 2 Diabetes Patients with and without Renal Dysfunction. *Int. J. Mol. Sci.* **2020**, *21*, 4236. [CrossRef]
26. Belzeaux, R.; Gorgievski, V.; Fiori, L.M.; Lopez, J.P.; Grenier, J.; Lin, R.; Nagy, C.; Ibrahim, E.C.; Gascon, E.; Courtet, P.; et al. GPR56/ADGRG1 is associated with response to antidepressant treatment. *Nat. Commun.* **2020**, *11*, 1635. [CrossRef]
27. Mehta, D.; Raison, C.L.; Woolwine, B.J.; Haroon, E.; Binder, E.B.; Miller, A.H.; Felger, J.C. Transcriptional signatures related to glucose and lipid metabolism predict treatment response to the tumor necrosis factor antagonist infliximab in patients with treatment-resistant depression. *Brain Behav. Immun.* **2013**, *31*, 205–215. [CrossRef]
28. Goh, W.W.B.; Wang, W.; Wong, L. Why Batch Effects Matter in Omics Data, and How to Avoid Them. *Trends Biotechnol.* **2017**, *35*, 498–507. [CrossRef]
29. Guo, Y.; Zhao, S.; Su, P.F.; Li, C.I.; Ye, F.; Flynn, C.R.; Shyr, Y. Statistical strategies for microRNAseq batch effect reduction. *Transl. Cancer Res.* **2014**, *3*, 260–265. [CrossRef]
30. Sims, A.H.; Smethurst, G.J.; Hey, Y.; Okoniewski, M.J.; Pepper, S.D.; Howell, A.; Miller, C.J.; Clarke, R.B. The removal of multiplicative, systematic bias allows integration of breast cancer gene expression—Improving meta-analysis and prediction of prognosis. *BMC Med. Genom.* **2008**, *1*, 42. [CrossRef]
31. Kim, H.; Golub, G.H.; Park, H. Missing value estimation for DNA microarray gene expression data: Local least squares imputation. *Bioinformatics* **2005**, *21*, 187–198. [CrossRef] [PubMed]
32. Wisniewski, J.R.; Hein, M.Y.; Cox, J.; Mann, M. A "proteomic ruler" for protein copy number and concentration estimation without spike-in standards. *Mol. Cell Proteom.* **2014**, *13*, 3497–3506. [CrossRef] [PubMed]
33. Andersen, C.L.; Jensen, J.L.; Orntoft, T.F. Normalization of real-time quantitative reverse transcription-PCR data: A model-based variance estimation approach to identify genes suited for normalization, applied to bladder and colon cancer data sets. *Cancer Res.* **2004**, *64*, 5245–5250. [CrossRef]
34. van der Maaten, L.; Hinton, G. Visualizing Data using t-SNE. *J. Mach. Learn. Res.* **2008**, *9*, 2579–2605.
35. Bodenhofer, U.; Kothmeier, A.; Hochreiter, S. APCluster: An R package for affinity propagation clustering. *Bioinformatics* **2011**, *27*, 2463–2464. [CrossRef] [PubMed]
36. Gutierrez-Sacristan, A.; Hernandez-Ferrer, C.; Gonzalez, J.R.; Furlong, L.I. psygenet2r: A R/Bioconductor package for the analysis of psychiatric disease genes. *Bioinformatics* **2017**, *33*, 4004–4006. [CrossRef] [PubMed]

37. Carvajal-Rodriguez, A.; de Una-Alvarez, J.; Rolan-Alvarez, E. A new multitest correction (SGoF) that increases its statistical power when increasing the number of tests. *BMC Bioinform.* **2009**, *10*, 209. [CrossRef]
38. Benjamini, Y.; Hochberg, Y. Controlling the False Discovery Rate—A Practical and Powerful Approach to Multiple Testing. *J. R. Stat. Soc. B* **1995**, *57*, 289–300. [CrossRef]
39. Legendre, P. Comparison of permutation methods for the partial correlation and partial Mantel tests. *J. Stat. Comput. Sim.* **2000**, *67*, 37–73. [CrossRef]
40. Wei, C.H.; Allot, A.; Leaman, R.; Lu, Z. PubTator central: Automated concept annotation for biomedical full text articles. *Nucleic Acids Res.* **2019**, *47*, W587–W593. [CrossRef]
41. Ahn, H.S.; Sohn, T.S.; Kim, M.J.; Cho, B.K.; Kim, S.M.; Kim, S.T.; Yi, E.C.; Lee, C. SEPROGADIC—Serum protein-based gastric cancer prediction model for prognosis and selection of proper adjuvant therapy. *Sci. Rep.* **2018**, *8*, 16892. [CrossRef]
42. Martinez-Aguilar, J.; Molloy, M.P. Label-free selected reaction monitoring enables multiplexed quantitation of S100 protein isoforms in cancer cells. *J. Proteome Res.* **2013**, *12*, 3679–3688. [CrossRef] [PubMed]
43. Schwenk, J.M.; Omenn, G.S.; Sun, Z.; Campbell, D.S.; Baker, M.S.; Overall, C.M.; Aebersold, R.; Moritz, R.L.; Deutsch, E.W. The Human Plasma Proteome Draft of 2017: Building on the Human Plasma PeptideAtlas from Mass Spectrometry and Complementary Assays. *J. Proteome Res.* **2017**, *16*, 4299–4310. [CrossRef] [PubMed]
44. Karpievitch, Y.V.; Dabney, A.R.; Smith, R.D. Normalization and missing value imputation for label-free LC-MS analysis. *BMC Bioinform.* **2012**, *13* (Suppl. 16), S5. [CrossRef]
45. Miller, A.H.; Raison, C.L. The role of inflammation in depression: From evolutionary imperative to modern treatment target. *Nat. Rev. Immunol.* **2016**, *16*, 22–34. [CrossRef] [PubMed]
46. Kuleshov, M.V.; Jones, M.R.; Rouillard, A.D.; Fernandez, N.F.; Duan, Q.; Wang, Z.; Koplev, S.; Jenkins, S.L.; Jagodnik, K.M.; Lachmann, A.; et al. Enrichr: A comprehensive gene set enrichment analysis web server 2016 update. *Nucleic Acids Res.* **2016**, *44*, W90–W97. [CrossRef] [PubMed]
47. Kennedy, J.J.; Abbatiello, S.E.; Kim, K.; Yan, P.; Whiteaker, J.R.; Lin, C.; Kim, J.S.; Zhang, Y.; Wang, X.; Ivey, R.G.; et al. Demonstrating the feasibility of large-scale development of standardized assays to quantify human proteins. *Nat. Methods* **2014**, *11*, 149–155. [CrossRef] [PubMed]
48. Kim, J.S.; Lee, Y.; Lee, M.Y.; Shin, J.; Han, J.M.; Yang, E.G.; Yu, M.H.; Kim, S.; Hwang, D.; Lee, C. Multiple reaction monitoring of multiple low-abundance transcription factors in whole lung cancer cell lysates. *J. Proteome Res.* **2013**, *12*, 2582–2596. [CrossRef]
49. Bhowmick, P.; Mohammed, Y.; Borchers, C.H. MRMAssayDB: An integrated resource for validated targeted proteomics assays. *Bioinformatics* **2018**, *34*, 3566–3571. [CrossRef]
50. Muth, C.; Bales, K.L.; Hinde, K.; Maninger, N.; Mendoza, S.P.; Ferrer, E. Alternative Models for Small Samples in Psychological Research: Applying Linear Mixed Effects Models and Generalized Estimating Equations to Repeated Measures Data. *Educ. Psychol. Meas.* **2016**, *76*, 64–87. [CrossRef]
51. Wang, M.; Long, Q. Modified robust variance estimator for generalized estimating equations with improved small-sample performance. *Stat. Med.* **2011**, *30*, 1278–1291. [CrossRef] [PubMed]
52. McNeish, D.; Stapleton, L.M. Modeling Clustered Data with Very Few Clusters. *Multivar Behav. Res.* **2016**, *51*, 495–518. [CrossRef]
53. Lopez-Vilchez, I.; Diaz-Ricart, M.; Navarro, V.; Torramade, S.; Zamorano-Leon, J.; Lopez-Farre, A.; Galan, A.M.; Gasto, C.; Escolar, G. Endothelial damage in major depression patients is modulated by SSRI treatment, as demonstrated by circulating biomarkers and an in vitro cell model. *Transl. Psychiatry* **2016**, *6*, e886. [CrossRef] [PubMed]
54. Fabbri, C.; Corponi, F.; Albani, D.; Raimondi, I.; Forloni, G.; Schruers, K.; Kasper, S.; Kautzky, A.; Zohar, J.; Souery, D.; et al. Pleiotropic genes in psychiatry: Calcium channels and the stress-related FKBP5 gene in antidepressant resistance. *Prog. Neuropsychopharmacol. Biol. Psychiatry* **2018**, *81*, 203–210. [CrossRef] [PubMed]
55. Bobinska, K.; Szemraj, J.; Galecki, P.; Talarowska, M. The role of MMP genes in recurrent depressive disorders and cognitive functions. *Acta Neuropsychiatr.* **2016**, *28*, 221–231. [CrossRef]

56. Fan, Y.; Chen, P.; Raza, M.U.; Szebeni, A.; Szebeni, K.; Ordway, G.A.; Stockmeier, C.A.; Zhu, M.Y. Altered Expression of Phox2 Transcription Factors in the Locus Coeruleus in Major Depressive Disorder Mimicked by Chronic Stress and Corticosterone Treatment In Vivo and In Vitro. *Neuroscience* **2018**, *393*, 123–137. [CrossRef]
57. Liu, J.; Zhang, H.X.; Li, Z.Q.; Li, T.; Li, J.Y.; Wang, T.; Li, Y.; Feng, G.Y.; Shi, Y.Y.; He, L. The YWHAE gene confers risk to major depressive disorder in the male group of Chinese Han population. *Prog. Neuropsychopharmacol. Biol. Psychiatry* **2017**, *77*, 172–177. [CrossRef]
58. Pope, H.G., Jr.; Kouri, E.M.; Hudson, J.I. Effects of supraphysiologic doses of testosterone on mood and aggression in normal men: A randomized controlled trial. *Arch. Gen. Psychiatry* **2000**, *57*, 133–140. [CrossRef]
59. Asselmann, E.; Kische, H.; Haring, R.; Hertel, J.; Schmidt, C.O.; Nauck, M.; Beesdo-Baum, K.; Grabe, H.J.; Pane-Farre, C.A. Prospective associations of androgens and sex hormone-binding globulin with 12-month, lifetime and incident anxiety and depressive disorders in men and women from the general population. *J. Affect. Disord.* **2019**, *245*, 905–911. [CrossRef]
60. Whalley, L.J.; Kutcher, S.; Blackwood, D.H.; Bennie, J.; Dick, H.; Fink, G. Increased plasma LH in manic-depressive illness: Evidence of a state-independent abnormality. *Br. J. Psychiatry* **1987**, *150*, 682–684. [CrossRef]
61. Cakici, N.; Bot, M.; Lamers, F.; Janssen, T.; van der Spek, P.J.; de Haan, L.; Bahn, S.; Penninx, B.; van Beveren, N.J.M. Increased serum levels of leptin and insulin in both schizophrenia and major depressive disorder: A cross-disorder proteomics analysis. *Eur. Neuropsychopharmacol.* **2019**, *29*, 835–846. [CrossRef] [PubMed]
62. Meltzer, H.Y.; Cho, H.W.; Carroll, B.J.; Russo, P. Serum dopamine-beta-hydroxylase activity in the affective psychoses and schizophrenia. Decreased activity in unipolar psychotically depressed patients. *Arch. Gen. Psychiatry* **1976**, *33*, 585–591. [CrossRef] [PubMed]
63. Paclt, I.; Koudelova, J.; Pacltova, D.; Kopeckova, M. Dopamine beta hydroxylase (DBH) plasma activity in childhood mental disorders. *Neuro Endocrinol. Lett.* **2009**, *30*, 604–609. [PubMed]
64. Puzynski, S.; Hauptmann, M.; Rode, A.; Kalinowski, A.; Bidzinska, E.; Beresewicz, M.; Bidzinski, A. Blood MAO/DBH index and the results of the treatment of endogenous depression. *Psychiatr. Pol.* **1990**, *24*, 202–208. [PubMed]
65. Yu, P.H.; O'Sullivan, K.S.; Keegan, D.; Boulton, A.A. Dopamine-beta-hydroxylase and its apparent endogenous inhibitory activity in the plasma of some psychiatric patients. *Psychiatry Res.* **1980**, *3*, 205–210. [CrossRef]
66. Zhou, Y.; Wang, J.; He, Y.; Zhou, J.; Xi, Q.; Song, X.; Ye, Y.; Ying, B. Association between dopamine beta-hydroxylase 19-bp insertion/deletion polymorphism and major depressive disorder. *J. Mol. Neurosci.* **2015**, *55*, 367–371. [CrossRef]
67. Zhan, Y.; Yang, Y.T.; You, H.M.; Cao, D.; Liu, C.Y.; Zhou, C.J.; Wang, Z.Y.; Bai, S.J.; Mu, J.; Wu, B.; et al. Plasma-based proteomics reveals lipid metabolic and immunoregulatory dysregulation in post-stroke depression. *Eur. Psychiatry* **2014**, *29*, 307–315. [CrossRef]
68. Wang, Q.; Su, X.; Jiang, X.; Dong, X.; Fan, Y.; Zhang, J.; Yu, C.; Gao, W.; Shi, S.; Jiang, J.; et al. iTRAQ technology-based identification of human peripheral serum proteins associated with depression. *Neuroscience* **2016**, *330*, 291–325. [CrossRef]
69. Stelzhammer, V.; Haenisch, F.; Chan, M.K.; Cooper, J.D.; Steiner, J.; Steeb, H.; Martins-de-Souza, D.; Rahmoune, H.; Guest, P.C.; Bahn, S. Proteomic changes in serum of first onset, antidepressant drug-naive major depression patients. *Int. J. Neuropsychopharmacol.* **2014**, *17*, 1599–1608. [CrossRef]
70. Ramsey, J.M.; Cooper, J.D.; Bot, M.; Guest, P.C.; Lamers, F.; Weickert, C.S.; Penninx, B.W.; Bahn, S. Sex Differences in Serum Markers of Major Depressive Disorder in the Netherlands Study of Depression and Anxiety (NESDA). *PLoS ONE* **2016**, *11*, e0156624. [CrossRef]
71. Moreira, E.G.; Correia, D.G.; Bonifacio, K.L.; Moraes, J.B.; Cavicchioli, F.L.; Nunes, C.S.; Nunes, S.O.V.; Vargas, H.O.; Barbosa, D.S.; Maes, M. Lowered PON1 activities are strongly associated with depression and bipolar disorder, recurrence of (hypo)mania and depression, increased disability and lowered quality of life. *World J. Biol. Psychiatry* **2019**, *20*, 368–380. [CrossRef] [PubMed]
72. Ullas Kamath, S.; Chaturvedi, A.; Bhaskar Yerrapragada, D.; Kundapura, N.; Amin, N.; Devaramane, V. Increased Levels of Acetylcholinesterase, Paraoxonase 1, and Copper in Patients with Moderate Depression- a Preliminary Study. *Rep. Biochem. Mol. Biol.* **2019**, *7*, 174–180. [PubMed]

73. Siwek, M.; Sowa-Kucma, M.; Styczen, K.; Misztak, P.; Nowak, R.J.; Szewczyk, B.; Dudek, D.; Rybakowski, J.K.; Nowak, G.; Maes, M. Associations of Serum Cytokine Receptor Levels with Melancholia, Staging of Illness, Depressive and Manic Phases, and Severity of Depression in Bipolar Disorder. *Mol. Neurobiol.* **2017**, *54*, 5883–5893. [CrossRef] [PubMed]
74. Kohler, C.A.; Freitas, T.H.; Maes, M.; de Andrade, N.Q.; Liu, C.S.; Fernandes, B.S.; Stubbs, B.; Solmi, M.; Veronese, N.; Herrmann, N.; et al. Peripheral cytokine and chemokine alterations in depression: A meta-analysis of 82 studies. *Acta Psychiatr. Scand.* **2017**, *135*, 373–387. [CrossRef]
75. Zhou, R.; Lu, Y.; Han, Y.; Li, X.; Lou, H.; Zhu, L.; Zhen, X.; Duan, S. Mice heterozygous for cathepsin D deficiency exhibit mania-related behavior and stress-induced depression. *Prog. Neuropsychopharmacol. Biol. Psychiatry* **2015**, *63*, 110–118. [CrossRef]
76. Heun, R.; Ptok, U.; Kolsch, H.; Maier, W.; Jessen, F. Contribution of apolipoprotein E and cathepsin D genotypes to the familial aggregation of Alzheimer's disease. *Dement. Geriatr. Cogn. Disord.* **2004**, *18*, 151–158. [CrossRef]
77. Zhao, F.; Yue, Y.; Jiang, H.; Yuan, Y. Shared genetic risk factors for depression and stroke. *Prog. Neuropsychopharmacol. Biol. Psychiatry* **2019**, *93*, 55–70. [CrossRef]
78. Tsang, R.S.; Mather, K.A.; Sachdev, P.S.; Reppermund, S. Systematic review and meta-analysis of genetic studies of late-life depression. *Neurosci. Biobehav. Rev.* **2017**, *75*, 129–139. [CrossRef]
79. Okada, M.; Nadanaka, S.; Shoji, N.; Tamura, J.; Kitagawa, H. Biosynthesis of heparan sulfate in EXT1-deficient cells. *Biochem. J.* **2010**, *428*, 463–471. [CrossRef]
80. Irie, F.; Badie-Mahdavi, H.; Yamaguchi, Y. Autism-like socio-communicative deficits and stereotypies in mice lacking heparan sulfate. *Proc. Natl. Acad. Sci. USA* **2012**, *109*, 5052–5056. [CrossRef]
81. Tulke, S.; Williams, P.; Hellysaz, A.; Ilegems, E.; Wendel, M.; Broberger, C. Nucleobindin 1 (NUCB1) is a Golgi-resident marker of neurons. *Neuroscience* **2016**, *314*, 179–188. [CrossRef]
82. Gupta, R.; Kapoor, N.; Raleigh, D.P.; Sakmar, T.P. Nucleobindin 1 caps human islet amyloid polypeptide protofibrils to prevent amyloid fibril formation. *J. Mol. Biol.* **2012**, *421*, 378–389. [CrossRef] [PubMed]
83. Kim, D.K.; Han, D.; Park, J.; Choi, H.; Park, J.C.; Cha, M.Y.; Woo, J.; Byun, M.S.; Lee, D.Y.; Kim, Y.; et al. Deep proteome profiling of the hippocampus in the 5XFAD mouse model reveals biological process alterations and a novel biomarker of Alzheimer's disease. *Exp. Mol. Med.* **2019**, *51*, 1–17. [CrossRef] [PubMed]
84. Woo, H.I.; Lim, S.W.; Myung, W.; Kim, D.K.; Lee, S.Y. Differentially expressed genes related to major depressive disorder and antidepressant response: Genome-wide gene expression analysis. *Exp. Mol. Med.* **2018**, *50*, 92. [CrossRef] [PubMed]
85. Mrdjen, D.; Pavlovic, A.; Hartmann, F.J.; Schreiner, B.; Utz, S.G.; Leung, B.P.; Lelios, I.; Heppner, F.L.; Kipnis, J.; Merkler, D.; et al. High-Dimensional Single-Cell Mapping of Central Nervous System Immune Cells Reveals Distinct Myeloid Subsets in Health, Aging, and Disease. *Immunity* **2018**, *48*, 380–395 e386. [CrossRef]
86. Paz, J.; Yao, H.; Lim, H.S.; Lu, X.Y.; Zhang, W. The neuroprotective role of attractin in neurodegeneration. *Neurobiol. Aging* **2007**, *28*, 1446–1456. [CrossRef]
87. English, J.A.; Lopez, L.M.; O'Gorman, A.; Focking, M.; Hryniewiecka, M.; Scaife, C.; Sabherwal, S.; Wynne, K.; Dicker, P.; Rutten, B.P.F.; et al. Blood-Based Protein Changes in Childhood Are Associated With Increased Risk for Later Psychotic Disorder: Evidence From a Nested Case-Control Study of the ALSPAC Longitudinal Birth Cohort. *Schizophr. Bull.* **2018**, *44*, 297–306. [CrossRef]
88. Surinova, S.; Schiess, R.; Huttenhain, R.; Cerciello, F.; Wollscheid, B.; Aebersold, R. On the development of plasma protein biomarkers. *J. Proteome Res.* **2011**, *10*, 5–16. [CrossRef]
89. Ahn, H.S.; Park, S.J.; Jung, H.G.; Woo, S.J.; Lee, C. Quantification of protein markers monitoring the pre-analytical effect of blood storage time before plasma isolation using (15) N metabolically labeled recombinant proteins. *J. Mass Spectrom.* **2018**, *53*, 1189–1197. [CrossRef]
90. Kaisar, M.; van Dullemen, L.F.A.; Thezenas, M.L.; Zeeshan Akhtar, M.; Huang, H.; Rendel, S.; Charles, P.D.; Fischer, R.; Ploeg, R.J.; Kessler, B.M. Plasma degradome affected by variable storage of human blood. *Clin. Proteom.* **2016**, *13*, 26. [CrossRef]
91. Rai, A.J.; Vitzthum, F. Effects of preanalytical variables on peptide and protein measurements in human serum and plasma: Implications for clinical proteomics. *Expert Rev. Proteom.* **2006**, *3*, 409–426. [CrossRef] [PubMed]

92. Pasella, S.; Baralla, A.; Canu, E.; Pinna, S.; Vaupel, J.; Deiana, M.; Franceschi, C.; Baggio, G.; Zinellu, A.; Sotgia, S.; et al. Pre-analytical stability of the plasma proteomes based on the storage temperature. *Proteome Sci.* **2013**, *11*, 10. [CrossRef]
93. Ferguson, R.E.; Hochstrasser, D.F.; Banks, R.E. Impact of preanalytical variables on the analysis of biological fluids in proteomic studies. *Proteom. Clin. Appl.* **2007**, *1*, 739–746. [CrossRef] [PubMed]

Publisher's Note: MDPI stays neutral with regard to jurisdictional claims in published maps and institutional affiliations.

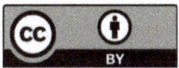

© 2020 by the authors. Licensee MDPI, Basel, Switzerland. This article is an open access article distributed under the terms and conditions of the Creative Commons Attribution (CC BY) license (http://creativecommons.org/licenses/by/4.0/).

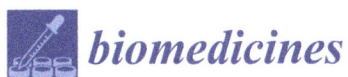

Article

Depression as a Risk Factor for Dementia and Alzheimer's Disease

Vanesa Cantón-Habas [1], Manuel Rich-Ruiz [1,2,*], Manuel Romero-Saldaña [1] and Maria del Pilar Carrera-González [1,3]

[1] Maimónides Institute for Biomedical Research (IMIBIC), University of Córdoba, Reina Sofia University Hospital, 14004 Córdoba, Spain; n92cahav@uco.es (V.C.-H.); z92rosam@uco.es (M.R.-S.); pcarrera@uco.es (M.d.P.C.-G.)
[2] Ciber Fragility and Healthy Aging (CIBERFES), 28001 Madrid, Spain
[3] Experimental and Clinical Physiopathology Research Group, Department of Health Sciences, Faculty of Experimental and Health Sciences, University of Jaén, E-23071 Jaén, Spain
* Correspondence: mrich@uco.es; Tel.: +34-69-542-4299

Received: 24 September 2020; Accepted: 26 October 2020; Published: 28 October 2020

Abstract: Preventing the onset of dementia and Alzheimer's disease (AD), improving the diagnosis, and slowing the progression of these diseases remain a challenge. The aim of this study was to elucidate the association between depression and dementia/AD and to identify possible relationships between these diseases and different sociodemographic and clinical features. In this regard, a case-control study was conducted in Spain in 2018–2019. The definition of a case was: A person ≥ 65 years old with dementia and/or AD and a score of 5–7 on the Global Deterioration Scale (GDS). The sample consisted of 125 controls; among the cases, 96 had dementia and 74 had AD. The predictor variables were depression, dyslipidemia, type 2 diabetes mellitus, and hypertension. The results showed that depression, diabetes mellitus, and older age were associated with an increased likelihood of developing AD, with an Odds Ratio (OR) of 12.9 (95% confidence interval (CI): 4.3–39.9), 2.8 (95% CI: 1.1–7.1) and 1.15 (95% CI: 1.1–1.2), respectively. Those subjects with treated dyslipidemia were less likely to develop AD (OR 0.47, 95% CI: 0.22–1.1). Therefore, depression and diabetes mellitus increase the risk of dementia, whereas treated dyslipidemia has been shown to reduce this risk.

Keywords: dementia; Alzheimer's disease; depression; diabetes mellitus; type 2; dyslipidemias; hypertension

1. Introduction

In recent decades, population aging has led to an increase in the number of people affected by cognitive impairment, this becoming a major problem both clinically and socially, especially in Western countries [1,2]. In this sense, while in 2016 there were 47.5 million people diagnosed with dementia, in 2050 it is expected to affect more than 135.5 million individuals [3], with Alzheimer's disease (AD) and vascular dementia (VD) the most common form of dementia [2,4,5].

However, the big problem with these diseases is not their frequency nor their growth forecasting, but their late diagnosis. The lack of differentiation between normal processes of cognitive impairment and disease states, coupled with the characteristic features of dementia—with an appearance that tends to be insidious and a development that tends to extend over time [6]—makes the first symptoms of dementia and AD easily go unnoticed [7,8]. Therefore, patients suffering from these diseases are diagnosed too late, when neurological symptoms are actually noticeable and the disease is already in very advanced stages [9]. In fact, previous studies point to how AD probably begins decades before the first symptoms appear [10]. As a result, the identification of risk/prodromal factors becomes essential to prevent the disease and, especially, to prevent late detection/diagnosis of the disease.

The association between this disease and many risk factors has been described. Some of them, such as dyslipidemia, hypertension, or tobacco use, have clear pathophysiological mechanisms because of their vascular component [11,12]. Nevertheless, this would not be the only association between dyslipidemia and AD since recent animal studies have shown how hypercholesterolemia may favor β-amyloid deposits characteristic of AD and therefore be related to neuroinflammation and loss of neuronal function [13]. However, despite being considered a risk factor for the development of AD, the pharmacological approach to this cardiovascular risk factor in older people would not prevent the onset of AD nor slow the course of neurodegenerative disease. This leads us to question the link described above between dyslipidemia and AD [14,15].

Other risk factors, such as type 2 diabetes mellitus (T2DM), seem to have a bidirectional relationship with AD, because it involves modifications in vascular function and structure, glucose metabolism, and insulin signaling, thus contributing to neurodegeneration [16–18]. In fact, both dementia and T2DM share symptoms, such as inflammation and altered insulin signaling mechanisms [19]. However, the relationship between the metabolism of tau and β-amyloid proteins has not yet been elucidated [20], so while some authors focus their research on understanding the link between this accumulation and the existence of other factors, such as amylin (protein co-secreted with insulin), others analyze whether the accumulation may be part of the diabetic phenotype [21,22].

Finally, others, such as anxiety and depression seem to be related to the appearance of dementia. However, while recent studies have described anxiety as a risk factor of AD, increasing the risk of this neurodegenerative disease by up to 50% [23], the exact link between depression and dementia is unknown and controversial, to the point of not knowing if depression is associated with a future development of AD and if it could be considered a risk factor for AD, or if, on the contrary, depression is a consequence of AD [24–26]. It appears that depressive symptoms in older adults with cognitive impairment may be related to the distinctive amyloid and tau signs of AD [27,28], thus establishing an association between depressive symptoms and cognitive impairment in older adults [29].

In this sense, the prevailing depressive symptoms among older adults could be considered modifiers of cognitive performance, but they could also be clinical indicators or early clinical signs and symptoms of AD [30,31], which would justify a comprehensive management of neuropsychological functioning in older people diagnosed with depression, regardless of the age of onset and the disease pattern (self-limiting, incident or persistent).

In this way, prevention of the onset of dementia would involve, first, assessing and adequately diagnosing this mental disorder and, second, addressing it with appropriate pharmacological and non-pharmacological treatment [32,33].

In this context, the aim of this study was to elucidate the association between depression and dementia/AD and to identify possible relationships between these diseases and different sociodemographic and clinical features.

2. Material and Methods

2.1. Study Design

This is a case-control study developed in four nursing homes and one dementia-specific facility in each of two urban areas of southern Spain between May 2018 and October 2019.

2.2. Participants and Selection Criteria

The study included a control group, consisting of 125 people without dementia, and a case group consisting of 96 participants with dementia, of whom 74 subjects had AD. This allowed a double epidemiological analysis to be carried out: firstly, between the control group ($n = 125$) and the dementia case group ($n = 96$); and secondly, between the control group and the AD case group ($n = 74$).

To ensure that patients actually had dementia or AD, strict criteria, including severity levels, were used. The inclusion criteria for participants with dementia were the following:

- Age ≥ 65 years.
- Medical diagnosis of dementia or AD with a global deterioration scale (GDS) score between 5 and 7 [34]. Patients received diagnosis of dementia if they met DSM-V clinical criteria and received a diagnosis of probable or possible AD according to NINCDS/ADRDA (National Institute of Neurological and Communicative Disorders and Stroke/Alzheimer's Disease and Related Disorders Association) criteria.
- Being included, at least, for three months in the listings of the dementia process. In the case of the institution dedicated to the care of patients with Alzheimer's disease, patients who had used this service for at least three months were included.
- Being unable to communicate verbally.
- Having a relative or legal representative that could sign the informed consent for the participation of the patient in the study.

People with AD who had comorbidity with other major clinical neurological illness were excluded. The inclusion criteria for participants without dementia (controls) were the following:

- Age ≥ 65 years.
- Being able to sign the informed consent for their participation in the study.
- Not presenting with a diagnosis of dementia or AD.

The recruitment of the individuals with dementia was conducted consecutively by the interventional nurses among the subjects they care for in their health care institution (lists of patients). The recruitment included all individuals (prevalent and incident cases) found during the study time in the mentioned settings. The controls were recruited, simultaneously, in the close environment of participants with dementia and/or in the area of influence of the centers involved in the recruitment of participants with dementia, among those within the same age range and who were willing to participate in this study.

The sample size was calculated for a 10% difference in the proportion of subjects presenting with diabetes mellitus (and 15% and 30% in subjects presenting with dyslipidemia and depression [35], respectively) in the group of subjects with and without dementia (calculated after a pilot study). An alpha risk of 5% and a beta risk of 20%, with a ratio of 1:1 and an estimated loss to follow-up of 10% were considered. The total number of subjects required was 219.

2.3. Study Measures

The main dependent variables were the diagnosis of dementia/AD and the scores of the GDS scale, whereas the main predictor variables were four chronic conditions related to dementia in previous studies: medical diagnosis of depression according to DSM-V, dyslipidemia, T2DM, and hypertension.

In addition, other study variables, such as sociodemographic characteristics (sex, age, and place of residence –rural or urban), were collected from the clinical record. Furthermore, the level of autonomy in basic activities of daily living was measured using the Barthel index. In this sense, the scales (GDS and Barthel Index) were administered by the research team at the time of data collection or, if collected from the medical record, were not more than three months old. The predictor variables (depression, dyslipidemia, T2DM, and hypertension) and the date of diagnosis of each of them were collected from the medical record to ensure the antecedents of these conditions.

2.4. Statistical Analysis

IBM SPSS Statistics 22.0 (SPSS/IBM, Chicago, IL, USA) and Epidat version 4.1 (Department of Sanida, Xunta de Galicia, Galicia, Spain) software was used for statistical and epidemiological treatment of the data.

Continuous variables were expressed as the mean ± standard deviation, while categorical variables were expressed as the frequency and proportion distribution. The Kolmogorov–Smirnov test with

Lilliefors correction and graphical representation tests, such as P–P and Q–Q plots, was applied to test the goodness of fit to a normal distribution of the data.

A Student's t test was used for variables with a normal distribution (using the Levene test for variance equality), whereas non-parametric tests, such as the U Mann–Whitney test (independent samples), were used for variables showing a non-normal distribution and were used for bivariate analysis. The Z test, chi squared test, and Fisher's exact test were used whenever necessary for each contingency tables of categorical variables.

Bivariate and multivariate analyses were performed by binary logistic regression. Goodness-of-fit tests for the model (2 loglikelihood, goodness-of-fit statistics, Nagelkerke R2, and Hosmer-Lemeshow test) were calculated to assess the global fit of the model. Exponentiation was used for the b-coefficients in the regression models to estimate the OR, and the standard error of the b-coefficients was used to calculate the 95% confidence interval (CI). The confounding effect was analyzed for those variables of the final model whose statistical significance value was between 0.05 and 0.2. It was considered a confounding effect when the crude and adjusted Beta coefficient variation was above 10%.

Receiver Operator Characteristic (ROC) curves were constructed, and the Area Under the Curve (AUC) was calculated to determine which explanatory variables best predicted the onset of dementia and AD. The diagnostic accuracy indicators, such as sensitivity, specificity, predictive values, and Youden and Validity Indices were analyzed.

The level of statistical significance was set at $p < 0.05$, and the confidence intervals were calculated at a 95% level.

2.5. Limitations

Firstly, it should be noted that no estimation of the incidence or prevalence of the events of interest (depression and dementia) could be performed because this study lacked a population base.

In addition, the design type involved constraints in establishing the temporary sequence of possible exposures (depression and others) and effects (dementia and AD, with GDS 5–7), since the onset (diagnosis) of chronic conditions/diseases is always uncertain.

By including prevalent cases (in addition to incident cases), we may have included the most surviving cases, so long-term cases may have been overrepresented ("Neyman fallacy").

For institutionalized older people, one type of selection bias, "Berkson's bias," should be considered, because a selection of cases from a nursing home or dementia-specific facility population could contain a higher proportion of older people with a secondary disease.

However, as an analytical observational study, the main limitation of this study is the possibility of confounding factors not covered by the design. However, efforts have been made to reduce the influence of these confounding factors by using multivariate data analysis techniques.

2.6. Ethical Aspects

The study was conducted in accordance with the precepts included in the Belmont report and the Helsinki Declaration (updated at the Seoul Assembly in 2008) for biomedical research. All candidates for entry into the study were informed through a Patient Information Sheet (PIS). Written informed consents were voluntarily signed by the patients. All participants were allowed to leave the study at any time. Subject anonymity and data confidentiality were guaranteed at all times. Finally, the study had the authorization of all participating centers and the permission of the Ethics Committee for Research of Andalusia (Acta n° 271, ref. 3672, approved on 5 December 2017).

3. Results

3.1. Sample Characteristics

A total of 221 participants were studied, of whom 168 (76%) were women. The overall mean age was 79.1 (8.6) years, 95% CI (78–80.3), and the range was 65–100 years. No significant differences in age between women and men were found.

A total of 48% of the sample were married, and 50% of the group of women were widows. With regard to institutionalization, 107 persons were admitted to one of two types of geriatric centers (48.4%), finding no sex differences. The sample consisted of 167 subjects living in an urban area (75.6%) compared with those living in a rural area.

A total of 96 participants had a diagnosis of dementia, 43.4% with a 95% CI (36.7–50.2) of the study subjects. Prevalence in women was 45.2% compared to 37.7% in men ($p = 0.42$). For AD ($n = 74$), the overall prevalence in the sample was 33.5% with a 95% CI (27–39.9), higher in women (35.7%) than in men (26.4%) $p = 0.28$. Finally, 22 participants were diagnosed with non-AD dementia.

With regard to the level of independence for performing basic daily life activities, the median Barthel Index score for people with dementia was 10 (max = 80 and min = 0). Consequently, 61.49% showed a total dependency, 31.25% showed a severe dependence, and 7.29% showed a moderate dependence.

Finally, the prevalence of other relevant clinical entities was: Depression (17.6%), T2DM (18.1%), hypertension (61.5%). In terms of dyslipidemia, the prevalence was 38.7%, and 74.4% of them were under treatment with statins. Table 1 shows the characteristics of the sample according to the study variables and sex.

3.2. Variables Associated with Dementia and AD

A double comparative analysis was carried out between the control group versus the group of cases with dementia and the group of cases with AD, by means of crude (unadjusted) binary logistic regression analysis, in order to know which study variables were associated with suffering from dementia in general, or AD in particular (Table 2).

Based on the results of Table 2, multivariate models were performed by binary logistic regression, for both dementia and Alzheimer's disease, including those independent variables with a statistical significance of $p \leq 0.2$ (all variables except sex and hypertension), and considering the parsimony of modeling (no more than five independent variables). The multivariate models performed were as follows:

- Model 1: Adjusted for age and depression.
- Model 2: Adjusted for age and dyslipidemias.
- Model 3: Adjusted for age, depression, dyslipidemias, and T2DM.

With regard to dementia, Table 3 shows the adjusted OR results for each explanatory variable in each of the proposed models. Table 3 shows that the age variable was involved in the three models with a high statistical significance ($p < 0.001$), as well as a stable adjusted OR value of approximately 1.16. That is, under equally adjusted variables, for each 1-year increase in the person's age, the risk of presenting dementia increases by 16%.

Table 1. Description of the sample according to sex.

Variable	Total n = 221	Women n = 168	Men n = 53	p Value
Age	79.1 (8.6)	79.1 (8.8)	79.1 (7.9)	0.99
Study Group				
Cases	96 (43.4%)	76 (45.2%)	20 (37.7%)	0.33
Controls	125 (56.6%)	92 (54.8%)	33 (62.3%)	
Marital Status				
Single	11 (5%)	9 (5.4%)	2 (3.8%)	
Married	106 (48%)	71 (42.3%)	35 (66%)	<0.05
Widowed	99 (44.8%)	84 (50%)	15 (28.3%)	
Divorced	5 (2.3%)	4 (2.4%)	1 (1.9%)	
Origin of Participants				
Health Center	114 (51.6%)	84 (50%)	30 (56.6%)	0.4
Nursing Home	107 (48.4%)	84 (50%)	23 (43.4%)	
Living area of the Sample				
Urban	167 (75.6%)	124 (73.8%)	43 (81.1%)	0.28
Rural	54 (24.4%)	44 (26.2%)	10 (18.9%)	
Clinical Variables				
Dementia	96 (43.4%)	76 (45.2%)	20 (37.7%)	0.42
Alzheimer's Disease	74 (77.1%)	60 (78.9%)	14 (70%)	
Vascular Dementia	8 (8.3%)	6 (7.9%)	2 (10%)	0.62
Senile Dementia	1 (1%)	1 (1.3%)	-	
Primary Dementia	2 (0.9%)	2 (1.2%)	-	
Mixed Dementia	11 (11.5%)	7 (9.2%)	4 (20%)	
Lewy Bodies Dementia	-	-	-	
Depression	39 (17.6%)	33 (19.6%)	6 (11.3%)	0.24
Hypertension	136 (61.5%)	105 (62.5%)	31 (58.5%)	0.72
T2DM [a]	40 (18.1%)	28 (16.7%)	12 (22.6%)	0.43
Dyslipidemia	86 (38.9%)	65 (38.7%)	21 (39.6%)	0.97
Statins (n = 86)	64 (74.4%)	50 (76.9%)	14 (66.7%)	0.51
Diagnosis Time (Years) Depression (n = 38)	14.7 (5.5)	15.3 (5.6)	11.2 (3.9)	0.09
Diagnosis Time (Years) Dementia (n = 33)	5.5 (3)	6 (2.9)	2.7 (1.5)	<0.05
Difference in Diagnosis Time (Years)	9 (4.2)	9.3 (4.4)	7.4 (2.1)	0.35

[a] Type 2 diabetes mellitus; - No subject met that condition.

Table 2. Crude logistic regression (unadjusted) for dementia and AD.

Variable	Dementia		Alzheimer's Disease	
	cOR 95% CI	p	cOR 95% CI	p
Age	1.15 (1.1–1.2)	<0.001	1.15 (1.1–1.2)	<0.001
Sex (Female)	1.4 (0.72–2.6)	0.34	1.5 (0.76–3.1)	0.23
Depression	10.4 (4.1–26.1)	<0.001	10.1 (3.9–26.2)	<0.001
Hypertension	1.25 (0.73–2.2)	0.41	1.35 (0.74–2.5)	0.33
T2DM	1.6 (0.79–3.1)	0.2	1.8 (0.87–3.7)	0.11
Dyslipidemia	0.52 (0.3–0.9)	<0.05	0.47 (0.26–0.88)	<0.05

cOR: crude Odds Ratio.

Table 3. Adjusted logistic regression models for dementia and AD outcome variables.

Model/Variables	Adjusted OR 95% CI	p Value
Dementia		
Model 1		
Age	1.16 (1.1–1.2)	<0.001
Depression	13.6 (4.8–38.7)	<0.001
Model 2		
Age	1.15 (1.1–1.2)	<0.001
Dyslipidemia	0.6 (0.3–1.1)	0.12 *
Model 3		
Age	1.16 (1.1–1.2)	<0.001
Depression	15.6 (5.3–45)	<0.001
Diabetes mellitus	2.6 (1.05–6.3)	<0.05
Dyslipidemia	0.54 (0.27–1.1)	0.089 **
AD		
Model 1		
Age	1.15 (1.1–1.2)	<0.001
Depression	11.7 (4–34.6)	<0.001
Model 2		
Age	1.15 (1.1–1.2)	<0.001
Dyslipidemia	0.53 (0.26–1.05)	0.07 ***
Model 3		
Age	1.15 (1.1–1.2)	<0.001
Depression	12.9 (4.3–39.9)	<0.001
Diabetes mellitus	2.8 (1.1–7.1)	<0.05
Dyslipidemia	0.47 (0.22–1.1)	0.056 ***

* Confounding effect was tested and did not remain in the final model. ** Confounding effector was tested and modified 12.5% of the Beta coefficient of the variable Diabetes Mellitus. *** were left in the final model due to their low p value.

The variable depression was included in models 1 and 3, and it was significantly associated with the presence of dementia in both models, its adjusted OR ranging between 13.6 (4.8–38.7) in Model 1 and 15.6 (5.3–45) in Model 3. This means that under equal variables included in the model, those subjects who suffered an episode of depression presented between 13.6- and 15.6-fold higher prevalence of dementia than subjects without depression.

The behavior of the dyslipidemia variable was not included in Model 2 ($p = 0.12$ and non-confounding effect), but was included in Model 3, obtaining an adjusted OR of 0.54 (0.27–1.1) $p = 0.089$, considering it as a confounding variable by causing a variation of the crude-adjusted value of the beta coefficient of the T2DM variable of 12.5%. This means that, under equal variables included in the model, those subjects with dyslipidemia have had a 1.85-fold (1/0.54) lower prevalence of dementia than subjects without dyslipidemia.

Finally, T2DM was associated with dementia, adjusted OR= 2.6 (1.05–6.3) $p < 0.05$. That is, under the equal variables of Model 3, subjects with diabetes suffered a 2.6-fold higher prevalence of dementia than subjects without T2DM.

Regarding AD as a dependent variable (Table 3), the results obtained were similar to those found in the multivariate models for dementia (partly explained by the collinearity between dementia-AD, being the latter part of dementia). Variables significantly associated with the outcome variables, as well as the sign and adjusted OR values, were very similar in dementia and AD models. The dyslipidemia variable was maintained in Models 2 and 3 due to its small alpha error ($p = 0.07$ and 0.056, respectively).

3.3. Diagnostic Accuracy of Dementia and AD

Table 4 shows the accuracy (diagnostic accuracy) and the safety and validity indicators of the multivariate logistic regression models for dementia and AD. For both variables, Model 3 adjusted for age, depression, dyslipidemia, and T2DM showed the highest goodness of fit (Nagelkerke $r^2 = 0.48$), i.e., the variables included accounted for 48% of the value of the result variable.

Table 4. Diagnostic accuracy of logistic regression models adjusted for dementia and AD.

Outcome Variable	Model	Goodness of Fit (Nagelkerke r^2)	Sensitivity	Specificity	Youden Index	PPV	NPV	Validity Index	AUC
Dementia	Model 1	0.45	71.9%	83.2%	0.55	76.7%	79.4%	78.3%	85%
Dementia	Model 2	0.32	67.7%	82.4%	0.5	74.7%	76.9%	76%	78.9%
Dementia	Model 3	0.48	77.1%	81.6%	0.59	76.3%	82.3%	79.6%	86%
AD	Model 1	0.43	63.5%	85.6%	0.49	72.3%	79.9%	77.4%	84.2%
AD	Model 2	0.32	64.9%	85.6%	0.5	72.7%	80.5%	77.9%	79.1%
AD	Model 3	0.48	66.2%	83.2%	0.49	70%	80.6%	76.9%	85.8%

Model 3 achieved for dementia an area under the curve of 86% (ROC curves in Figure 1), a sensitivity of 77.1%, and a specificity of 81.6%, which resulted in a Youden index of 0.59, with a positive predictive value (PPV) of 76.3% and a negative predictive value (NPV) of 82.3%. The percentage of correctly classified persons (validity index) was 79.6%.

Model 3 obtained an area under the curve of 85.8% and a diagnostic validity index of 76.9% for AD. Sensitivity was 66.2%, and specificity was 83.2%, with a Youden index of 0.48. PPV and NPV were 70% and 80.6%, respectively.

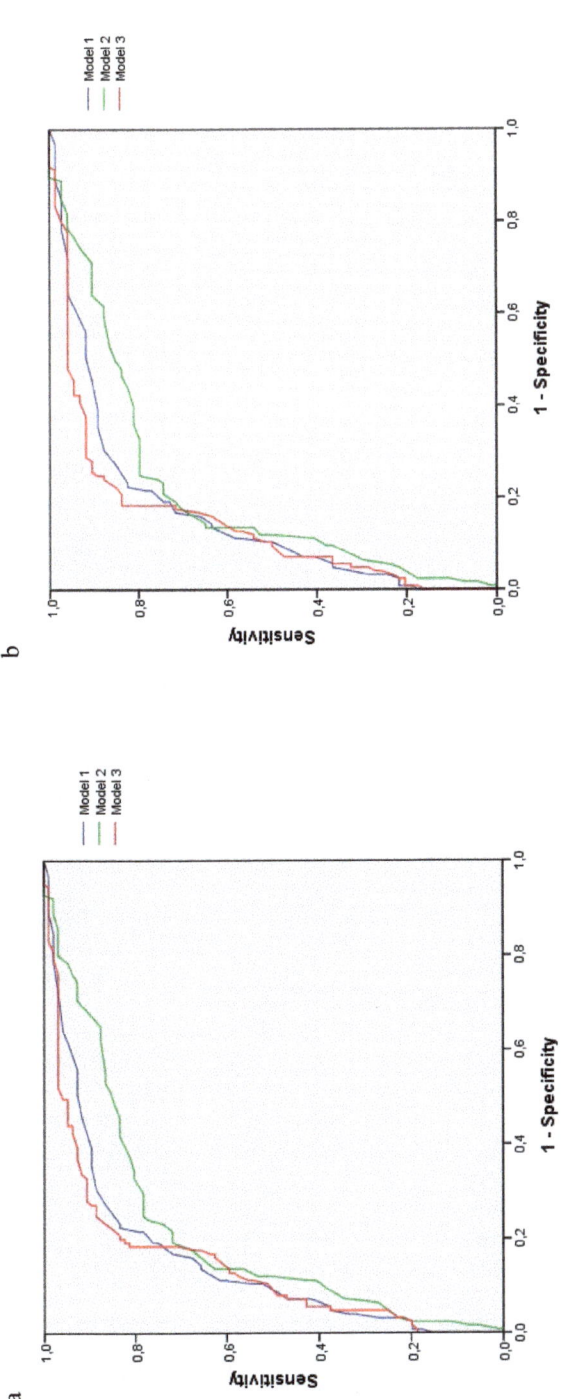

Figure 1. ROC curves for multivariate logistic regression models for dementia and AD outcome variables. (a). Outcome Variable: Dementia; (b). Outcome Variable: AD.

4. Discussion

Recent research, consistent with the results of the present study, indicates that dementia and depression are diseases with a high prevalence and with a remarkable overlap in their epidemiological data [36,37].

However, the temporary sequence of this association is controversial. On the one hand, several authors point out that the presence of late depressive symptoms in older people could be the first manifestation of dementia, so depression, in this case, would be a prodromal factor of dementia [38,39]. On the other hand, some authors state that people with depression have an increased risk of being diagnosed with dementia and/or AD in old ages [40,41], results that are consistent with the present study, where those subjects with a diagnosis of depression had between 13.6 and 15.6 times higher prevalence of dementia than subjects without depression.

Nevertheless, this association between the two diseases, based on the existing literature, will be determined by the severity of the depressive symptoms, the recurrence of episodes, the general state of health of the person, and the presence of depression in adulthood [42–45].

With regard to the latter point, multiple studies indicate that the link between the two diseases would be limited by the time of onset of depression [46,47]. Therefore, age must be understood as a factor of great importance in this relationship, even more when thanks to the development of imaging techniques, it has been possible to compare the causal relationship between these two clinical entities from the pathophysiological point of view, because in people diagnosed with depression at an old age, the presence of β-amyloid plaques and accumulation of tau protein in the brain years before the presentation of dementia have been verified [48,49].

Thus, the onset of these symptoms in old ages can be understood as a prodromal factor, and in turn, the appearance of early depression can be understood as a risk factor for developing dementia and/or AD in both early and old ages [50,51].

In addition, the consideration of depressive symptoms as a prodromal factor would be higher in people diagnosed with dementia with Lewy bodies or VD than in those affected by AD [52,53].

Regarding the pathophysiological link between the two diseases, it appears to be centered on microglia activation as the basis of the process of cerebral neuroinflammation described in both diseases [54]. In this sense, the studies developed by Gathel et al., (2019) take on special relevance, because their objectives were to try to establish a relationship between depressive symptoms, cognition, and cortical amyloid in community-dwelling older adults [29].

Despite the evident relationship between these diseases, health professionals often treat these two diseases independently, focusing the treatment of dementia, particularly in the case of AD, on memory decline and forgetting to include the care of the depressive behavioral symptoms that these patients present as a key element [55]. This inadequate approach to depression in people with dementia increases functional and cognitive impairment, especially if the person also suffers from anxiety as it seems to accentuate the cognitive decline [56], thus intensifying the loss of independence of the person, and ultimately it is associated with an increase in the institutionalization of these patients [57].

Moreover, beyond depression, and as our results show, older age is a risk factor itself for developing dementia and/or AD [58,59]. If the other variables are equal, for every 1-year increase in the person's age, the risk of developing dementia increases by 16%.

Another of the diseases described in the scientific literature due to its potential relationship with the development of dementia, and as has been proven in the results of the present study, is T2DM, which must be understood as a risk factor for dementia [60]. Specifically, the findings of the present study estimate that those with T2DM experienced 2.6 times higher prevalence of dementia than subjects without T2DM. However, this decrease in cognitive functions, particularly memory and reasoning, and therefore the development of dementia seems to depend, according to the existing literature, on two factors in people with TMD2: The duration of the disease and the glycemic control [61].

In addition, T2DM has also been defined as a risk factor specifically for patients with AD with depression, because increased serum levels of glycosylated hemoglobin favor a worsening of depressive symptoms in patients with AD. This is why adequate control of T2DM, through hygienic-dietary measures and appropriate pharmacological treatment, can reduce the severity of depression in patients with this neurodegenerative disease [62].

With regard to the influence of dyslipidemia, and in accordance with our results, it should be noted that low levels of HDL increase the risk of AD [63], as well as a greater progression of the disease [64], whereas high serum HDL levels are associated with improved memory function [65]. In this sense, according to Ward et al. (2010), there is a positive relationship between HDL levels and gray matter volume in the temporal area, and consequently with de cognitive function [66], with this relationship limited by the fact that HDL contains apolipoprotein E (APOE) [67]. In addition, recent studies indicate that increased serum LDL levels are associated with higher deposits of β-amyloid protein in the brain, resulting in increased risk of developing AD [64,68].

However, in addition to the described metabolic relationship between APOE, HDL, and AD, brain neuroinflammation is a fundamental connection point between dyslipidemia and dementia [69]. Thus, the pharmacological approach to dyslipidemia using drugs, such as statins, could not only reduce serum lipid levels, a widely recognized function of this treatment, but would help to mitigate the inflammatory process, thus benefiting all patients with AD, although the progression of this positive effect over time is still unknown [70,71].

In this regard, some studies suggest that treatment of dyslipidemia with statins decreases the risk of dementia and AD [72,73], which would support the results of the present study. Similarly, the use of statins is associated with a decrease in the incidence of all types of dementia, except VD [74]. However, it is not recommended to systematically use statin therapy in all people with dyslipidemia because of its controversial interference with cognitive function [75,76].

Health professionals will be responsible for discerning which subjects may benefit from the dual function of this pharmacological treatment because they present other risk factors contributing to the development of dementia or because they already have cognitive impairment [77,78].

5. Conclusions

Depression should be considered a risk factor for dementia, and especially AD. Moreover, people with diabetes are at higher risk of dementia than those without this chronic condition, so the appropriate approach to diabetes could significantly decrease this causal relationship. In addition, properly treated dyslipidemia may reduce the risk of dementia.

Regarding sociodemographic variables, age appears to be a decisive risk factor, even more relevant than depression.

Author Contributions: V.C.-H., M.d.P.C.-G. and M.R.-R. conceptualized the project and conceived the study design. V.C.-H. and M.d.P.C.-G. performed the data collection. M.R.-R. analyzed the data. V.C.-H. drafted the manuscript. M.d.P.C.-G., M.R.-R. and M.R.-S. reviewed and edited the draft manuscript. All authors have read and agreed to the published version of the manuscript.

Funding: This study was supported by the Health Department of the Regional Government of Andalusia (PI-0357–2017).

Acknowledgments: We would like to thank the patients and families who participated in the recruitment process, as well as the institutions "Asociación San Rafael de Alzheimer y otrasdemencias" (Córdoba), Residencia de mayores de fundaciónGerón de Villaharta (Córdoba), Residencia de Jesús Nazareno (Córdoba) and Residencia de Mayores Altos del Jontoya (Jaén).

Conflicts of Interest: The authors declare no conflict of interest.

References

1. Prince, M.; Ali, G.-C.; Guerchet, M.; Prina, A.M.; Albanese, E.; Wu, Y.-T. Recent global trends in the prevalence and incidence of dementia, and survival with dementia. *Alzheimer's Res. Ther.* **2016**, *8*. [CrossRef] [PubMed]
2. Alzheimer's Association. 2020 Alzheimer's disease facts and figures. *Alzheimer's Dement.* **2020**, *16*, 391–460. [CrossRef] [PubMed]

3. Beard, J.R.; Officer, A.M.; Cassels, A.K. The World Report on Ageing and Health. *GERONT* **2016**, *56*, S163–S166. [CrossRef] [PubMed]
4. Ferreira, D.; Perestelo-Pérez, L.; Westman, E.; Wahlund, L.-O.; Sarría, A.; Serrano-Aguilar, P. Meta-Review of CSF Core Biomarkers in Alzheimer's Disease: The State-of-the-Art after the New Revised Diagnostic Criteria. *Front. Aging Neurosci.* **2014**, *6*, 47. [CrossRef]
5. Wortmann, M. Dementia: A global health priority—Highlights from an ADI and World Health Organization report. *Alzheimer's Res. Ther.* **2012**, *4*, 40. [CrossRef]
6. Harada, C.N.; Natelson Love, M.C.; Triebel, K. Normal Cognitive Aging. *Clin. Geriatr. Med.* **2013**, *29*, 737–752. [CrossRef]
7. Gale, S.A.; Acar, D.; Daffner, K.R. Dementia. *Am. J. Med.* **2018**, *131*, 1161–1169. [CrossRef]
8. Arvanitakis, Z.; Shah, R.C.; Bennett, D.A. Diagnosis and Management of Dementia: Review. *JAMA* **2019**, *322*, 1589–1599. [CrossRef]
9. Shao, Y.; Zeng, Q.T.; Chen, K.K.; Shutes-David, A.; Thielke, S.M.; Tsuang, D.W. Detection of probable dementia cases in undiagnosed patients using structured and unstructured electronic health records. *BMC Med. Inform. Decis. Mak.* **2019**, *19*, 128. [CrossRef]
10. Sperling, R.A.; Aisen, P.S.; Beckett, L.A.; Bennett, D.A.; Craft, S.; Fagan, A.M.; Iwatsubo, T.; Jack, C.R.; Kaye, J.; Montine, T.J.; et al. Toward defining the preclinical stages of Alzheimer's disease: Recommendations from the National Institute on Aging-Alzheimer's Association workgroups on diagnostic guidelines for Alzheimer's disease. *Alzheimer's Dement.* **2011**, *7*, 280–292. [CrossRef]
11. Anstey, K.J.; von Sanden, C.; Salim, A.; O'Kearney, R. Smoking as a risk factor for dementia and cognitive decline: A meta-analysis of prospective studies. *Am. J. Epidemiol.* **2007**, *166*, 367–378. [CrossRef] [PubMed]
12. Jia, L.; Quan, M.; Fu, Y.; Zhao, T.; Li, Y.; Wei, C.; Tang, Y.; Qin, Q.; Wang, F.; Qiao, Y.; et al. Dementia in China: Epidemiology, clinical management, and research advances. *Lancet Neurol.* **2020**, *19*, 81–92. [CrossRef]
13. Oliveira, B.C.D.L.; Bellozi, P.M.Q.; Reis, H.J.; De Oliveira, A.C.P. Inflammation as a Possible Link Between Dyslipidemia and Alzheimer's Disease. *Neuroscience* **2018**, *376*, 127–141. [CrossRef] [PubMed]
14. Mejías-Trueba, M.; Pérez-Moreno, M.A.; Fernández-Arche, M. Ángeles Systematic review of the efficacy of statins for the treatment of Alzheimer's disease. *Clin. Med.* **2018**, *18*, 54–61. [CrossRef]
15. McGuinness, B.; Craig, D.; Bullock, R.; Passmore, P. Statins for the prevention of dementia. *Cochrane Database Syst. Rev.* **2009**, CD003160. [CrossRef]
16. Shinohara, M.; Sato, N. Bidirectional interactions between diabetes and Alzheimer's disease. *Neurochem. Int.* **2017**, *108*, 296–302. [CrossRef]
17. Tumminia, A.; Vinciguerra, F.; Parisi, M.; Frittitta, L. Type 2 Diabetes Mellitus and Alzheimer's Disease: Role of Insulin Signalling and Therapeutic Implications. *Int. J. Mol. Sci.* **2018**, *19*, 3306. [CrossRef]
18. Moran, C.; Beare, R.; Phan, T.; Starkstein, S.; Bruce, D.; Romina, M.; Srikanth, V. Neuroimaging and its Relevance to Understanding Pathways Linking Diabetes and Cognitive Dysfunction. *J. Alzheimer's Dis.* **2017**, *59*, 405–419. [CrossRef]
19. Martins, R.N. Understanding the Link between Dementia and Diabetes. *J. Alzheimer's Dis.* **2017**, *59*, 389–392. [CrossRef]
20. Biessels, G.J.; Despa, F. Cognitive decline and dementia in diabetes mellitus: Mechanisms and clinical implications. *Nat. Rev. Endocrinol.* **2018**, *14*, 591–604. [CrossRef]
21. Bharadwaj, P.; Wijesekara, N.; Liyanapathirana, M.; Newsholme, P.; Ittner, L.; Fraser, P.; Verdile, G. The Link between Type 2 Diabetes and Neurodegeneration: Roles for Amyloid-β, Amylin, and Tau Proteins. *J. Alzheimer's Dis.* **2017**, *59*, 421–432. [CrossRef] [PubMed]
22. Miklossy, J.; Qing, H.; Radenovic, A.; Kis, A.; Vileno, B.; Làszló, F.; Miller, L.; Martins, R.N.; Waeber, G.; Mooser, V.; et al. Beta amyloid and hyperphosphorylated tau deposits in the pancreas in type 2 diabetes. *Neurobiol. Aging* **2010**, *31*, 1503–1515. [CrossRef]
23. Santabárbara, J.; Lipnicki, D.; Bueno-Notivol, J.; Olaya-Guzmán, B.; Villagrasa, B.; López-Antón, R. Updating the evidence for an association between anxiety and risk of Alzheimer's disease: A meta-analysis of prospective cohort studies. *J. Affect. Disord.* **2020**, *262*, 397–404. [CrossRef] [PubMed]
24. Norton, S.; Matthews, F.E.; Barnes, D.E.; Yaffe, K.; Brayne, C. Potential for primary prevention of Alzheimer's disease: An analysis of population-based data. *Lancet Neurol.* **2014**, *13*, 788–794. [CrossRef]

25. Rosenberg, P.B.; Mielke, M.M.; Appleby, B.S.; Oh, E.S.; Geda, Y.E.; Lyketsos, C.G. The association of neuropsychiatric symptoms in MCI with incident dementia and Alzheimer disease. *Am. J. Geriatr. Psychiatry* **2013**, *21*, 685–695. [CrossRef]
26. Bennett, S.; Thomas, A.J. Depression and dementia: Cause, consequence or coincidence? *Maturitas* **2014**, *79*, 184–190. [CrossRef] [PubMed]
27. Donovan, N.J.; Locascio, J.J.; Marshall, G.A.; Gatchel, J.R.; Hanseeuw, B.J.; Rentz, D.M.; Johnson, K.A.; Sperling, R.A.; for the Harvard Aging Brain Study. Longitudinal Association of Amyloid Beta and Anxious-Depressive Symptoms in Cognitively Normal Older Adults. *Am. J. Psychiatry* **2018**, *175*, 530–537. [CrossRef] [PubMed]
28. Krell-Roesch, J.; Lowe, V.J.; Neureiter, J.; Pink, A.; Roberts, R.O.; Mielke, M.M.; Vemuri, P.; Stokin, G.B.; Christianson, T.J.; Jack, C.R.; et al. Depressive and anxiety symptoms and cortical amyloid deposition among cognitively normal elderly persons: The Mayo Clinic Study of Aging. *Int. Psychogeriatr.* **2017**, *30*, 245–2512018. [CrossRef] [PubMed]
29. Gatchel, J.R.; Rabin, J.S.; Buckley, R.F.; Locascio, J.J.; Quiroz, Y.T.; Yang, H.-S.; Vannini, P.; Amariglio, R.E.; Rentz, D.M.; Properzi, M.; et al. Longitudinal Association of Depression Symptoms With Cognition and Cortical Amyloid Among Community-Dwelling Older Adults. *JAMA Netw. Open* **2019**, *2*, e198964. [CrossRef]
30. Capogna, E.; Manca, R.; De Marco, M.; Hall, A.; Soininen, H.; Venneri, A. Understanding the effect of cognitive/brain reserve and depression on regional atrophy in early Alzheimer's disease. *Postgrad. Med.* **2019**, *131*, 533–538. [CrossRef]
31. Olaya, B.; Moneta, M.V.; Miret, M.; Ayuso-Mateos, J.L.; Haro, J.M. Course of depression and cognitive decline at 3-year follow-up: The role of age of onset. *Psychol. Aging* **2019**, *34*, 475–485. [CrossRef]
32. Kuring, J.K.; Mathias, J.L.; Ward, L. Prevalence of Depression, Anxiety and PTSD in People with Dementia: A Systematic Review and Meta-Analysis. *Neuropsychol. Rev.* **2018**, *28*, 393–416. [CrossRef] [PubMed]
33. Perna, L.; Wahl, H.W.; Weberpals, J.; Jansen, L.; Mons, U.; Schöttker, B.; Brenner, H. Incident depression and mortality among people with different types of dementia: Results from a longitudinal cohort study. *Soc. Psychiatry Psychiatr. Epidemiol.* **2019**, *54*, 793–801. [CrossRef] [PubMed]
34. Reisberg, B.; Ferris, S.H.; de Leon, M.J.; Crook, T. The Global Deterioration Scale for assessment of primary degenerative dementia. *Am. J. Psychiatry* **1982**, *139*, 1136–1139. [CrossRef] [PubMed]
35. Lee, H.J.; Seo, H.I.; Cha, H.Y.; Yang, Y.J.; Kwon, S.H.; Yang, S.J. Diabetes and Alzheimer's Disease: Mechanisms and Nutritional Aspects. *Clin. Nutr. Res.* **2018**, *7*, 229. [CrossRef]
36. Arthur, A.; Savva, G.M.; Barnes, L.E.; Borjian-Boroojeny, A.; Dening, T.; Jagger, C.; Matthews, F.E.; Robinson, L.; Brayne, C.; the Cognitive Function and Ageing Studies Collaboration; et al. Changing prevalence and treatment of depression among older people over two decades. *Br. J. Psychiatry* **2019**, *216*, 49–54. [CrossRef]
37. Helvik, A.-S.; Barca, M.L.; Bergh, S.; Šaltytė-Benth, J.; Kirkevold, Ø.; Borza, T. The course of depressive symptoms with decline in cognitive function—A longitudinal study of older adults receiving in-home care at baseline. *BMC Geriatr.* **2019**, *19*, 231. [CrossRef] [PubMed]
38. Burke, S.L.; Cadet, T.; Alcide, A.; O'Driscoll, J.; Maramaldi, P. Psychosocial risk factors and Alzheimer's disease: The associative effect of depression, sleep disturbance, and anxiety. *Aging Ment. Health* **2017**, *22*, 1577–1584. [CrossRef]
39. Mirza, S.S.; Wolters, F.J.; Swanson, S.A.; Koudstaal, P.J.; Hofman, A.; Tiemeier, H.; Ikram, M.A. 10-year trajectories of depressive symptoms and risk of dementia: A population-based study. *Lancet Psychiatry* **2016**, *3*, 628–635. [CrossRef]
40. Burke, S.L.; Maramaldi, P.; Cadet, T.; Kukull, W. Associations between depression, sleep disturbance, and apolipoprotein E in the development of Alzheimer's disease: Dementia. *Int. Psychogeriatr.* **2016**, *28*, 1409–1424. [CrossRef]
41. Liu, Y.-C.; Meguro, K.; Nakamura, K.; Akanuma, K.; Nakatsuka, M.; Seki, T.; Nakaaki, S.; Mimura, M.; Kawakami, N. Depression and Dementia in Old-Old Population: History of Depression May Be Associated with Dementia Onset. The Tome Project. *Front. Aging Neurosci.* **2017**, *9*, 335. [CrossRef]
42. Graziane, J.A.; Beer, J.C.; Snitz, B.E.; Chang, C.-C.H.; Ganguli, M. Dual Trajectories of Depression and Cognition: A Longitudinal Population-Based Study. *Am. J. Geriatr. Psychiatry* **2016**, *24*, 364–373. [CrossRef] [PubMed]
43. Valkanova, V.; Ebmeier, K.P.; Allan, C.L. Depression is linked to dementia in older adults. *Practitioner* **2017**, *261*, 11–15. [PubMed]

44. García, P.G.; De-La-Cámara, C.; Santabárbara, J.; López-Antón, R.; Quintanilla, M.Á.; Ventura, T.; Marcos, G.; Campayo, A.; Saz, P.; Lyketsos, C.; et al. Depression and incident Alzheimer disease: The impact of disease severity. *Am. J. Geriatr. Psychiatry* **2013**, *23*, 119–129. [CrossRef]
45. Santabárbara Serrano, J.; Sevil Pérez, A.; Olaya, B.; Gracia García, P.; López Antón, R. Depresión tardía clínicamente relevante y riesgo de demencia: Revisión sistemática y metaanálisis de estudios prospectivos de cohortes. *Rev. Neurol.* **2019**, *68*, 493. [CrossRef]
46. Jamieson, A.; Goodwill, A.M.; Termine, M.; Campbell, S.; Szoeke, C. Depression related cerebral pathology and its relationship with cognitive functioning: A systematic review. *J. Affect. Disord.* **2019**, *250*, 410–418. [CrossRef]
47. Leyhe, T.; Reynolds, C.F.; Melcher, T.; Linnemann, C.; Klöppel, S.; Blennow, K.; Zetterberg, H.; Dubois, B.; Lista, S.; Hampel, H. A common challenge in older adults: Classification, overlap, and therapy of depression and dementia. *Alzheimer's Dement.* **2016**, *13*, 59–71. [CrossRef] [PubMed]
48. Goukasian, N.; Hwang, K.S.; Romero, T.; Grotts, J.; Do, T.M.; Groh, J.R.; Bateman, D.R.; Apostolova, L.G. Association of brain amyloidosis with the incidence and frequency of neuropsychiatric symptoms in ADNI: A multisite observational cohort study. *BMJ Open* **2019**, *9*, e031947. [CrossRef] [PubMed]
49. Linnemann, C.; Lang, U.E. Pathways Connecting Late-Life Depression and Dementia. *Front. Pharmacol.* **2020**, *11*, 279. [CrossRef]
50. Brzezińska, A.; Bourke, J.; Rivera-Hernández, R.; Tsolaki, M.; Woźniak, J.; Kaźmierski, J. Depression in Dementia or Dementia in Depression? Systematic Review of Studies and Hypotheses. *Curr. Alzheimer Res.* **2020**, *17*, 16–28. [CrossRef]
51. Peakman, G.; Karunatilake, N.; Seynaeve, M.; Perera, G.; Aarsland, D.; Stewart, R.; Mueller, C. Clinical factors associated with progression to dementia in people with late-life depression: A cohort study of patients in secondary care. *BMJ Open* **2020**, *10*, e035147. [CrossRef] [PubMed]
52. Anor, C.J.; O'Connor, S.; Saund, A.; Tang-Wai, D.F.; Keren, R.; Tartaglia, M.C. Neuropsychiatric Symptoms in Alzheimer Disease, Vascular Dementia, and Mixed Dementia. *Neurodegener. Dis.* **2017**, *17*, 127–134. [CrossRef]
53. Chiu, P.-Y.; Wang, C.-W.; Tsai, C.-T.; Li, S.-H.; Lin, C.-L.; Lai, T.-J. Depression in dementia with Lewy bodies: A comparison with Alzheimer's disease. *PLoS ONE* **2017**, *12*, e0179399. [CrossRef] [PubMed]
54. Santos, L.E.; Beckman, D.; Ferreira, S.T. Microglial dysfunction connects depression and Alzheimer's disease. *Brain Behav. Immun.* **2016**, *55*, 151–165. [CrossRef]
55. Goodarzi, Z.; Mele, B.; Guo, S.; Hanson, H.; Jette, N.; Patten, S.; Pringsheim, T.; Holroyd-Leduc, J. Guidelines for dementia or Parkinson's disease with depression or anxiety: A systematic review. *BMC Neurol.* **2016**, *16*, 244. [CrossRef]
56. Sinoff, G.; Werner, P. Anxiety disorder and accompanying subjective memory loss in the elderly as a predictor of future cognitive decline. *Int. J. Geriat. Psychiatry* **2003**, *18*, 951–959. [CrossRef] [PubMed]
57. Deardorff, W.J.; Grossberg, G.T. Behavioral and psychological symptoms in Alzheimer's dementia and vascular dementia. In *Handbook of Clinical Neurology*; Elsevier: Amsterdam, The Netherlands, 2019; Volume 165, pp. 5–32, ISBN 9780444640123.
58. Livingston, G.; Sommerlad, A.; Orgeta, V.; Costafreda, S.G.; Huntley, J.; Ames, D.; Ballard, C.; Banerjee, S.; Burns, A.; Cohen-Mansfield, J.; et al. Dementia prevention, intervention, and care. *Lancet* **2017**, *390*, 2673–2734. [CrossRef]
59. Wahl, D.; Solon-Biet, S.M.; Cogger, V.C.; Fontana, L.; Simpson, S.J.; Le Couteur, D.G.; Ribeiro, R.V. Aging, lifestyle and dementia. *Neurobiol. Dis.* **2019**, *130*, 104481. [CrossRef]
60. Su, M.; Naderi, K.; Samson, N.; Youssef, I.; Fülöp, L.; Bozso, Z.; Laroche, S.; Delatour, B.; Davis, S. Mechanisms Associated with Type 2 Diabetes as a Risk Factor for Alzheimer-Related Pathology. *Mol. Neurobiol.* **2019**, *56*, 5815–5834. [CrossRef]
61. Tuligenga, R.H.; Dugravot, A.; Tabák, A.G.; Elbaz, A.; Brunner, E.J.; Kivimäki, M.; Singh-Manoux, A. Midlife type 2 diabetes and poor glycaemic control as risk factors for cognitive decline in early old age: A post-hoc analysis of the Whitehall II cohort study. *Lancet Diabetes Endocrinol.* **2014**, *2*, 228–235. [CrossRef]
62. Yang, H.; Hong, W.; Chen, L.; Tao, Y.; Peng, Z.; Zhou, H. Analysis of risk factors for depression in Alzheimer's disease patients. *Int. J. Neurosci.* **2020**, *130*, 1136–1141. [CrossRef] [PubMed]

63. Ancelin, M.-L.; Ripoche, E.; Dupuy, A.-M.; Barberger-Gateau, P.; Auriacombe, S.; Rouaud, O.; Berr, C.; Carrière, I.; Ritchie, K. Sex Differences in the Associations Between Lipid Levels and Incident Dementia. *J. Alzheimer's Dis.* **2013**, *34*, 519–528. [CrossRef] [PubMed]
64. Ereed, B.; Villeneuve, S.; Mack, W.J.; DeCarli, C.; Chui, H.C.; Jagust, W.J. Associations between serum cholesterol levels and cerebral amyloidosis. *JAMA Neurol.* **2014**, *71*, 195–200. [CrossRef]
65. Kinno, R.; Mori, Y.; Kubota, S.; Nomoto, S.; Futamura, A.; Shiromaru, A.; Kuroda, T.; Yano, S.; Ishigaki, S.; Murakami, H.; et al. High serum high-density lipoprotein-cholesterol is associated with memory function and gyrification of insular and frontal opercular cortex in an elderly memory-clinic population. *NeuroImage: Clin.* **2019**, *22*, 101746. [CrossRef]
66. Ward, M.A.; Bendlin, B.B.; McLaren, D.G.; Hess, T.M.; Gallagher, C.L.; Kastman, E.K.; Rowley, H.A.; Asthana, S.; Carlsson, C.M.; Sager, M.A.; et al. Low HDL cholesterol is associated with lower gray matter volume in cognitively healthy adults. *Front. Aging Neurosci.* **2010**. [CrossRef] [PubMed]
67. Raber, J.; Huang, Y.; Ashford, J. ApoE genotype accounts for the vast majority of AD risk and AD pathology. *Neurobiol. Aging* **2004**, *25*, 641–650. [CrossRef]
68. Sáiz-Vazquez, O.; Puente-Martínez, A.; Ubillos-Landa, S.; Pacheco-Bonrostro, J.; Santabárbara, J. Cholesterol and Alzheimer's Disease Risk: A Meta-Meta-Analysis. *Brain Sci.* **2020**, *10*, 386. [CrossRef]
69. Petek, B.; Villa-Lopez, M.; Loera-Valencia, R.; Gerenu, G.; Winblad, B.; Kramberger, M.G.; Ismail, M.-A.-M.; Eriksdotter, M.; Garcia-Ptacek, S. Connecting the brain cholesterol and renin-angiotensin systems: Potential role of statins and RAS-modifying medications in dementia. *J. Intern. Med.* **2018**, *284*, 620–642. [CrossRef]
70. Armitage, J.; Baigent, C.; Barnes, E.; Betteridge, D.J.; Blackwell, L.; Blazing, M.; Bowman, L.; Braunwald, E.; Byington, R.; Cannon, C.; et al. Efficacy and safety of statin therapy in older people: A meta-analysis of individual participant data from 28 randomised controlled trials. *Lancet* **2019**, *393*, 407–415. [CrossRef]
71. Bagheri, H.; Ghasemi, F.; Barreto, G.E.; Sathyapalan, T.; Jamialahmadi, T.; Sahebkar, A. The effects of statins on microglial cells to protect against neurodegenerative disorders: A mechanistic review. *BioFactors* **2020**, *46*, 309–325. [CrossRef]
72. Geifman, N.; Brinton, R.D.; Kennedy, R.E.; Schneider, L.S.; Butte, A.J. Evidence for benefit of statins to modify cognitive decline and risk in Alzheimer's disease. *Alzheimer's Res. Ther.* **2017**, *9*, 1–10. [CrossRef]
73. Huang, C.-N.; Li, H.-H.; Lin, C.-L. Neuroprotective effects of statins against amyloid β-induced neurotoxicity. *Neural Regen. Res.* **2018**, *13*, 198–206. [CrossRef] [PubMed]
74. Chu, C.-S.; Tseng, P.-T.; Stubbs, B.; Chen, T.-Y.; Tang, C.-H.; Li, D.-J.; Yang, W.-C.; Chen, Y.-W.; Wu, C.-K.; Veronese, N.; et al. Use of statins and the risk of dementia and mild cognitive impairment: A systematic review and meta-analysis. *Sci. Rep.* **2018**, *8*, 5804. [CrossRef]
75. Sahebzamani, F.M. Examination of the FDA Warning for Statins and Cognitive Dysfunction. *J. Pharmacovigil.* **2014**, *2*. [CrossRef]
76. Crum, J.; Wilson, J.R.; Sabbagh, M.N. Does taking statins affect the pathological burden in autopsy-confirmed Alzheimer's dementia? *Alzheimer's Res. Ther.* **2018**, *10*, 104. [CrossRef] [PubMed]
77. Schultz, B.G.; Patten, D.K.; Berlau, D.J. The role of statins in both cognitive impairment and protection against dementia: A tale of two mechanisms. *Transl. Neurodegener.* **2018**, *7*, 5. [CrossRef] [PubMed]
78. Zissimopoulos, J.M.; Barthold, D.; Brinton, R.D.; Joyce, G. Sex and Race Differences in the Association between Statin Use and the Incidence of Alzheimer Disease. *JAMA Neurol.* **2017**, *74*, 225. [CrossRef] [PubMed]

Publisher's Note: MDPI stays neutral with regard to jurisdictional claims in published maps and institutional affiliations.

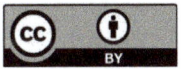

© 2020 by the authors. Licensee MDPI, Basel, Switzerland. This article is an open access article distributed under the terms and conditions of the Creative Commons Attribution (CC BY) license (http://creativecommons.org/licenses/by/4.0/).

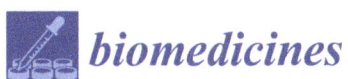

Article

Early Depression Independently of Other Neuropsychiatric Conditions, Influences Disability and Mortality after Stroke (Research Study—Part of PROPOLIS Study)

Katarzyna Kowalska [1], Łukasz Krzywoszański [2], Jakub Droś [3], Paulina Pasińska [4], Aleksander Wilk [5] and Aleksandra Klimkowicz-Mrowiec [1,*]

1. Department of Neurology, Faculty of Medicine, Jagiellonian University Medical College, 31-008 Kraków, Poland; katarzyna.olga.kowalska@gmail.com
2. Institute of Psychology, Pedagogical University of Krakow, 30-084 Kraków, Poland; lukasz.krzywoszanski@up.krakow.pl
3. Doctoral School in Medical and Health Sciences, Jagiellonian University Medical College, 31-008 Kraków, Poland; jakub.dros@gmail.com
4. Department of Medical Didactics, Faculty of Medicine, Jagiellonian University Medical College, 31-008 Kraków, Poland; paulina.potoczek@gmail.com
5. Department of Neurosurgery, University Hospital, 30-688 Kraków, Poland; wialeksander@gmail.com
* Correspondence: Aleksandra.Klimkowicz@mp.pl; Tel.: +48-12-424-86-35

Received: 19 October 2020; Accepted: 15 November 2020; Published: 17 November 2020

Abstract: Post-stroke depression (PSD) is the most frequent neuropsychiatric consequence of stroke. The nature of the relationship between PSD and mortality still remains unknown. One hypothesis is that PSD could be more frequent in those patients who are more vulnerable to physical disability, a mediator variable for higher level of physical damage related to higher risk of mortality. Therefore, the authors' objective was to explore the assumption that PSD increases disability after stroke, and secondly, that mortality is higher among patients with PSD regardless of stroke severity and other neuropsychiatric conditions. We included 524 consecutive patients with acute stroke or transient ischemic attack, who were screened for depression between 7–10 days after stroke onset. Physical impairment and death were the outcomes measures at evaluation check points three and 12 months post-stroke. PSD independently increased the level of disability three (OR = 1.94, 95% CI 1.31–2.87, $p = 0.001$), and 12 months post-stroke (OR = 1.61, 95% CI 1.14–2.48, $p = 0.009$). PSD was also an independent risk factor for death three (OR = 5.68, 95% CI 1.58–20.37, $p = 0.008$) and 12 months after stroke (OR = 4.53, 95% CI 2.06–9.94, $p = 0.001$). Our study shows the negative impact of early PSD on the level of disability and survival rates during first year after stroke and supports the assumption that depression may act as an independent mediator for disability leading to death in patients who are more vulnerable for brain injury.

Keywords: post-stroke depression; disability level; mortality

1. Introduction

Stroke is not only a leading cause of permanent functional disability, but also often causes severe impairment of mental health. Post-stroke depression (PSD) is the most frequent neuropsychiatric complication of stroke. In the meta-analysis by Hackett and Pickles [1], the pooled data showed that depression was present in 31% of stroke survivors at any time up to five-years post stroke, however its frequency varied across studies from 5% at two to five days after stroke to 84% at three months after stroke. Our data on PSD, among Polish patients with stroke, showed that PSD occurs in 54.58% of patients at the hospital, in 58.51% three months, and in 54.75% 12 months after the stroke [2].

It is important to recognize that depression is not a normal consequence of stroke, and still a lot of patients with stroke and physical impairment will not develop depression. Depression often coexist with other neuropsychiatric conditions which also increase the risk of negative prognosis, like apathy, anxiety, dementia, or delirium, and which often are misdiagnosed with depression. Sorting them out is essential for both, a correct risk assessment and for proper interventions.

Depressive symptoms occurring early after stroke increase the risk of negative consequences including death [3]. The rate of mortality among patients with PSD differs at different time points after stroke, also different risk factors are identified to increase the risk of death in this population [3–5]. Despite the fact that many studies have dealt with PSD, the nature of the relationship between PSD and mortality remains unknown and requires further analysis in order to draw a convincing conclusion. Among different hypothesis about the relationship between PSD and mortality one states that depression could be more frequent in those patients who are more vulnerable to physical disability [6] and PSD could act as a mediator variable for severe physical damage related to higher risk of mortality. A better understanding of this association would strengthen the evidence for causality, improve the therapeutic approach to patients with PSD, and provide prognostic information on survival. To check this hypothesis, we assumed that PSD negatively influences disability after stroke, regardless of stroke severity, other neuropsychiatric conditions, and higher mortality among patients with PSD.

Therefore, the objective of this study was to assess the change in the level of disability over a year in patients with PSD and their risk of death compared to depression-free patients by controlling other neuropsychiatric conditions and the severity of stroke.

2. Materials and Methods

This study was conducted as part of a larger prospective study, known as the PROPOLIS (PRospective Observational POLish Study on post-stroke delirium). Testing took place in the stroke unit at the University Hospital and Outpatient Clinic at the Neurology Department, University Hospital, Krakow. All procedures performed in this study involving human participants were in accordance with the ethical standards of the institutional and national research committee and with the 1964 Helsinki declaration and its later amendments. Informed written consent was provided by each participant or caregiver. The Local Bioethics Committee of Jagiellonian University approved the study (KBET/63/B/2014).

2.1. Population and Design

The consecutive patients admitted to the Stroke Unit at the University Hospital in Krakow, with stroke (ischemic or hemorrhagic) or transient ischemic attack (TIA) met inclusion criteria (Patients > 18 years of age, admitted within 48 h from the first stroke symptoms, speaking Polish, without serious communication deficits), were included into this sub-study. All patients had neuroimaging (CT/MRI) performed on admission. Stroke was defined as a sudden onset of neurological deficit lasting longer than 24 h. All patients were treated according to standard protocols of international guidelines [7].

Data regarding socio-demographic factors and comorbidities was collected. The Cumulative Illness Rating Scale (CIRS) was used as a general indicator of health status [8]. The severity of clinical deficit after stroke was graded by the National Institutes of Health Stroke Scale (NIHSS) [9] and the disability prior to admission was assessed by the modified Rankin Scale (mRS) [10].

Depression symptoms were assessed between 7 and 10 days after admission with Polish version of Patient Health Questionnaire-9 (PHQ-9) [11]. This questionnaire queries symptoms present using 4-point Likert scale with item scores ranging from 0 (symptoms not present) to 3 (symptoms present nearly every day). The score ranges from 0 (no depressive symptoms) to 27 (all symptoms occurring nearly every day) and can be used to determine depression severity (0–4 indicates no depression,

5–9 mild depression, 10 to 14 moderate depression, 15–19 moderately severe depression and 20–27 severe depression). PHQ-9 shows good reliability, validity and clinical utility when used in stroke patients [12]. Patients enrolled in the study completed the questionnaire on their own or with the help of a psychologist when filling out was impossible or difficult (e.g., the patient could not hold the pen because of a paresis or had a visual impairment). Depression was diagnosed if the patient received 5 or more points on the PHQ-9 scale [13].

To evaluate post-stroke apathy (PSA), the Apathy Evaluation Scale-C (AES-C) [14] was used. AES is an 18-item questionnaire with a clinician rated version that was applied in this study. The questions address patient's activities, interest in doing things, relationship with others and feelings over the past two to three weeks. Each item is rated on a 4-point Likert scale with item scoring ranging from 1 (not at all true) to 4 (very true). The total AES-C score ranges from 18 to 72, with higher scores indicating greater apathy. The AES has good reliability and validity and was frequently used in studies on post-stroke apathy [14]. Apathy was diagnosed with AES score of ≥ 37 points [15].

Anxiety was measured with Polish adaptation of State Trait Anxiety Inventory (STAI) [16,17], the 40-item instrument, measuring, respectively, transient and enduring levels of anxiety. The state scale used in the present study administered as a self-completion questionnaire by the interviewer, assessed how the patients felt at the moment or in the recent past and how they anticipate their feelings to be in a specific, hypothetic situation in the future. The STAI scale is scored on four levels of anxiety intensity from 1 (not at all) to 4 (very much) and with a sum score between 20 and 80. The raw results are interpreted by referring to a relevant sten scores and then categorized into three levels of anxiety: low (1–4 sten), moderate (5–6 sten) and high (7–10 sten) [17].

Patients were screened for delirium with the abbreviated version of Confusion Assessment Method (bCAM) or the Intensive Care Units version (CAM-ICU), specifically in patients with motor aphasia or those who could not communicate for other reasons [18,19]. The final diagnosis of delirium was based on both clinical observation and structural assessment. The diagnostic criteria for delirium were based on the DSM-5 classification [20].

To screen for pre-stroke depression (pre-SD), a member of family/spouse or a close informant of the patient's household filled out the Neuropsychiatric Inventory [21]. In addition, patients were asked about previous treatment for depression, and medical records were checked for antidepressants among the medications currently taken by the patient.

In order to diagnose patients with pre-stroke dementia, a Polish version of Informant Questionnaire on Cognitive Decline in the Elderly (IQCODE) was used [22].

2.2. Outcome Assessment

We assessed the following outcome measures: presence of depression between 7–10th day after admission to the hospital, degree of disability in daily activities and mortality after stroke 3 and 12 months after stroke during the follow-up visit. Patients who did not attend a follow-up visit were contacted by phone and the information was gathered. A neurologist and a psychologist, both uninvolved in the baseline assessment of patients, were responsible for data acquisition.

2.3. Statistics

Statistical analysis was performed using Statistica 13.3 software (StatSoft®, Kraków, Poland). Qualitative variables were compared using the chi-squared test with or without Yates' correction, as appropriate. Quantitative values were presented as medians with interquartile ranges (IQRs) and compared with the Mann-Whitney U test due to non-normal distribution in each case. Correlations were statistically evaluated using Pearson's correlation tests and correlation coefficients (r) were obtained.

Associations between PSD (based on the PHQ-9 cut-off point) and 3-month and 12-month mortality were found using univariate logistic regression models. Predictive values were presented as odds ratios (ORs) with 95% confidence intervals (CIs). Similarly, associations between PSD and disability (increase in mRS of ≥1) were evaluated. Then, multivariate logistic regression models were adjusted for age, gender, and comorbidities (CIRS score). *p*-values < 0.05 were considered statistically significant.

3. Results

From 750 patients included into PROPOLIS study 524 filled out the PHQ-9. After three and 12 months after stroke 514 and 487 patients were available for examination, respectively. A flowchart (Figure 1) and a timeline (Figure 2) show the study design.

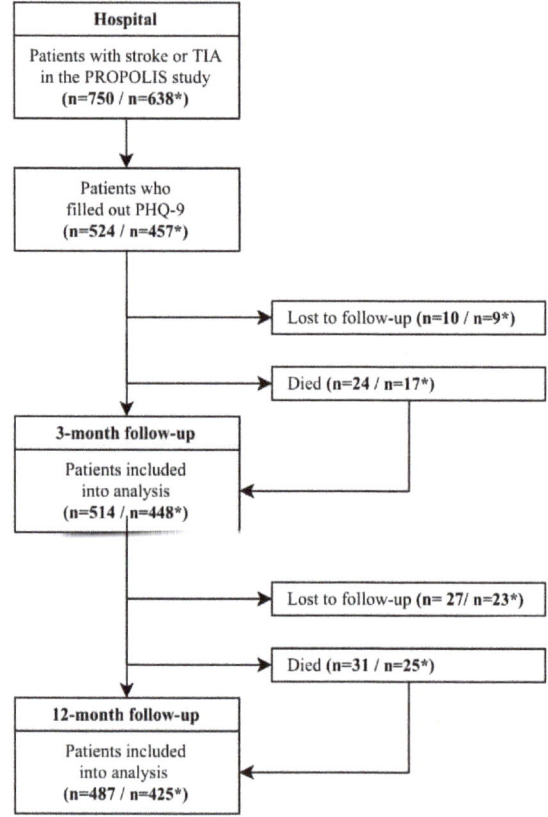

* number of cases after exclusion of patients with pre-stroke depression

Figure 1. Study flowchart.

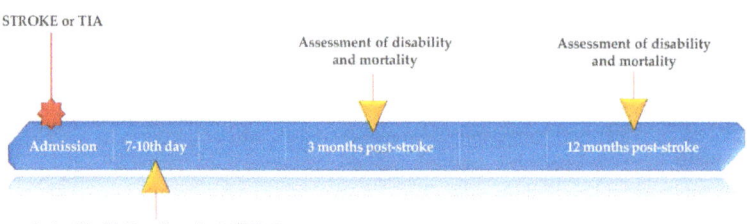

Figure 2. Study timeline.

When compared to controls, patients with PSD were significantly older, more often females, less often had left hemispheres stroke and treatment with recombinant tissue plasminogen activator (rt-PA), suffered from pneumonia, and had higher C-reactive protein (CRP) levels during hospitalization. Also, they were significantly more physically disabled prior to admission, more often had TIA or stroke in the past and had more comorbidities at baseline comparisons. Early depression was significantly more often accompanied by other neuropsychiatric conditions: apathy, anxiety, delirium, and dementia. Table 1 shows the details.

After three months, 24 patients died, 10 were lost from the follow-up and mRS score was not obtained in 18 patients. After 12 months, 31 persons died, and another 27 patients were lost from the follow-up. Patients who were lost from the follow-up did not differ significantly from those analyzed. Table 2 shows the results.

In the first step, we compared patients with PHQ-9 ≥ 5 points with those who scored 4 or less. After 3 and 12 months after stroke, PSD was an independent risk factor for death in multivariable logistic regression analysis. Also, PSD independently increased the level of disability of 1 point on mRS among patients with PSD three and 12 months post-stroke. Table 3 and Figures 3 and 4 show the final results.

In the second step, we excluded patients with pre-SD from further analyses. The general characteristic of patients with PSD and controls, after exclusion of patients with pre-SD, are shown in Table 4. The final results were very similar to those obtained in first analysis. Only the side of stroke lost its significance.

In regression analyses, PSD was still an independent variable for mortality and increased level of disability measured by mRS three and 12 months after stroke. Table 5 shows the results.

Patients that were lost from the follow-up in this sub-analysis did not differ significantly from analyzed group. Table 6 shows the details.

In the third step, we compared only pre-SD with patients without depression (pre- or post-stroke). Patients with pre-SD were significantly more often women, had more comorbidities and had higher level of disability prior to admission. Table 7 shows the details.

Pre-SD increased the level of disability on mRS of 1 point at three and 12 months post-stroke and predicted mortality within 12 months after stroke. Table 8 shows the results.

Patients with pre-SD significantly more often had PSD and they also had significantly more severe depression when compared to other individuals. There was no relationship between NIHSS score and PHQ-9 score. Tables 9 and 10 show the results.

Table 1. Baseline characteristics of patients without and with post-stroke depression in hospital. (All included patients).

Variable	Data	No Depression n = 238 (45.42%)	Depression n = 286 (54.58%)	p-Value
Male gender *	524	143/238 (60.08)	122/286 (42.66)	<0.001
Age [years] **	524	68 (60–78)	71 (62–80)	0.022
Higher education *	518	49/235 (20.85)	49/283 (17.31)	0.306
Length of education [years] **	515	11 (10–14)	11 (10–13)	0.122
Hemorrhagic stroke *	524	12/238 (5.04)	16/286 (5.59)	0.780
TOAST classification:				
- large-artery atherosclerosis *	457	27/210 (12.86)	28/247 (11.34)	0.618
- cardioembolism *	457	11/210 (5.24)	15/247 (6.07)	0.701
- small-vessel occlusion *	457	63/210 (30.00)	79/247 (31.98)	0.648
- other determined etiology *	457	107/210 (50.95)	122/247 (49.39)	0.740
- undetermined etiology *	457	2/210 (0.95)	3/247 (1.21)	0.855
Side of stroke:				
- right hemisphere *	524	93/238 (39.09)	136/286 (47.55)	0.051
- left hemisphere *	524	112/238 (47.06)	105/286 (36.71)	0.017
- posterior part *	524	31/238 (13.03)	35/286 (12.24)	0.787
- more than one localization *	524	2/238 (0.84)	10/286 (3.50)	0.084
rt-Pa treatment *	524	68/238 (28.57)	52/286 (18.18)	0.007
Thrombectomy *	524	12/238 (5.04)	12/286 (4.20)	0.645
Medical history:				
- hypertension *	524	158/238 (66.39)	206/286 (72.03)	0.163
- diabetes *	524	49/238 (20.59)	92/286 (32.17)	0.003
- atrial fibrillation *	524	39/238 (16.39)	54/286 (18.88)	0.457
- myocardial infraction *	524	33/238 (13.87)	40/286 (13.99)	0.968
- PCI or CABG *	524	22/238 (9.24)	25/286 (8.74)	0.841
- smoking—ever *	523	118/237 (49.79)	149/286 (52.10)	0.599
- smoking—current *	523	62/237 (26.16)	86/286 (30.07)	0.323
- previous stroke or TIA *	522	32/237 (13.50)	60/285 (21.05)	0.024
CIRS, total score **	524	7 (5–11)	10 (6–13)	<0.001
Pneumonia *	524	8/238 (3.36)	23/286 (8.04)	0.038
Urinary tract infections *	505	58/232 (25.00)	81/273 (29.67)	0.242
Length of hospital stay [days] **	524	9 (8–10)	9 (8–11)	0.320
Aphasia in hospital *	524	53/238 (22.27)	50/286 (17.48)	0.170
Neglect in hospital *	524	22/238 (9.24)	34/286 (11.89)	0.329
Vision deficits in hospital *	524	59/238 (24.79)	89/286 (31.12)	0.109
Delirium in hospital *	524	25/238 (10.50)	66/286 (23.08)	<0.001
AES score at 7–10th day in hospital **	480	29 (20–38)	34 (25–43)	<0.001
STAI-S score at 7–10th day in hospital **	520	32 (27–39)	42 (33–52)	<0.001
STAI-T score at 7–10th day in hospital **	519	35 (30–41.5)	47 (40–54)	<0.001
NIHSS at admission **	524	4 (2–8)	4 (2–9)	0.649
Pre-hospital mRS **	524	0 (0–0)	0 (0–1)	0.002
Pre-hospital IQCODE **	436	78 (78–79)	78 (78–83)	0.007
CRP level in hospital [mg/l] **	507	3.82 (1.63–10.34)	5.75 (2.04–18.60)	0.003

* n (%); ** median (IQR); TOAST—Trial of Org 10172 in Acute Stroke Treatment; rt-Pa—recombinant tissue plasminogen activator; PCI—percutaneous coronary interventions; CABG—coronary artery bypass graft; TIA—transient ischemic attack; CIRS—Cumulative Illness Rating Scale; AES—Apathy Evaluation Scale; STAI—State-Trait Anxiety Inventory (S—state scale, T—trait scale); NIHSS—National Institutes of Health Stroke Scale; mRS—Modified Rankin Scale; IQCODE—Informant Questionnaire on Cognitive Decline in the Elderly; CRP—C-reactive protein.

Table 2. Comparison of analyzed and lost to follow-up cases. (All included patients).

Variable	Data	Analyzed Cases	Lost to Follow-Up	p-Value
Comparison of Analyzed (n = 514) and Lost to Follow-Up (n = 10) Cases for 3-Month Mortality				
Male gender *	524	259/514 (50.39)	6/10 (60.00)	0.777
Age (years) **	524	69 (61–79)	69.5 (62–77)	0.581
CIRS, total score **	524	8.5 (5–12)	7 (5–10)	0.441
NIHSS at admission **	524	4 (2–9)	3 (0–10)	0.428
Pre-hospital mRS **	524	0 (0–0)	0 (0–0)	0.834
Comparison of Analyzed (n = 496) and Lost to Follow-Up (n = 28) Cases for 3-Month mRS				
Male gender *	524	250/496 (50.40)	15/28 (53.57)	0.744
Age (years) **	524	69 (61–79)	71 (62–79.5)	0.662
CIRS, total score **	524	9 (5–12)	7.5 (5–11.5)	0.374
NIHSS at admission **	524	4 (2–9)	3 (0–7)	0.113
Pre-hospital mRS **	524	0 (0–0)	0 (0–0.5)	0.858
Comparison of Analyzed (n = 487) and Lost to Follow-Up (n = 37) Cases for 12-Month Mortality and mRS				
Male gender *	524	244/487 (50.10)	21/37 (56.76)	0.435
Age (years) **	524	69 (61–79)	71 (63–78)	0.639
CIRS, total score **	524	9 (5–12)	7 (4–11)	0.130
NIHSS at admission **	524	4 (2–8)	4 (2–12)	0.317
Pre-hospital mRS **	524	0 (0–0)	0 (0–0)	0.871

* n (%); ** median (IQR); CIRS—Cumulative Illness Rating Scale; NIHSS—National Institutes of Health Stroke Scale; mRS—Modified Rankin Scale.

Table 3. Influence of post-stroke depression on mortality and disability 3 and 12 months after stroke. (All included patients).

Variable	Data	Incidence, n (%)		Univariate Logistic Regression Model		Multivariate Logistic Regression Model *	
		No Depression	Depression	OR (95CI)	p-Value	OR (95CI)	p-Value
3 months:							
Mortality	514	3/234 (1.28)	21/230 (7.50)	6.243 (1.838–21.204)	0.003	5.685 (1.586–20.378)	0.008
Increase in mRS of ≥1	496	121/228 (53.07)	191/268 (71.27)	2.194 (1.514–3.179)	<0.001	1.944 (1.315–2.876)	0.001
12 months:							
Mortality	487	9/220 (4.09)	46/267 (17.23)	4.880 (2.331–10.216)	<0.001	4.535 (2.065–9.964)	<0.001
Increase in mRS of ≥1	487	112/220 (50.91)	178/267 (66.67)	1.929 (1.336–2.783)	<0.001	1.681 (1.141–2.478)	0.009

* adjusted for age, gender and CIRS (Cumulative Illness Rating Scale); mRS—Modified Rankin Scale.

Table 4. Baseline characteristics of patients without and with post-stroke depression in hospital. (Only patients without Pre-Stroke Depression).

Variable	Data	No Depression n = 223 (48.80%)	Depression n = 234 (51.20%)	p-Value
Male gender *	457	139/223 (62.33)	104/234 (44.44)	<0.001
Age (years) **	457	67 (60–78)	73 (62–80)	0.011
Higher education *	451	47/220 (21.36)	40/231 (17.32)	0.276
Length of education (years) **	449	12 (10–14)	11 (9–13)	0.064
Hemorrhagic stroke *	457	12/223 (5.38)	12/234 (5.13)	0.904
TOAST classification:				
- large-artery atherosclerosis *	398	24/197 (12.18)	22/201 (10.95)	0.699
- cardioembolism *	398	11/197 (5.58)	11/201 (5.47)	0.961
- small-vessel occlusion *	398	59/197 (29.95)	65/201 (32.34)	0.607
- other determined etiology *	398	101 (51.27)	101/201 (50.25)	0.839
- undetermined etiology *	398	2/197 (1.02)	2/201 (1.00)	0.630
Side of stroke:				
- right hemisphere *	457	88/223 (39.46)	108/234 (46.15)	0.149
- left hemisphere *	457	102/223 (45.74)	88/234 (37.61)	0.079
- posterior part *	457	31/223 (13.90)	30/234 (12.82)	0.734
- more than one localization *	457	2/223 (0.90)	8/23 (3.42)	0.128
rt-Pa treatment *	457	61/223 (27.35)	41/234 (17.52)	0.012
Thrombectomy *	457	11/223 (4.93)	9/234 (3.85)	0.570
Medical history:				
- hypertension *	457	148/223 (66.37)	172/234 (73.50)	0.096
- diabetes *	457	44/223 (19.73)	76/234 (32.48)	0.002
- atrial fibrillation *	457	35/223 (15.70)	44/234 (18.80)	0.380
- myocardial infraction *	457	32/223 (14.35)	32/234 (13.68)	0.836
- PCI or CABG *	457	22/223 (9.87)	20/234 (8.55)	0.626
- smoking—ever *	456	112/222 (50.45)	118/234 (50.43)	0.996
- smoking—current *	456	59/222 (26.58)	66/234 (28.21)	0.697
- previous stroke or TIA *	455	30/222 (13.51)	49/233 (21.03)	0.036
CIRS, total score **	457	7 (4–11)	9 (6–12)	<0.001
Pneumonia *	457	7/223 (3.14)	21/234 (8.97)	0.009
Urinary tract infections *	442	52/218 (23.85)	68/224 (30.36)	0.124
Length of hospital stay [days] **	457	9 (8–10)	9 (8–11)	0.472
Aphasia in hospital *	457	48/223 (21.52)	40/234 (17.09)	0.230
Neglect in hospital *	457	20/223 (8.97)	28/234 (11.97)	0.296
Vision deficits in hospital *	457	53/223 (23.77)	71/234 (30.34)	0.114
Delirium in hospital *	457	20/223 (8.97)	53/234 (22.65)	<0.001
AES score at 7–10th day in hospital **	411	28 (20–36)	32.5 (24–42)	<0.001
STAI-S score at 7–10th day in hospital **	453	31 (27–39)	41 (32–51)	<0.001
STAI-T score at 7–10th day in hospital **	452	35 (30–41)	45 (39–53)	<0.001
NIHSS at admission **	457	4 (2–7)	4 (2–9)	0.673
Pre-hospital mRS **	457	0 (0–1)	0 (0–1)	0.003
Pre-hospital IQCODE **	377	78 (78–79)	78 (78–81)	0.019
CRP level in hospital [mg/L] **	442	3.74 (1.59–10.77)	5.44 (1.97–17.25)	0.010

* n (%); ** median (IQR); TOAST—Trial of Org. 10172 in Acute Stroke Treatment; rt-Pa—recombinant tissue plasminogen activator; PCI—percutaneous coronary interventions; CABG—coronary artery bypass graft; TIA—transient ischemic attack; CIRS—Cumulative Illness Rating Scale; AES—Apathy Evaluation Scale; STAI—State-Trait Anxiety Inventory (S—state scale, T—trait scale); NIHSS—National Institutes of Health Stroke Scale; mRS—Modified Rankin Scale; IQCODE—Informant Questionnaire on Cognitive Decline in the Elderly; CRP—C-reactive protein.

Table 5. Influence of post-stroke depression on mortality and disability 3 and 12 months after stroke. (Only patients without Pre-stroke depression).

Variable	Data	Incidence, n (%)		Univariate Logistic Regression Model		Multivariate Logistic Regression Model *	
		No Depression	Depression	OR (95CI)	p-Value	OR (95CI)	p-Value
3 months:							
Mortality	448	3/219 (1.37)	14/229 (6.11)	4.688 (1.328–16.548)	0.016	4.447 (1.184–16.707)	0.027
Increase in mRS of ≥1	432	109/213 (51.17)	151/219 (68.95)	2.119 (1.431–3.137)	<0.001	1.856 (1.227–2.806)	0.003
12 months:							
Mortality	425	9/208 (4.33)	33/217 (15.21)	3.966 (1.847–8.512)	<0.001	3.712 (1.644–8.381)	0.002
Increase in mRS of ≥1	425	104/208 (50.00)	140/217 (64.52)	1.818 (1.232–2.682)	0.003	1.588 (1.056–2.387)	0.026

* adjusted for age, gender and CIRS (Cumulative Illness Rating Scale); mRS—Modified Rankin Scale.

Table 6. Comparison of analyzed and lost to follow-up cases. (Only patients without Pre-Stroke Depression).

Variable	Data	Analyzed Cases	Lost to Follow-Up	p-Value
Comparison of Analyzed (n = 448) and Lost to Follow-Up (n = 9) Cases for 3-Month Mortality				
Male gender *	457	237/448 (52.90)	5/9 (66.67)	0.629
Age (years) **	457	69.5 (61–79)	68 (62–71)	0.366
CIRS, total score **	457	8 (5–12)	6 (5–10)	0.276
NIHSS at admission **	457	4 (2–8)	3 (0–10)	0.496
Pre-hospital mRS **	457	0 (0–0)	0 (0–0)	0.991
Comparison of Analyzed (n = 432) and Lost to Follow-Up (n = 25) Cases for 3-Month mRS				
Male gender *	457	229/432 (53.01)	14/25 (56.00)	0.771
Age (years) **	457	69 (61–79)	71 (62–78)	0.909
CIRS, total score **	457	8 (5–12)	6 (5–10)	0.278
NIHSS at admission **	457	4 (2–8)	3 (0–7)	0.216
Pre-hospital mRS **	457	0 (0–0)	0 (0–1)	0.573
Comparison of Analyzed (n = 425) and Lost to Follow-Up (n = 32) Cases for 12-Month Mortality and mRS				
Male gender *	457	223/425 (52.47)	20/32 (62.50)	0.273
Age (years) **	457	69 (61–79)	69.5 (62–78)	0.874
CIRS, total score **	457	8 (5–12)	7 (3–11)	0.122
NIHSS at admission **	457	4 (2–8)	4 (2–12)	0.364
Pre-hospital mRS **	457	0 (0–0)	0 (0–0)	0.575

* n (%); ** median (IQR); CIRS—Cumulative Illness Rating Scale; NIHSS—National Institutes of Health Stroke Scale; mRS—Modified Rankin Scale.

Table 7. Baseline characteristics of patients without depression and with pre-stroke depression.

Variable	Data	No Depression n = 223 (79.08%)	Pre-Stroke Depression n = 59 (20.92%)	p-Value
Male gender *	282	139/223 (62.33)	20/59 (33.90)	<0.001
Age (years) **	282	67 (60–78)	68 (61–79)	0.302
Previous stroke or TIA *	281	30/222 (13.51)	13/59 (22.03)	0.106
CIRS, total score **	282	7 (4–11)	11 (6–15)	<0.001
NIHSS at admission **	282	4 (2–7)	5 (2–11)	0.264
Pre-hospital mRS **	282	0 (0–0)	0 (0–1)	0.034

* n (%); ** median (IQR); TIA—transient ischemic attack; CIRS—Cumulative Illness Rating Scale; NIHSS—National. Institutes of Health Stroke Scale; mRS—Modified Rankin Scale.

Table 8. Influence of pre-stroke depression on mortality and disability 3 and 12 months after stroke.

Variable	Incidence, n (%)			Univariate Logistic Regression Model		Multivariate Logistic Regression Model *	
	Data	No Depression	Pre-Stroke Depression	OR (95CI)	p-Value	OR (95CI)	p-Value
3 months:							
Mortality	277	3/219 (1.37)	6/58 (10.34)	8.308 (2.011–34.322)	0.003	2.414 (0.376–15.497)	0.353
Increase in mRS of ≥1	270	109/213 (51.17)	47/57 (82.46)	4.484 (2.153–9.338)	<0.001	3.965 (1.826–8.610)	<0.001
12 months:							
Mortality	264	9/208 (4.33)	12/56 (21.43)	6.030 (2.394–15.191)	<0.001	3.406 (1.064–10.904)	0.039
Increase in mRS of ≥1	264	104/208 (50.00)	42/56 75.00)	3.000 (1.546–5.823)	0.001	2.395 (1.171–4.897)	0.017

* adjusted for age, gender and CIRS (Cumulative Illness Rating Scale); mRS—Modified Rankin Scale.

Table 9. Association of incidence of pre-stroke depression with post-stroke depression and median PHQ-9 score.

Variable	Data	Pre-Stroke Depression n = 59 (20.92%)	No Pre-Stroke Depression n = 457 (88.57%)	p-Value
Post-stroke depression *	516	48/59 (81.36)	234/457 (51.20)	<0.001
PHQ-9 score **	516	9 (6–12)	5 (2–9)	<0.001

* n (%); ** median (IQR); PHQ-9—The Patient Health Questionnaire-9.

Table 10. Correlations between NIHSS and PHQ-9 at the hospital.

Group	Data	Pearson's Correlation Coefficient (r)	p-Value
All patients	524	−0.0128	0.770
Pre-stroke depression excluded	457	−0.0384	0.413

NIHSS—National Institutes of Health Stroke Scale; PHQ-9—The Patient Health Questionnaire-9.

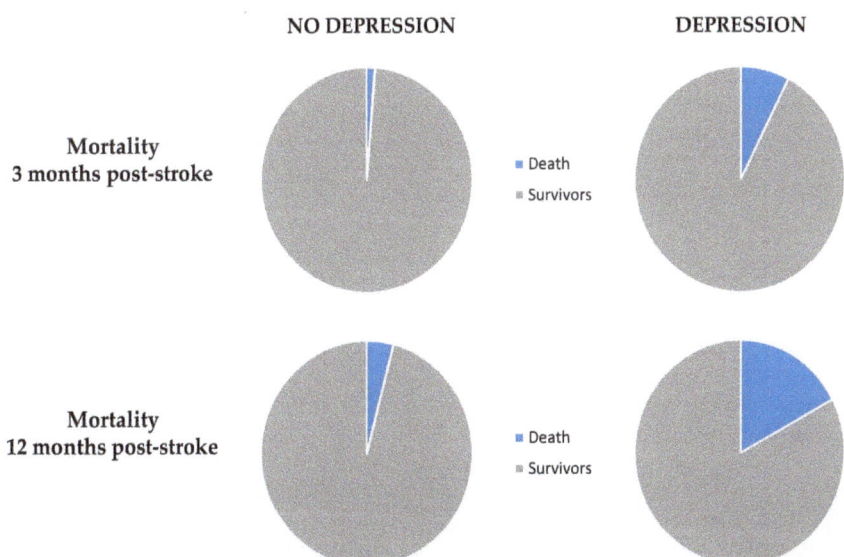

Figure 3. A pie chart presenting the influence of post-stroke depression on mortality.

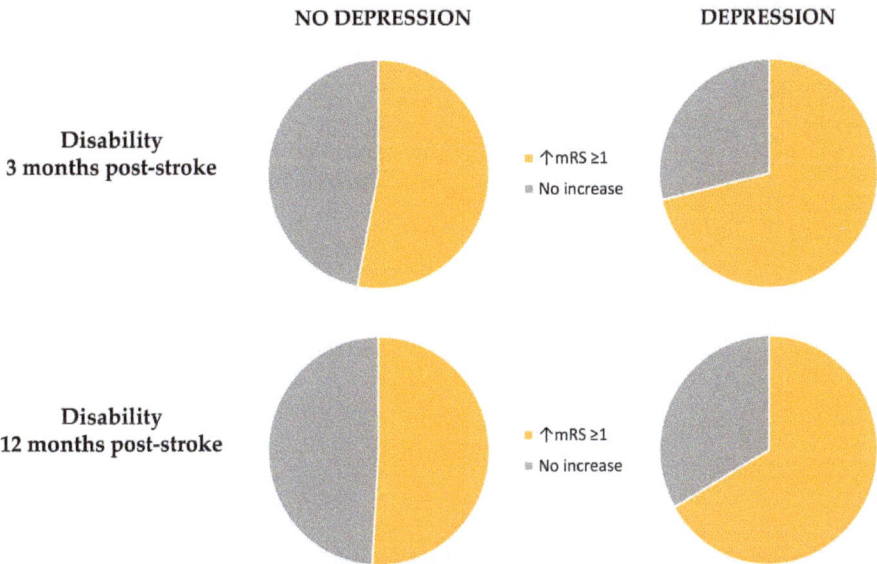

Figure 4. A pie chart presenting the influence of post-stroke depression on disability.

4. Discussion

In our cohort, depression was diagnosed in 54.58% of patients between seven and 10 days after stroke. Patients who developed depressive symptoms in acute phase of stroke had about six times higher risk of death three months after stroke and nearly 4.5 times higher risk after 12 months, when compared to patients without depression. PSD negatively influenced level of disability and mortality rate at three and 12 months after stroke. Both outcomes were independent from stroke severity and concomitant neuropsychiatric conditions.

Other studies have also reported an association between PSD and mortality after stroke. In study by Williams et al. [23], among total of 51,119 patients hospitalized with an ischemic stroke, those diagnosed with PSD had a higher three-year mortality risk, even despite being younger and having fewer chronic conditions. Previous meta-analysis [4–6], also showed that mortality was an independent outcome of depression after stroke and patients with early PSD had a risk of death about 1.5 higher as compared with non-depressed individuals, considering both short- and long-term mortality. In a study by Razmara et al. [24], the combination of depression and stroke was associated with all—cause mortality, with the highest risk of death in those aged 65–74 years. Patients with depressive symptoms were about 35 times more likely to die when compared to stroke survivors without depression.

Our study found that PSD increases the level of disability both three and 12 months after stroke. In earlier studies [25,26], depressed patients have been found more dependent in activities of daily living at three and 15-month follow-up than patients without depression. Paolucci et al. [27] estimated that PSD is a relevant factor that is responsible for about 15% of the increased disability observed in post—stroke depressive patient.

As was shown, pre-SD was associated with higher stroke morbidity and mortality [28]. In our cohort, pre-SD was independently related to increased mortality 12 months post-stroke but not three months. The number of patients with pre-SD was small which can explain this lack of association for the three-month observation.

Pre-SD, which is due to many factors, e.g., social, degenerative, or vascular, also negatively influenced the level of disability both three and 12 months after stroke. Results of this study suggest, that regardless of etiology, depression increases negative outcomes after stroke.

The association between stroke and depression is well established as well as between stroke and poor functional outcome. The connecting factor between depression, physical impairment, and mortality in patients with stroke can be brain-derived neurotrophic factor (BDNF), a member of the neurotrophin family, involved in neuronal development, differentiation, and survival.

There is a general agreement that etiology of mood disorders is multifactorial. Hypotheses about the participation and interrelationship of down regulation of neurotrophins, inflammation, hypothalamic-pituitary-adrenal axis hyperactivity and stress in pathophysiology of depression have an important support in literature [29].

Recent findings have reported that BDNF is a key regulator in the neuro-immune axis regulation, but its potential mechanism in depression remains unclear [30]. Lower BDNF levels were found to be a significant risk factor for PSD [31] as well as in clinically depressed individuals [32]. BDNF could intermediate between depression and the level of disability after stroke. Stroke activates microglia, which are brain guards and the first non-neuronal cells to respond to various acute brain injuries [33]. An inflammatory state can contribute to the development and progression of depression pathology, influencing alterations of the neuroplasticity caused by reduced BDNF expression, activity, and affinity to a receptor [30,34,35]. Moreover, BDNF levels are mediated by physical exercise enhancing its levels in the brain [36]. Activity-driven increases in BDNF have also been shown to promote motor recovery after stroke [37]. Physical rehabilitation may be impaired by depressions, and depressed patients are less likely to exercise what lowers the level of BDNF and intensify functional impairment. For the time being, there is not enough evidence of a definitive link between BDNF and depression, disability and mortality, and their potential interrelationships need to be confirmed in future studies.

Immunological mechanisms, as mentioned, are implicated in the pathogenesis of depressive symptoms. C-reactive protein is the inflammatory biomarker, an acute phase protein that increases in level during the acute phase of inflammation. Patients with depression exhibit increased peripheral blood concentrations of CRP [38,39]. Elevated CRP along with other peripheral blood markers of inflammation have been found to predict development of depression [40] and resistance to antidepressant therapy [41]. A few studies have examined the relationship between circulating CRP and risk of post-stroke depression with conflicting results [42–44]. In the previous sub-study, we found that this association was significant for depression diagnosed during hospitalization, but there was no association between depression diagnosed three months post-stroke and CRP levels [45]. Interestingly, in this present, much larger study, patients with depression, diagnosed at the hospital, had significantly higher level of CRP than dementia-free patients, thus supporting the hypothesis of the role of immunological mechanisms in development of depressive symptoms.

In the pathophysiology of depression, a dysregulated kynurenine pathway has also been implicated. In this pathway, tryptophan is broken down into kynurenine and then to neurotoxic quinolinic acid and decreases the availability of tryptophan for serotonin synthesis. The altered levels of kynurenines have been implicated in psychiatric [46] and neurodegenerative diseases [47]. Preliminary data from one small study among patients with stroke also suggest that the kynurenine pathway may be implicated in PSD and disability [48]. Kynurenic acid seems to be useful not only in process of diagnosis but also in prediction of the treatment response [49].

Research shows that inflammation is an important, multi-directional factor in the etiology of depression, but further research is still needed on its role in diagnosing depression, guiding decision making on clinical treatment and monitoring the course of the disease and the risk of its relapse.

Strengths and Weaknesses of the Study

The first step in arriving at a correct diagnosis of mental health problems is to distinguish depression from other psychiatric syndromes that can cause confusion, such as delirium, dementia, apathy, or anxiety. Evaluating different mental problems concurrently is also important to distinguish between the right diagnoses, given the overlap between them. Careful and broad evaluation of mental health problems at the hospital is a strong side of PROPOLIS.

Prior psychiatric illness can influence mental status post-stroke, i.e., represents either recurrence or continuation of a preexisting psychiatric illness. Therefore, in PROPOLIS, we carefully screened for neuro-psychiatric conditions including depression, dementia, delirium, anxiety, and apathy pre-stroke.

This study had prospective design and included a large number of patients at the baseline, which helped to sustain a reasonably large number of patients during all follow-ups. Patients that were lost in the follow-up didn't differ significantly from those followed-up.

A variety of raters; neurologist and psychologist assessed patients at baseline and during follow-up visits. This is considered as the strength of this study, because follow-up raters were blind for the patients' previous performance and behavior. On the other hand, patients who are more familiar to assessors are more willing to ask for help if they have problems with understanding the questions from the questionnaire and therefore provide more adequate answers. Therefore, a variety of raters can be also considered as a weakness of the study.

Some limitations of our study and bias inducers should also be addressed. Firstly, the PROPOLIS was designed to determine frequency, predictors, and clinical consequences of post-stroke delirium. Depressive symptoms were considered as a secondary endpoint of the study. Secondly, we used questionnaires to describe symptoms of depression, since using interviews with mental health professional was not feasible. Thirdly, the first evaluation for depressive disorders took place before the 14th day after stroke, which may have overestimated the prevalence of depression in the acute phase of stroke. Fourthly, during the follow-up visits, we observed, most depressed patients did not have formal diagnosis of depression and were not treated, but data on the treatment with antidepressants were not collected during the follow-ups. Because treatment with antidepressants might influence the study outcome, this is considered as a limitation. Fifth, as this was a single center study, the generalizability of our results may be limited.

5. Conclusions

Depression can act as a mediator variable for a higher disability level and mortality in patients more vulnerable to brain injury, independently of other neuropsychiatric mental health problems.

A high prevalence of depression after stroke should stress the need for future research exploring its possible pathomechanism and testing, if an early management of depression may change life expectancy after stroke and improve the outcome, even if functional deficits remain.

Author Contributions: Conceptualization, K.K. and A.K.-M.; methodology, K.K., P.P. and A.K.-M.; validation, K.K., Ł.K., J.D., A.W. and A.K.-M.; formal analysis, K.K., Ł.K. and A.W.; investigation, K.K. and P.P.; writing—original draft preparation, K.K. and A.K.-M.; writing—review and editing, J.D., Ł.K., A.W., P.P. and A.K.-M.; supervision A.K.-M.; project administration, A.K.-M.; funding acquisition, A.K.-M. All authors have read and agreed to the published version of the manuscript.

Funding: Faculty of Medicine of Jagiellonian University Medical College (Leading National Research Centre 2012–2017) funded the collection of data for the study. Grant number KNOW-9000474.

Acknowledgments: We thank Małgorzata Mazurek for manuscript editing, and Elżbieta Klimiec for data collection.

Conflicts of Interest: The authors declare no conflict of interest.

References

1. Hackett, M.L.; Pickles, K. Part I: Frequency of depression after stroke: An updated systematic review and meta-analysis of observational studies. *Int. J. Stroke* **2014**, *9*, 1017–1025. [CrossRef]
2. Kowalska, K.; Droś, J.; Mazurek, M.; Pasińska, P.; Gorzkowska, A.; Klimkowicz-Mrowiec, A. Delirium Post-Stroke: Short- and Long-Term Effect on Depression, Anxiety, Apathy and Aggression (Research Study—Part of PROPOLIS Study). *J. Clin. Med.* **2020**, *9*, 2232. [CrossRef]
3. Bartoli, F.; Di Brita, C.; Crocamo, C.; Clerici, M.; Carrà, G. Early Post-stroke Depression and Mortality: Meta-Analysis and Meta-Regression. *Front. Psychiatry* **2018**, *9*, 530. [CrossRef]
4. Ayerbe, L.; Ayis, S.; Wolfe, C.D.A.; Rudd, A.G. Natural history, predictors and outcomes of depression after stroke: Systematic review and meta-analysis. *Br. J. Psychiatry* **2013**, *202*, 14–21. [CrossRef]
5. Bartoli, F.; Lillia, N.; Lax, A.; Crocamo, C.; Mantero, V.; Carra, G.; Agostini, E.; Clerici, M. Depression after Stroke and Risk of Mortality: A Systematic Review and Meta-Analysis. *Stroke Res. Treat.* **2013**, *2013*, 862978. [CrossRef]
6. Hackett, M.L.; Anderson, C.S. Predictors of depression after stroke: A systematic review of observational studies. *Stroke* **2005**, *36*, 2296–2301. [CrossRef]
7. Intercollegiate Stroke Working Party. *National Clinical Guideline for Stroke*, 4th ed.; Royal College of Physicians: London, UK, 2012.
8. de Groot, V.; Beckerman, H.; Lankhorst, G.J.; Bouter, L.M. How to measure comorbidity. a critical review of available methods. *J. Clin. Epidemiol.* **2003**, *56*, 221–229. [CrossRef]
9. Meyer, B.C.; Lyden, P.D. The modified national institutes of health stroke scale: Its time has come. *Int. J. Stroke* **2009**, *4*, 267–273. [CrossRef] [PubMed]
10. Broderick, J.P.; Adeoye, O.; Elm, J. Evolution of the Modified Rankin Scale and Its Use in Future Stroke Trials. *Stroke* **2017**, *48*, 2007–2012. [CrossRef]
11. Tomaszewski, K.; Zarychta, M.; Bieńkowska, A.; Chmurowicz, E.; Nowak, W.; Skalska, A. Validation of the Patient Health Questionnaire-9 Polish version in the hospitalised elderly population. *Psychiatr. Pol.* **2011**, *45*, 223–233.
12. de Man-van Ginkel, J.M.; Gooskensm, F.; Schepers, V.P.; Schuurmans, M.J.; Lindeman, E.; Hafsteinsdóttir, T.B. Screening for poststroke depression using the patient health questionnaire. *Nurs. Res.* **2012**, *61*, 333–341. [CrossRef] [PubMed]
13. Kroenke, K.; Spitzer, R.L.; Williams, J.B.W. The PHQ-9: Validity of a Brief Depression Severity Measure. *J. Gen. Intern. Med.* **2001**, *16*, 606–613. [CrossRef] [PubMed]

14. Marin, R.S.; Biedrzycki, R.C.; Firinciogullari, S. Reliability and Validity of the Apathy Evaluation Scale. *Psychiatry Res.* **1991**, *38*, 143–162. [CrossRef]
15. Brodaty, H.; Sachdev, P.S.; Withall, A.; Altendorf, A.; Valenzuela, M.J.; Lorentz, L. Frequency and clinical, neuropsychological and neuroimaging correlates of apathy following stroke—The Sydney Stroke Study. *Psychol. Med.* **2005**, *35*, 1707–1716. [CrossRef]
16. Spielberger, C.D.; Gorsuch, R.L.; Lushene, P.R.; Vagg, P.R.; Jacobs, G.A. *Manual for the State-Trait Anxiety Inventory*; Consulting Psychologists Press, Inc.: Palo Alto, CA, USA, 1983.
17. Wrześniewski, K.; Sosnowski, T.; Jaworowska, A.; Fecenec, D. *STAI. State-Trait Anxiety Inventory. Polish Adaptation STAI*, 4th ed.; Pracownia Testów Psychologicznych Polskiego Towarzystwa Psychologicznego: Warszawa, Poland, 2011.
18. Inouye, S.K.; Van Dyck, C.H.; Alessi, C.A.; Balkin, S.; Siegal, A.P.; Horwitz, R.I. Clarifying confusion: The confusion assessment method. A new method for detection of delirium. *Ann. Intern. Med.* **1990**, *113*, 941–948. [CrossRef]
19. Ely, E.W.E.; Inouye, S.K.; Bernard, G.R.; Gordon, S.; Francis, J.; May, L.; Truman, B.; Speroff, T.; Gautam, S.; Margolin, R.; et al. Delirium in mechanically ventilated patients: Validity and reliability of the confusion assessment method for the intensive care unit (CAM-ICU). *JAMA* **2001**, *286*, 2703–2710. [CrossRef] [PubMed]
20. American Psychiatric Association. *Diagnostic and Statistical Manual of Mental Disorders*, 5th ed.; DSM-5; American Psychiatric Association: Arlington, MA, USA, 2013.
21. Cummings, J.L.; Mega, M.; Gray, K.; Rosenberg-Thompson, S.; Carusi, D.A.; Gornbein, J. The Neuropsychiatric Inventory: Comprehensive assessment of psychopathology in dementia. *Neurology* **1994**, *44*, 2308–2314. [CrossRef] [PubMed]
22. Klimkowicz, A.; Dziedzic, T.; Slowik, A.; Szczudlik, A. Incidence of pre-and poststroke dementia: Cracow stroke registry. *Dement. Geriatr. Cogn. Disord.* **2002**, *14*, 137–140. [CrossRef]
23. Williams, L.S.; Ghose, S.S.; Swindle, R.W. Depression and other mental health diagnoses increase mortality risk after ischemic stroke. *Am. J. Psych.* **2004**, *161*, 1090–1095. [CrossRef]
24. Razmara, A.; Valle, N.; Markovic, D.; Sanossian, N.; Ovbiagele, B.; Dutta, T.; Towfighi, A. Depression Is Associated with a Higher Risk of Death among Stroke Survivors. *J. Stroke Cerebrovasc. Dis.* **2017**, *26*, 2870–2879. [CrossRef]
25. Pohjasvaara, T.; Vataja, R.; Leppävuori, A.; Kaste, M.; Erkinjuntti, T. Depression is an independent predictor of poor long-term functional outcome post-stroke. *Eur. J. Neurol.* **2001**, *8*, 315–319. [CrossRef]
26. Pohjasvaara, T.; Leppävuori, A.; Siira, I.; Vataja, R.; Kaste, M.; Erkinjuntti, T. Frequency and clinical determinants of poststroke depression. *Stroke* **1998**, *29*, 2311–2317. [CrossRef]
27. Paolucci, S.; Iosa, M.; Coiro, P.; Venturiero, V.; Savo, A.; De Angelis, D.; Morone, G. Post-stroke Depression Increases Disability More Than 15% in Ischemic Stroke Survivors: A Case-Control Study. *Front. Neurol.* **2019**, *10*, 926. [CrossRef]
28. Pan, A.; Sun, Q.; Okereke, O.I.; Rexrode, K.M.; Hu, F.B. Depression and risk of stroke morbidity and mortality: A meta-analysis and systematic review. *JAMA* **2011**, *306*, 1241–1249. [CrossRef]
29. Verduijn, J.; Milaneschi, Y.; Schoevers, R.A.; van Hemert, A.M.; Beekman, A.T.F.; Penninx, B.W.J.H. Pathophysiology of major depressive disorder: Mechanisms involved in etiology are not associated with clinical progression. *Transl. Psychiatry* **2015**, *5*, e649. [CrossRef]
30. Jin, Y.; Sun, L.H.; Yang, W.; Cui, R.J.; Xu, S.B. The role of BDNF in the neuroimmune axis regulation of mood disorders. *Front. Neurol.* **2019**, *10*, 515. [CrossRef]
31. Noonan, K.; Carey, L.M.; Crewther, S.G. Meta-analyses indicate associations between neuroendocrine activation, deactivation in neurotrophic and neuroimaging markers in depression after stroke. *J. Stroke Cerebrovasc. Dis.* **2013**, *22*, e124–e135. [CrossRef]
32. Bocchio-Chiavetto, L.; Bagnardi, V.; Zanardini, R.; Molteni, R.; Nielsen, M.G.; Placentino, A.; Giovannini, C.; Rillosi, L.; Ventriglia, M.; Riva, M.A.; et al. Serum and plasma BDNF levels in major depression: A replication study and meta-analyses. *World J. Biol. Psychiatry* **2010**, *11*, 763–773. [CrossRef]
33. Lan, X.; Liu, R.; Sun, L.; Zhang, T.; Du, G. Methyl salicylate 2-O-β-D-lactoside, a novel salicylic acid analogue, acts as an anti-inflammatory agent on microglia and astrocytes. *J. Neuroinflammation* **2011**, *8*, 98. [CrossRef]
34. Pariante, C.M. Why are depressed patients inflamed? A reflection on 20 years of research on depression, glucocorticoid resistance and inflammation. *Eur. Neuropsychopharmacol.* **2017**, *27*, 554–559. [CrossRef]

35. Wohleb, E.S.; Franklin, T.; Iwata, M.; Duman, R.S. Integrating neuroimmune systems in the neurobiology of depression. *Nat. Rev. Neurosci.* **2016**, *17*, 497–511. [CrossRef] [PubMed]
36. Bathina, S.; Das, U.N. Brain-derived neurotrophic factor and its clinical implications. *Arch. Med. Sci.* **2015**, *11*, 1164–1178. [CrossRef] [PubMed]
37. Clarkson, A.N.; Overman, J.J.; Zhong, S.; Mueller, R.; Lynch, G.; Carmichael, S.T. AMPA receptor-induced local brain-derived neurotropic factor signaling mediates motor recovery after stroke. *J. Neurosci.* **2011**, *31*, 3766–3775. [CrossRef] [PubMed]
38. Howren, M.B.; Lamkin, D.M.; Suls, J. Associations of depression with C-reactive protein, IL-1, and IL-6: A meta-analysis. *Psychosom. Med.* **2009**, *71*, 171–186. [CrossRef]
39. Haapakoski, R.; Mathieu, J.; Ebmeier, K.P.; Alenius, H.; Kivimaki, M. Cumulative meta-analysis of interleukins 6 and 1beta, tumour necrosis factor alpha and C-reactive protein in patients with major depressive disorder. *Brain Behav. Immun.* **2015**, *49*, 206–215. [CrossRef]
40. Gimeno, D.; Kivimaki, M.; Brunner, E.J.; Elovainio, M.; De Vogli, R.; Steptoe, A.; Kumari, M.; Lowe, G.D.O.; Rumley, A.; Marmot, M.G.; et al. Associations of C-reactive protein and interleukin-6 with cognitive symptoms of depression: 12-year follow-up of the Whitehall II study. *Psychol. Med.* **2009**, *39*, 413–423. [CrossRef]
41. Strawbridge, R.; Arnone, D.; Danese, A.; Papadopoulos, A.; Herane Vives, A.; Cleare, A.J. Inflammation and clinical response to treatment in depression: A meta-analysis. *Eur. Neuropsychopharmacol.* **2015**, *25*, 1532–1543. [CrossRef]
42. Jiménez, I.; Sobrino, T.; Rodríguez-Yáñez, M.; Pouso, M.; Cristobo, I.; Sabucedo, M.; Blanco, M.; Castellanos, M.; Leira, R.; Castillo, J. High serum levels of leptin are associated with post-stroke depression. *Psychol. Med.* **2009**, *39*, 1201–1209. [CrossRef]
43. Yang, R.R.; Lu, B.C.; Li, T.; Du, Y.F.; Wang, X.; Jia, Y.X. The relationship between high-sensitivity C-reactive protein at admission and post stroke depression: A 6-month follow-up study. *Int. J. Geriatr. Psychiatry* **2016**, *31*, 231–239. [CrossRef]
44. Cheng, L.S.; Tu, W.J.; Shen, Y.; Zhang, L.J.; Ji, K. Combination of high-sensitivity C-reactive protein and homocysteine predicts the post-stroke depression in patients with ischemic stroke. *Mol. Neurobiol.* **2018**, *55*, 2952–2958. [CrossRef]
45. Kowalska, K.; Pacinolta, P.; Klimiec-Moskal, E.; Pera, J.; Słowik, A.; Klimkowicz-Mrowiec, A.; Dziedzic, T. C-reactive protein and post-stroke depressive symptoms. *Sci. Rep.* **2020**, *10*, 1431. [CrossRef] [PubMed]
46. Hunt, C.; Macedo e Cordeiro, T.; Suchting, R.; de Dios, C.; Cuellar Leal, V.A.; Soares, J.C.; Dantzer, R.; Teixeira, A.L.; Selvaraj, S. Effect of immune activation on the kynurenine pathway and depression symptoms—A systematic review and meta-analysis. *Neurosci. Biobeha. Rev.* **2020**, *118*, 514–523. [CrossRef] [PubMed]
47. Tanaka, M.; Toldi, J.; Vécsei, L. Exploring the Etiological Links behind Neurodegenerative Diseases: Inflammatory Cytokines and Bioactive Kynurenines. *Int. J. Mol. Sci.* **2020**, *21*, 2431. [CrossRef] [PubMed]
48. Carrillo-Mora, P.; Pérez-De la Cruz, V.; Estrada-Cortés, B.; Toussaint-González, P.; Martínez-Cortéz, J.A.; Rodríguez-Barragán, M.; Quinzaños-Fresnedo, J.; Rangel-Caballero, F.; Gamboa-Coria, G.; Sánchez-Vázquez, I.; et al. Serum Kynurenines Correlate with Depressive Symptoms and Disability in Poststroke Patients: A Cross-sectional Study. *Neurorehabilit. Neural Repair* **2020**, *34*, 936–944. [CrossRef] [PubMed]
49. Erabi, H.; Okada, G.; Shibasaki, C.; Setoyama, D.; Kang, D.; Takamura, M.; Yoshino, A.; Fuchikami, M.; Kurata, A.; Kato, T.A.; et al. Kynurenic acid is a potential overlapped biomarker between diagnosis and treatment response for depression from metabolome analysis. *Sci. Rep.* **2020**, *10*, 16822. [CrossRef] [PubMed]

Publisher's Note: MDPI stays neutral with regard to jurisdictional claims in published maps and institutional affiliations.

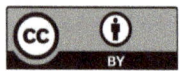

© 2020 by the authors. Licensee MDPI, Basel, Switzerland. This article is an open access article distributed under the terms and conditions of the Creative Commons Attribution (CC BY) license (http://creativecommons.org/licenses/by/4.0/).

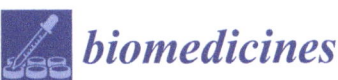

Review

Crosstalk between Depression and Dementia with Resting-State fMRI Studies and Its Relationship with Cognitive Functioning

Junhyung Kim [1,2] and Yong-Ku Kim [3,*]

1. Department of Psychiatry, Korea University Guro Hospital, Korea University College of Medicine, Seoul 08308, Korea; jhcabilover@gmail.com
2. Department of Psychiatry, Yonsei University College of Medicine, Seoul 03080, Korea
3. Department of Psychiatry, Korea University Ansan Hospital, Korea University College of Medicine, Ansan 15355, Korea
* Correspondence: yongku@korea.edu; Tel.: +82-10-9270-3259

Abstract: Alzheimer's disease (AD) is the most common type of dementia, and depression is a risk factor for developing AD. Epidemiological studies provide a clinical correlation between late-life depression (LLD) and AD. Depression patients generally remit with no residual symptoms, but LLD patients demonstrate residual cognitive impairment. Due to the lack of effective treatments, understanding how risk factors affect the course of AD is essential to manage AD. Advances in neuroimaging, including resting-state functional MRI (fMRI), have been used to address neural systems that contribute to clinical symptoms and functional changes across various psychiatric disorders. Resting-state fMRI studies have contributed to understanding each of the two diseases, but the link between LLD and AD has not been fully elucidated. This review focuses on three crucial and well-established networks in AD and LLD and discusses the impacts on cognitive decline, clinical symptoms, and prognosis. Three networks are the (1) default mode network, (2) executive control network, and (3) salience network. The multiple properties emphasized here, relevant for the hypothesis of the linkage between LLD and AD, will be further developed by ongoing future studies.

Keywords: depression; late-life depression; dementia; Alzheimer's disease; neuroimaging; resting-state functional magnetic resonance imaging; default mode network; executive control network; salience network

1. Introduction

Dementia, one of the most common neurodegenerative disorders, is a devastating illness characterized by significant cognitive decline that induces interference in daily life and behavioral disturbances [1]. Alzheimer's disease (AD) is the most common dementia type, with worldwide patients expected to increase from 82 million in 2030 to 152 million in 2050 [2]. One in every 2–3 people over the age of 85 will develop AD-related dementia [3], and most AD patients experience mild cognitive impairment (MCI), which is the preclinical status of dementia with modest cognitive decline without dysfunction in daily life [4,5]. Several studies have established that the accumulation of amyloid β, hyperphosphorylation of tau proteins, and neuroinflammation affect the neurodegeneration seen in AD [6,7]. However, there is no effective drug for both delaying onset and restoring cognitive function. Therefore, delaying disease onset or progression could provide a significant reduction in the social and economic burden of these diseases [8]. For delaying or preventing AD, previous studies have found several modifiable risk factors, including diet, midlife hypertension, type 2 diabetes mellitus, smoking, cognitive/physical inactivity, traumatic brain injury, and depression [9–11].

Depression is the most prevalent coexisting noncognitive feature that occurs along with cognitive deficits and is associated with neurodegenerative disorders and cognitive decline [12–14]. Because a major depressive disorder (MDD) is a heterogeneous diagnostic category that features differences in symptom profiles, comorbidities, and the course of disease [15,16], late-life depression (LLD) with an age of depression onset over 60 years has received a great deal of attention [17,18]. Moreover, the global number of individuals with LLD has increased by 27.1% from 2007 to 2017 [19]. Therefore, elucidating the link between the two disorders will help doctors and families understand and manage AD. Epidemiologic data have shown that LLD increases the risk of AD [20,21], and LLD is a risk factor that affects the progression of dementia from the normal cognition to MCI and from MCI to dementia [12,21–23]. Additionally, the risk of conversion from MCI to AD may vary due to the symptom severity of LLD or its successful treatment [24]. Individuals with LLD and high amyloid β levels exhibited a shortened conversion time than those without depression and with high amyloid β levels [25,26]. Altered levels and metabolism of amyloid β seen in AD were also reported in individuals with LLD [27]. Although these findings support previously suggested mechanisms that connect depression and dementia [28], a previous systematic review pointed out that these results are not consistent with other studies [29]. This discrepancy may be due to the study population differences or methodologic differences between the various studies [30]. Therefore, it is necessary to subdivide the study population and conduct research associated with more specific criteria.

Cognitive impairments in individuals with depression have been consistently reported in meta-analyses and reviews [31–34]. Based on these results, difficulties with concentration and making decisions have been described as part of major depressive disorder (MDD) [1]. Cognitive impairments in MDD were reported across most domains [35,36]. These cognitive impairments in MDD patients are usually normalized after remission of the MDD [35,36]. However, studies using a comprehensive neuropsychological battery have reported that cognitive impairment in remitted LLD patients persisted in executive function and episodic memory compared to healthy controls [37–39]. In addition, a longitudinal study has reported that LLD patients exhibit a significant decline in all domains, and three-month remitters also exhibited a significant decline in verbal fluency and executive function [17], suggesting that certain aspects of executive functioning are associated with the traits of LLD. Although other studies reported inconsistent results with no difference in LLD [40–42], these inconsistent results may be attributed to the differences in cognitive tests. Episodic memory is the other main impaired cognitive domain in individuals with MCI [43]. Impairment in these cognitive domains was usually exhibited to a greater extent in individuals with LLD+MCI (and those with AD), relative to individuals with LLD [44–47].

In recent years, using improved neuroimaging technology, we can investigate brain structure and function through neuroimaging tools, magnetic resonance imaging (MRI), computed tomography, and positron emission tomography (PET). Among them, functional MRI (fMRI) can provide information about the properties of functional connectivity (FC)—that is, collections of brain regions that are coactivated to support shared functions—during a task or rest (i.e., in the absence of stimuli) through measuring the blood oxygenation level-dependent (BOLD) signal [48,49]. More specifically, previous studies have suggested resting-state (rs)-fMRI as a promising method for investigating the behavioral characteristics including psychological states: sustained attention [50], personality [51], temperament traits [52], creative ability [53], and cognitive ability, such as working memory and motor performance [54]. These newer methods provide reproducible results and reflect stable trait-like neurobiological signatures [55,56]. Recent work also presents that the patterns of resting-state FC are uniquely related both to specific symptoms and to respond to different forms of treatment [57,58]. Thus, reviewing rs-fMRI results seems to be suitable for understanding the links between AD/MCI and LLD.

2. Methodological Overview of Resting-State fMRI (rs-fMRI) Studies

Various analytical strategies are available to study resting-state network connectivity [59]. (1) Seed-based analysis is a hypothesis-driven approach when researchers initially select the seed region of interest based on their hypothesis and a calculated brain connectivity map by detecting temporal correlation [48]. Seed-based analyses are attractive for assessing FC changes in small samples with good statistical power; however, whole-brain analyses are required to address a more comprehensive understandings on changes in rs-fMRI [60]. (2) Regional homogeneity (ReHo) evaluates the similarity or synchronization between different time series given a region or given regions and their neighbors [61]. (3) Independent component analysis (ICA) is a more complex approach that decomposes the whole brain into a set of independent components as a functional map [62,63]. (4) Graph theory constructs models of interrelationships (represented by edges) between brain regions (represented by nodes) and assesses the state of the brain network using various measures [64,65]. (5) To address directional interaction within and between functional networks, incorporating resting-state effective connectivity have been conducted [66]. Data-driven techniques such as Granger causal analysis and Bayesian network analysis provide new insights into effective connectivity [66,67]. (6) The amplitude of low-frequency fluctuation (ALFF) and fractional ALFF (fALFF) techniques were developed to assess the spontaneous low frequency (0.01–0.08 Hz) fluctuations in the fMRI signal intensity at rest, which could reflect the intensity of regional brain spontaneous neural activity [68,69].

Several rs-fMRI studies, aiming to unravel the neurobiological mechanisms of depression and dementia, have investigated abnormalities in various structures, including the frontal gyrus, precuneus, cingulate gyrus, parahippocampal cortex, cerebellum, or putamen [70–72]. However, recent meta-analyses of these studies did not reveal any significant regional convergence of neuroimaging findings for depression [73,74], suggesting that no single brain region is exclusively responsible for LLD's heterogeneous symptoms. A behavior or a clinical symptom typically involves synchronizing many brain regions in a network-based fashion [75]. Experiments have identified three major functional networks in LLD, AD, and MCI: (1) the default mode network (DMN), (2) executive control network (ECN), and (3) salience network (SN) [41,76–78]. Below, we review rs-fMRI studies in LLD, AD, and MCI patients according to individual neural networks for ease of interpretation of the results associated with cognitive function. The analysis methods for resting-state functional connectivity, reference anatomy used for brain parcellation, types of scanners, and characteristics of groups included in the study are essential pieces of information to understand the study results clearly. Therefore, we presented the table which summarizes sample size, age, study type, scanner type, reference space, and analysis method of each section's key studies in Supplementary materials.

3. The Default Mode Network (DMN)

3.1. Overview of DMN

The DMN was initially described as brain regions that consistently showed synchronized deactivation during tasks and activation during rest [79]. This network now generally includes the medial prefrontal cortices (mPFCs), the posterior cingulate cortex (PCC), precuneus, inferior parietal lobule, lateral temporal cortex, and hippocampal formation [80,81]. The DMN is known to be normally deactivated during complex cognitive processing and active during rest, and further studies found that DMN activity is associated with internal processes, such as self-referential thinking [82], autobiographical memory [83], or thinking about the future [84]. Previous meta-analyses, including studies measuring ReHo, ALFF, and fALFF, suggested that altered DMN connectivity seems robust to the choice of analytical methods [85]. The DMN is generally divided into an anterior subdivision centered on the mPFC and a posterior subdivision centered on the PCC and the precuneus cortex [80,86]. Although both the anterior and posterior parts of the DMN are related to spontaneous or self-generated cognition, they seem to be different according to their specific functions [86,87]. Generally, the anterior DMN is more related to self-referential processing and emotion regulation, partly through its strong connections with limbic areas, and the posterior DMN has been implicated in both consciousness and memory processing through its relation to the hippocampal formation [87,88].

3.2. rs-fMRI Studies Associated with DMN in Late-Life Depression (LLD)

The fact that DMN is related to processes mostly employed during rest, such as self-generated thought, has gained significant attention, especially with studies related to depression [89]. DMN activity is considered to be negatively correlated to the ECN activity because reducing the brain's perspective processes seems necessary to focus on the imminent task [84]. In this line, failure to reduce DMN activity has been suggested as a sign of an inability to quiet or inhibit internal mentation or emotional processing [90]. Although not the focus of this review, the relative increases in DMN connectivity during tasks has been consistently reported in various task-based fMRI studies in individuals with depression [91,92]. Several rs-fMRI studies have also reported a relative increase in DMN connectivity [93].

In addition, the difference of connectivity pattern between the anterior and the posterior DMNs in individuals with LLD has been reported. Decreased FC in the posterior DMN have been reported in individuals with LLD compared to healthy controls by rs-fMRI studies using ReHo and ALFF [94–96]. Opposing elevation of FC in the anterior DMN was also observed in LLD patients [96]. This difference of FC between the anterior and the posterior DMNs, increased in the anterior DMN and decreased in the posterior DMN, has been also reported in rs-fMRI studies in younger adults with depressed moods compared to healthy controls [77,97]. Although the results in the elderly were not presented, several studies reported that the anterior and the posterior DMNs were associated with different depressive symptoms, rumination, and autobiographical memory, respectively [98]. Moreover, this difference persisted after 12 weeks of antidepressant treatment in young subjects who recovered from MDD [99].

Seed-based analysis that used seed regions of the PCC and precuneus reported interesting results. Unmedicated LLD patients presented with decreased PCC connectivity with increased connectivity in the anterior DMN at baseline. This decrease in connectivity was partly restored after 12 weeks of treatment with paroxetine [100], suggesting that connectivity between the anterior and posterior DMN regions reflects treatment effects. Seed-based analysis presented that the dissociation between the posterior DMN and ECN was also reported in LLD individuals with current depression compared to the healthy control group [92]. During the restoration of this dissociation after antidepressant treatment, it was also reported that the connectivity between PCC and MFG decreased at baseline, then the FC from PCC to the bilateral medial frontal gyrus increased after 12 weeks of antidepressant treatment in LLD patients [101]. In the seed-based analysis using mPFC as a seed region, the dissociation between the anterior and posterior DMNs in depression has been consistently reported in young adults [102,103]. Van Tol et al. (2014) reported increased connectivity between the mPFC and left anterior insula, indicating increased connectivity between the anterior DMN and the SN [103]. We presented key findings associated with LLD in Table 1 and characteristics of main rs-fMRI studies in Supplementary Table S1.

Table 1. Summary of key findings of resting-state functional MRI (rs-fMRI) studies associated with the default mode network (DMN) in late-life depression (LLD) patients included in the review.

Summary of Key Findings	Key Studies
Relative increase in DMN functional connectivity	[92]
Dissociation within DMN network - decreased posterior DMN functional connectivity - elevation anterior DMN functional connectivity	[94–96]
Restoration of dissociation within DMN network was associated with antidepressant treatment	[100,101]

Abbreviations: DMN, Default mode network.

3.3. rs-fMRI Studies Associated with DMN in Alzheimer's Disease (AD) and Mild Cognitive Impairment (MCI)

The DMN has garnered considerable attention in rs-fMRI studies of neurodegenerative diseases, and the findings have been rather consistent. Early rs-fMRI studies focused on the hippocampus [104], because amyloidosis and tau pathology initially appear in the hippocampus [105–107], and hippocampal volume loss during the progression of AD is directly associated with cognitive decline in longitudinal studies [108,109]. Various seed-based analyses have reported that less hippocampal FC was found in a broad spectrum of cortical and subcortical regions in AD patients than in healthy individuals [110–112]. This altered hippocampal FC has been replicated in more recent seed-based analyses [113–117].

Various rs-fMRI studies that used ICA, fALFF, and ALFF to assess broader networks have also reported consistent results. While there are some inconsistent results in the exact regions reported as being affected by decreased connectivity, there are common significant regions that are nodes of the DMN in AD, including the precuneus and PCC [118–132]. Decreased connectivity within the DMN is often accompanied by increased connectivity in the frontoparietal network and SN [133]. In addition to these well-established results of the entire DMN, further studies addressed the dissociation between subdivisions of the DMN (anterior and posterior), suggested by ICA studies in AD patients [120]. There are both results with connectivity reductions mainly in the posterior DMN [134], but with altered connectivity to the anterior DMN [135,136]. In the dissociation between subdivisions of the DMN, an interesting result was reported in longitudinal studies. Findings from patients with early-onset Alzheimer's disease revealed an increase in the anterior DMN and decreased posterior DMN connectivity [120].

Analysis based on graph theory to assess the alteration of brain networks in AD has shown impressive results. The degree of centrality and clustering coefficients represent the density of a network that is reduced in AD patients [137–140], and networks in AD had longer distances than healthy controls with the loss of edges [141–143]. These studies also reported a negative correlation between small-worldness that reflected a balance between local processing and global integration in the human brain and disease severity [138–140]. Similar to overall network changes, small-worldness has been consistently reported in AD patients, asymptomatic apolipoprotein Apo ε4 mutation carriers, and the aging elderly [140,144]. However, inconsistent results have reported an increase in the clustering coefficient in AD compared to healthy subjects [128,143].

Alteration of DMN connectivity is associated with a genetic mutation in AD. In particular, autosomal-dominant mutation carriers (PSEN1, PSEN2, or APP), who were young and asymptomatic, presented with altered DMN connectivity [145–147]. Regarding the Apo ε4 allele, various studies have reported diminished DMN connectivity in carriers of at least one Apo ε4 allele in all age ranges [144,146–151]. These results suggest some potential for the use of DMN connectivity for early identification of AD in young adults who carry relevant genetic mutations. Moreover, rs-fMRI studies have also reported DMN connectivity changes before the amyloidosis detected by Pittsburgh compound B [152–154], which can support the potential of DMN connectivity as an early marker of AD.

The clinical implication of DMN connectivity has been investigated in various areas. Altered DMN connectivity was correlated with the extent of cognitive decline in middle-aged and elderly Apo ε4 allele carriers [155–157]. This association has been shown consistently in AD or MCI patients related to global cognition and episodic memory performance [127,158–161]. With consistent results of altered DMN connectivity in rs-fMRI studies, attention has been focused on how these alterations can be counteracted by treatment [78]. Studies on donepezil's effect on the resting-state networks in AD have found that the application of donepezil leads to an increase in previously reduced connectivity with no differences in study groups at baseline [162,163].

Additionally, altered connectivity between the anterior and posterior DMNs is associated with aging and age-related cognitive decline [147,164]. This dissociation in DMN subdivision has also been shown in the cognitively normal elderly who presented with abnormal cerebrospinal fluid amyloid or tau proteins [165], or cerebral amyloidosis detected by PET [166]. These results are congruent with the idea that AD patients have a long preclinical period with functional alterations before the onset of disease symptoms. For the network connectivity changes in the progression of AD, longitudinal studies reported decreased connectivity between the precuneus and ECN [167], different local aging patterns in the FC between the left hippocampus and the PCC [168], and decreased global connectivity associated with the striatum [169]. Based on the suggested potential of DMN to provide biomarkers, several rs-fMRI studies have addressed early detection, classification, and prediction in AD and MCI. These studies have shown relatively high performances: ICA [161,170–173], seed-based analysis [174], and graph theory [175]. We presented key findings associated with AD and MCI in Table 2 and characteristics of main rs-fMRI studies in Supplementary Tables S2 and S3.

Table 2. Summary of key findings of rs-fMRI studies associated with the default mode network (DMN) in Alzheimer's disease (AD) and mild cognitive impairment (MCI) patients included in the review.

Summary of Key Findings	Key Studies
Decreased in DMN functional connectivity	[112,118,123,126–128,131]
Dissociation within DMN network; - decreased posterior DMN functional connectivity - elevation anterior DMN functional connectivity	[134,135]
DMN networks had longer distances with the loss of edges	[138,141,142]
Altered DMN functional connectivity was associated with decline of cognition	[143,158,160]
Altered DMN functional connectivity was associated with genetic mutation	[146,149,152,154,157,163]

Abbreviations: DMN, default mode network.

4. The Executive Control Network (ECN)

4.1. Overview of ECN

The ECN, a functionally linked system, consists of brain structure cores that include the dorsolateral prefrontal cortex (dlPFC), medial frontal cortex, lateral parietal cortex, cerebellum, and supplementary motor area [176]. Initially, studies investigating executive function using task-based fMRI identified the coactivation patterns of an ECN during executive function tasks [177]. Beyond task-based fMRI, rs-fMRI studies, and structural MRI studies have also identified an ECN [176,178]. Moreover, a close correlation between executive function changes with aging and alterations in the ECN have been reported [179]. This correlation has been reported in studies that used the ECN to study the functional mechanisms of executive function changes in patients with psychiatric disorders, Parkinson's disease [180], MCI [181], AD [182], and LLD [183].

4.2. rs-fMRI Studies Associated with ECN in LLD

Disruption of the ECN in LLD patients with current depression symptoms has been consistently reported compared to healthy controls [184,185]. Particularly, seed-based analyses using the dlPFC as the seed region demonstrated decreased FC in the frontoparietal areas in LLD individuals with current depression [41]. Other studies using the cerebellum as a seed region reported decreased FC in ECN nodes, including in dlPFC and the parietal cortex, as well as DMN nodes [186,187]. Studies using ICA analysis presented different connectivity patterns for each region in the ECN, with increased FC in the inferior parietal but decreased FC in the dlPFC and superior frontal areas [39]. This decreased connectivity associated with the ECN has been consistently presented in other rs-fMRI studies using ReHo [94,188] and ALFF [40]. Additionally, LLD remitters also demonstrated decreased FC in the frontal-parietal cortex 3 months after remission [189]. After 21 months, individuals with remitted LLD presented a return to decreased FC.

Executive dysfunction is a common symptom in LLD patients. About 30 to 40% of nondemented elders with LLD demonstrate executive dysfunction during neuropsychological tests [190]. Disruption of the ECN was associated with executive dysfunction that included susceptibility to distraction, an inability to sustain attention, poor multitasking, organizational difficulties, and concrete or rigid thinking [191]. A recent study reported that LLD patients' FC between the dlPFC and other bilateral regions was negatively associated with executive function in LLD subjects [192]. Researchers reported that executive dysfunction is associated with greater functional disability levels in LLD [193,194]. Deficits in word-list generation and response inhibition that represent executive function predict poor and slow antidepressant responses and relapses [195,196]. In this regard, the ECN seems to be related to the LLD's clinical prognosis associated with executive dysfunction. We presented key findings associated with LLD in Table 3 and characteristics of main rs-fMRI studies in Supplementary Table S4.

Table 3. Summary of key findings of rs-fMRI studies associated with the executive control network (ECN) in late-life depression (LLD) patients included in the review.

Summary of Key Findings	Key Studies
Decreased in ECN functional connectivity	[186,188]
Restoration of ECN functional connectivity after remission	[189]
Decreased in ECN functional connectivity was associated with executive dysfunction	[192]

Abbreviations: ECN, executive control network.

4.3. rs-fMRI studies associated with the ECN in AD and MCI

Additionally, in AD and MCI, rs-fMRI studies using the ICA analysis identified a significant difference in ECN connectivity across AD and MCI patients and normal controls [197]. In the case of intraconnectivity of the ECN, results seem inconclusive, with some studies reporting no changes in AD patients and others reporting increased connectivity [121,127,198]. However, studies using seed-based analysis consistently reported abnormal FCs between the hippocampus and nodes of the ECN. Previous studies have demonstrated that functional brain activity within portions of the ECN was abnormal in patients with MCI and AD [182,199]. Specifically, the directed FCs from the left hippocampus to the right superior frontal gyrus (SFG) and left medial frontal gyrus (MFG) to the right hippocampus were significantly decreased in MCI or AD patients. The SFG [175] and the MFG [200,201] are essential components of the dlPFC that play essential roles in the ECN.

Moreover, Cai et al. (2017) reported different effective connectivity patterns for the ECN in normal controls and three subgroups of MCI: (1) MCI-R—MCI reverted to the normal functioning state and stabilized to the normal state in 24 months; (2) MCI-S—MCI patients who remained in a stable disease state for 24 months; (3) MCI-P—MCI that progressed to AD and stabilized to AD in 24 months. In this study, the effective connectivity patterns in the ECN were less disrupted and less obvious among MCI-R and MCI-S to MCI-P. In addition, ECN connectivity strengths were not changed in MCI-R patients and normal controls compared to MCI-S and MCI-P patients [181]. These results suggest the importance of the ECN in dementia progression from MCI to AD. We presented key findings associated with AD and MCI in Table 4 and characteristics of main rs-fMRI studies in Supplementary Table S5.

Table 4. Summary of key findings of rs-fMRI studies associated with the executive control network (ECN) in Alzheimer's disease (AD) and mild cognitive impairment (MCI) patients included in the review.

Summary of Key Findings	Key Studies
Decreased in ECN functional connectivity	[197]
Inconclusive result was also reported (increased ECN functional connectivity in AD)	[198]
ECN functional connectivity was associated with AD progression	[181]

Abbreviations: ECN, executive control network; AD, Alzheimer's disease.

5. The Salience Network (SN)

5.1. Overview of SN

The SN is the brain network that detects and filters external stimuli and recruits relevant functional networks [202]. This network is essential for detecting and integrating emotional and sensory stimuli, allocating attention, and switching between internally directed cognition and externally directed cognition [203]. The SN's hub is the ventral anterior insula [204], and the SN also includes nodes in the amygdala, hypothalamus, ventral striatum, and thalamus [203]. The SN was suggested to be functionally subdivided into dorsal and ventral components that support cognitive and emotional controls, respectively [205]. The key SN regions activated during cognitive tasks consist of dorsal components: the dorsal anterior cingulate cortex and the right anterior insula [205,206]. For example, the SN engages the ECN and disengages the DMN during cognitive tasks but does the opposite during rest [207]. Regarding cognitive function, the extent of dissociation between the ECN and SN is related to cognitive task performance [208]. Additionally, the structural connectivity shown by diffusion tensor image analysis is also positively correlated with SN intraconnectivity (right anterior insula to dorsal anterior cingulate cortex) and deactivation of the DMN during tasks, which is in turn related to cognitive function [209].

5.2. rs-fMRI Studies Associated with the SN in LLD

A disrupted standard pattern of SN connectivity is suggested to be one of the key traits of the pathogenesis of depression, particularly in the insula and amygdala [210]. Elevated connectivity between the insula and DMN was enhanced in MDD patients, which may hinder the above standard pattern [91]. The FC from the amygdala, another important SN node, to the hippocampus was decreased in adolescents with depression and at a high risk of depression [211,212]. Additionally, seed-based analysis in younger adults using the amygdala as a seed region was positively associated with increased amygdala FC with DMN nodes and long-term negative emotions [213]. One study that addressed apathy in LLD patients found that LLD patients with apathy exhibit increased FC between the SN and DMN compared with nonapathetic elders with depression [77]. Overall, these results may suggest that increased FC between the SN and DMN may predispose individuals to depression and is further correlated with vegetative symptoms in LLD [186]. However, inconsistent results for decreased FC between the amygdala and precuneus in depressed patients compared with controls have been reported [214].

Network analysis reported that elders with LLD also demonstrate a decreased negative FC between the SN and ECN compared to nondepressed age-matched controls [39]. Another study that compared correlation patterns among significant brain networks in LLD patients compared to nondepressed elderly controls reported dissociation patterns among the ECN/SN, and DMN observed in controls [215]. These results represent a failure of internetwork cohesiveness in LLD [185]. Moreover, decreased negative FC between the ECN and the SN was associated with cognitive impairment and severity of depression symptoms in LLD patients [39]. In addition, a worse treatment response to antidepressants was also associated with this disrupted standard SN pattern [216]. We presented key findings associated with LLD in Table 5 and characteristics of main rs-fMRI studies in Supplementary Table S6.

Table 5. Summary of key findings of rs-fMRI studies associated with the salience network (SN) in late-life depression (LLD) patients included in the review.

Summary of Key Findings	Key Studies
Decreased SN functional connectivity	[39]
Increased functional connectivity between SN and DMN	[77,215]
Disrupted SN pattern was associated with worse treatment response	[216]

Abbreviations: DMN, default mode network; SN, salience network.

5.3. rs-fMRI Studies Associated with SN in AD and MCI

SN connectivity has increasingly gained attention from researchers who address neurodegenerative disease [133]. Although intensified SN connectivity was observed in AD patients compared to healthy controls in ICA studies [130,170], another ICA study in AD patients found contradictory evidence of a decrease in dorsal SN [121]. This increased SN connectivity has been consistently reported in cognitively normal individuals with elevated amyloid levels [166,217], Apo ε4 carriers [156,218], and MCI patients [74]. Moreover, studies that have addressed both amyloid and tau within the DMN and SN reported interesting results, with increased connectivity in the SN and DMN in individuals with elevated amyloid but little evidence of tau, but decreased connectivity in the SN and DMN in individuals with both elevated tau and amyloid levels [219]. These findings highlight the point that SN connectivity changes occur in preclinical dementia, and SN connectivity may change with disease progression. We presented key findings associated with AD and MCI in Table 6 and characteristics of main rs-fMRI studies in Supplementary Table S7.

Table 6. Summary of key findings of main rs-fMRI studies associated with the salience network (SN) in Alzheimer's disease (AD) and mild cognitive impairment (MCI) patients included in the review.

Summary of Key Findings	Key Studies
Intensified SN functional connectivity was observed in AD patients	[170]
Increased SN functional connectivity was associated with - elevation of amyloid level, Apo ε4 carriers, and elevation of tau	[166,217–219]

Abbreviations: SN, salience network; AD, Alzheimer's disease.

6. Conclusions

Alteration in brain networks during the resting state contributes to the symptoms and progression of LLD and AD. Above, we described LLD and AD, focusing on key networks known to be necessary for the network-level description of these two diseases: the DMN, ECN, and SN (Figure 1). A growing body of literature suggests an opposite direction for overall DMN alterations in LLD and AD, with increased connectivity of the DMN in LLD but decreased DMN connectivity in AD. However, the dissociation between the anterior DMN and posterior DMN provides insight into the link between depression and dementia. In the early stage of AD, the alteration in the DMN is different between its anterior and posterior subdivisions, with increased anterior DMN connectivity, and decreased posterior DMN connectivity [120]. Similar dissociation patterns were also observed in individuals with depression, and this increased anterior DMN persists after antidepressant treatments [99]. Additionally, a posterior DMN connectivity reduction was observed in individuals with LLD + MCI compared to LLD only [46,188] and also in LLD patients with an inadequate response to treatment [101]. Additionally, the PCC, the hub of the posterior DMN, is a marker of very early AD progression, as consistently seen with T1-weighted imaging, postmortems, and PET studies [220–222]. Although this association between the dissociation of DMN connectivity and AD and LLD remains to be explored, severe depression may induce the clinical manifestation of cognitive impairment or the onset of eventual cognitive decline, a signal of intrinsic network dysfunction.

Regarding the ECN, both AD and LLD exhibit disrupted ECN connectivity. As discussed, executive dysfunction associated with disrupted ECN connectivity seems to be related to the clinical prognosis of LLD with poor and slow antidepressant responses and a high relapse rate. The findings that the degree of ECN disruption is associated with cognitive decline 24 months after MCI is also covered above. With the hypothesis that depression precedes cognitive decline or induces cognitive decline [223], these results suggest the possibility that the ECN is a target that can modify the impact of LLD on cognitive declines. A noninvasive treatment is being conducted with the ECN as a target [224].

Another interesting issue seen in rs-fMRI studies is associated with the pathogenic process. Several studies using rs-fMRI associated with AD, tau, and amyloid pathology consistently reported that the spreading of these pathologies throughout the brain correlates to brain network disruption, as discussed in this review. Because the DMN, ECN, and SN are multimodal networks that are metabolically expensive and display high rates of cerebral blood flow, aerobic glycolysis, and oxidative glucose metabolism [225], these networks may be vulnerable to AD-associated pathogenic processes. Although spatial deposition patterns have been not convergent, there has been a recent observation that tau and amyloid plaques overlap with brain tissue loss in hub regions of these discussed brain networks [226]. Another review also points to this correlation and suggests that AD-associated pathophysiological processes may explain changes in these networks [133].

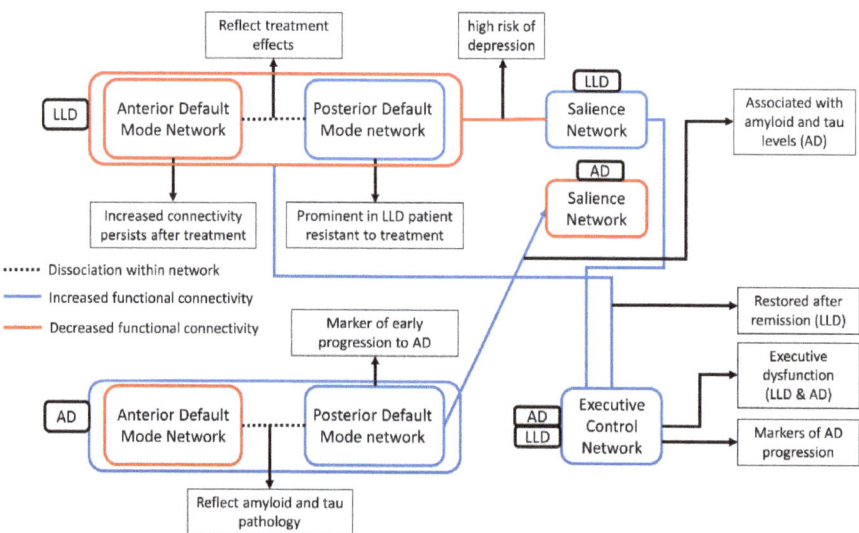

Figure 1. The figure presents the aberrant functional connectivity between three networks in AD and LLD and its clinical implication. Blue line and red line indicate the decreased functional connectivity and the increased functional connectivity compared with healthy control, respectively. Decreased functional connectivity of the executive control network was commonly observed in AD and LLD [192,197]. In contrast, the functional connectivity of the salience network and the default mode network were differently altered. The default mode network connectivity decreased in AD and increased in LLD [90,127], and the salience network increased in AD and decreased in LLD [130,215]. However, dissociated functional connectivity pattern in DMN, increased in the anterior DMN and decreased in the posterior DMN, was commonly observed in both AD and LLD [96,166]. This dissociation reflects treatment effects in LLD and amyloid/tau pathology in AD [100,165]. This similarity of dissociation seems to be a possible mechanism of association between LLD and AD highlighted in epidemiological studies.

Despite the consistent findings across studies, several critical knowledge gaps remain. The lack of standardized protocol for addressing the brain using rs-fMRI has not been adequately addressed. Regarding preprocessing steps of fMRI for dealing with noise, preprocessing steps for rs-fMRI data have evolved to be more diverse than preprocessing for task-based fMRI data. With the diversity of statistical approaches applied to the purified data, these nonstandardized various methods make comparisons across studies extremely difficult. Even if the same terms are used to describe results such as network strength or connectivity, one method's results cannot be compared well with the results of studies using other technologies.

Additionally, our literature did not include task-based fMRI studies in AD and LDD, which clearly expressed the need for additional research. Compared to rs-fMRI studies, a task-based fMRI study is a relatively conventional approach and is challenging to perform due to the needs of involving tasks. Nevertheless, preprocessing steps and statistical methods for task-based fMRI have been more standardized than those for rs-fMRI and have less influenced results, where an external behavioral standard is available. Because task-based fMRI studies are more clinically interpretable, future studies that include tailored tasks concerning specific cognitive, emotional, and social functions would expand our knowledge of AD and LLD.

Recent studies using directed graph theory or combining multiple imaging tools have presented promising results in the field of diagnosis and prediction [227,228]. Therefore, future studies combining multimodal imaging tools such as PET, MRI, and fMRI in AD and LLD patients samples with special considerations such as age, sex, age of onset, treatment outcomes, the severity of illness, and cognitive impairment would help us understand the fundamental functional pathological changes in AD and LLD. Longitudinal studies that include various treatment tools would also help uncover the association between depression and AD-associated pathophysiological processes. Standardized protocols in fMRI data collection and analysis would be helpful to reduce heterogeneity across these physiological states.

Supplementary Materials: The following are available online at https://www.mdpi.com/2227-9059/9/1/82/s1.

Author Contributions: J.K. reviewed and summarized articles, prepared figures, and wrote the manuscript. Y.-K.K. conceived the structure of the paper, supervised the review, organized the figures, and wrote the manuscript. All authors contributed to the critical reading and writing of the manuscript. All authors have read and agreed to the published version of the manuscript.

Funding: This research received no external funding.

Institutional Review Board Statement: Not applicable.

Informed Consent Statement: Not applicable.

Data Availability Statement: No new data were created or analyzed in this study. Data sharing is not applicable to this article.

Conflicts of Interest: The author declares no conflict of interest.

References

1. Association, A.P. *Diagnostic and Statistical Manual of Mental Disorders (DSM-5®)*; American Psychiatric Pub: Washington, DC, USA, 2013; ISBN 0890425574.
2. World Health Organization. Dementia. Available online: https://www.who.int/news-room/fact-sheets/detail/dementia (accessed on 21 December 2020).
3. Hebert, L.E.; Weuve, J.; Scherr, P.A.; Evans, D.A. Alzheimer disease in the United States (2010–2050) estimated using the 2010 census. *Neurology* **2013**, *80*, 1778–1783. [CrossRef] [PubMed]
4. Petersen, R.C.; Stevens, J.C.; Ganguli, M.; Tangalos, E.G.; Cummings, J.L.; DeKosky, S.T. Practice parameter: Early detection of dementia: Mild cognitive impairment. *Neurology* **2001**, *56*, 1133–1142. [CrossRef] [PubMed]
5. Association, A. 2018 Alzheimer's disease facts and figures. *Alzheimer's Dement.* **2018**, *14*, 367–429. [CrossRef]
6. Greenberg, S.M.; Bacskai, B.J.; Hernandez-Guillamon, M.; Pruzin, J.; Sperling, R.; van Veluw, S.J. Cerebral amyloid angiopathy and Alzheimer disease—One peptide, two pathways. *Nat. Rev. Neurol.* **2020**, *16*, 30–42. [CrossRef]
7. Ozben, T.; Ozben, S. Neuro-inflammation and anti-inflammatory treatment options for Alzheimer's disease. *Clin. Biochem.* **2019**, *72*, 87–89. [CrossRef]
8. Brookmeyer, R.; Johnson, E.; Ziegler-Grahamm, K.; Arrighi, H.M. Forecasting the global prevalence and burden of Alzheimer's disease. *Alzheimer's Dement.* **2007**, *3*, 186–191. [CrossRef]
9. Baumgart, M.; Snyder, H.M.; Carrillo, M.C.; Fazio, S.; Kim, H.; Johns, H. Summary of the evidence on modifiable risk factors for cognitive decline and dementia: A population-based perspective. *Alzheimer's Dement.* **2015**, *11*, 718–726. [CrossRef]
10. Xu, W.; Tan, L.; Wang, H.-F.; Jiang, T.; Tan, M.-S.; Tan, L.; Zhao, Q.-F.; Li, J.-Q.; Wang, J.; Yu, J.-T. Meta-analysis of modifiable risk factors for Alzheimer's disease. *J. Neurol.* **2015**, *86*, 1299–1306. [CrossRef]
11. Clare, L.; Wu, Y.-T.; Teale, J.C.; MacLeod, C.; Matthews, F.; Brayne, C.; Woods, B.; Team, C.-W. study Potentially modifiable lifestyle factors, cognitive reserve, and cognitive function in later life: A cross-sectional study. *PLoS Med.* **2017**, *14*, e1002259. [CrossRef]
12. Chi, S.; Wang, C.; Jiang, T.; Zhu, X.-C.; Yu, J.-T.; Tan, L. The Prevalence of Depression in Alzheimer's Disease: A Systematic Review and Meta-Analysis. *Curr. Alzheimer Res.* **2015**, *12*, 189–198. [CrossRef]
13. Fuchs, E. Neurogenesis in the adult brain: Is there an association with mental disorders? *Eur. Arch. Psychiatry Clin. Neurosci.* **2007**, *257*, 247–249. [CrossRef] [PubMed]
14. Herbert, J.; Lucassen, P.J. Depression as a risk factor for Alzheimer's disease: Genes, steroids, cytokines and neurogenesis—What do we need to know? *Front. Neuroendocrinol.* **2016**, *41*, 153–171. [CrossRef] [PubMed]
15. Goldberg, D. The heterogeneity of "major depression". *World Psychiatry* **2011**, *10*, 226–228. [CrossRef] [PubMed]
16. Lynch, C.J.; Gunning, F.M.; Liston, C. Causes and Consequences of Diagnostic Heterogeneity in Depression: Paths to Discovering Novel Biological Depression Subtypes. *Biol. Psychiatry* **2020**, *88*, 83–94. [CrossRef]

17. Riddle, M.; Potter, G.G.; McQuoid, D.R.; Steffens, D.C.; Beyer, J.L.; Taylor, W.D. Longitudinal Cognitive Outcomes of Clinical Phenotypes of Late-Life Depression. *Am. J. Geriatr. Psychiatry* **2017**, *25*, 1123–1134. [CrossRef]
18. Leggett, A.; Zarit, S.H.; Hoang, C.N.; Nguyen, H.T. Correlates of cognitive impairment in older Vietnamese. *Aging Ment. Health* **2013**, *17*, 915–923. [CrossRef]
19. Tedros, A.G.; Christopher, J.L.M. Global Burden of Disease Study 2017. *Lancet* **2017**, *5*, 1–27.
20. Ownby, R.L.; Crocco, E.; Acevedo, A.; John, V.; Loewenstein, D. Depression and Risk for Alzheimer Disease: Systematic Review, Meta-analysis, and Metaregression Analysis. *Arch. Gen. Psychiatry* **2006**, *63*, 530–538. [CrossRef]
21. Diniz, B.S.; Sibille, E.; Ding, Y.; Tseng, G.; Aizenstein, H.J.; Lotrich, F.; Becker, J.T.; Lopez, O.L.; Lotze, M.T.; Klunk, W.E.; et al. Plasma biosignature and brain pathology related to persistent cognitive impairment in late-life depression. *Mol. Psychiatry* **2015**, *20*, 594–601. [CrossRef]
22. Brailean, A.; Aartsen, M.J.; Muniz-Terrera, G.; Prince, M.; Prina, A.M.; Comijs, H.C.; Huisman, M.; Beekman, A. Longitudinal associations between late-life depression dimensions and cognitive functioning: A cross-domain latent growth curve analysis. *Psychol. Med.* **2017**, *47*, 690–702. [CrossRef]
23. Ismail, Z.; Elbayoumi, H.; Fischer, C.E.; Hogan, D.B.; Millikin, C.P.; Schweizer, T.; Mortby, M.E.; Smith, E.E.; Patten, S.B.; Fiest, K.M. Prevalence of Depression in Patients with Mild Cognitive Impairment: A Systematic Review and Meta-analysis. *JAMA Psychiatry* **2017**, *74*, 58–67. [CrossRef] [PubMed]
24. Almeida, O.P.; Hankey, G.J.; Yeap, B.B.; Golledge, J.; Flicker, L. Depression as a modifiable factor to decrease the risk of dementia. *Transl. Psychiatry* **2017**, *7*, e1117. [CrossRef] [PubMed]
25. Brendel, M.; Pogarell, O.; Xiong, G.; Delker, A.; Bartenstein, P.; Rominger, A. Depressive symptoms accelerate cognitive decline in amyloid-positive MCI patients. *Eur. J. Nucl. Med. Mol. Imaging* **2015**, *42*, 716–724. [CrossRef] [PubMed]
26. Mahgoub, N.; Alexopoulos, G.S. Amyloid Hypothesis: Is There a Role for Antiamyloid Treatment in Late-Life Depression? *Am. J. Geriatr. Psychiatry* **2016**, *24*, 239–247. [CrossRef] [PubMed]
27. Do Nascimento, K.K.F.; Silva, K.P.; Malloy-Diniz, L.F.; Butters, M.A.; Diniz, B.S. Plasma and cerebrospinal fluid amyloid-β levels in late-life depression: A systematic review and meta-analysis. *J. Psychiatr. Res.* **2015**, *69*, 35–41. [CrossRef] [PubMed]
28. Butters, M.A.; Young, J.B.; Lopez, O.; Aizenstein, H.J.; Mulsant, B.H.; Reynolds, C.F., 3rd; DeKosky, S.T.; Becker, J.T. Pathways linking late-life depression to persistent cognitive impairment and dementia. *Dialogues Clin. Neurosci.* **2008**, *10*, 345–357.
29. Geerlings, M.I.; Gerritsen, L. Late-Life Depression, Hippocampal Volumes, and Hypothalamic-Pituitary-Adrenal Axis Regulation: A Systematic Review and Meta-analysis. *Biol. Psychiatry* **2017**, *82*, 339–350. [CrossRef] [PubMed]
30. Edwards Iii, G.A.; Gamez, N.; Escobedo, G., Jr.; Calderon, O.; Moreno-Gonzalez, I. Modifiable Risk Factors for Alzheimer's Disease. *Front. Aging Neurosci.* **2019**, *11*, 146–163. [CrossRef]
31. Epp, A.M.; Dobson, K.S.; Dozois, D.J.A.; Frewen, P.A. A systematic meta analysis of the Stroop task in depression. *Clin. Psychol. Rev.* **2012**, *32*, 316–328. [CrossRef]
32. Monteiro, S.; Monteiro, B.; Candida, M.; Adler, N.; Campos, C.; Rocha, N.B.F.; Paes, F.; Nardi, A.E.; Machado, S. Association between depression severity and executive functioning in late-life depression: A systematic review. *Med. Express* **2016**, *3*, 1–9. [CrossRef]
33. Roca, M.; Vives, M.; López-Navarro, E.; García-Campayo, J.; Gili, M. Cognitive impairments and depression: A critical review. *Actas Esp. Psiquiatr.* **2015**, *43*, 187–193. [PubMed]
34. Weisenbach, S.L.; Kumar, A. Current Understanding of the Neurobiology and Longitudinal Course of Geriatric Depression. *Curr. Psychiatry Rep.* **2014**, *16*, 463–471. [CrossRef] [PubMed]
35. Rock, P.L.; Roiser, J.P.; Riedel, W.J.; Blackwell, A.D. Cognitive impairment in depression: A systematic review and meta-analysis. *Psychol. Med.* **2014**, *44*, 2029–2040. [CrossRef]
36. Ahern, E.; Semkovska, M. Cognitive functioning in the first-episode of major depressive disorder: A systematic review and meta-analysis. *Neuropsychology* **2017**, *31*, 52–72. [CrossRef] [PubMed]
37. Liao, W.; Zhang, X.; Shu, H.; Wang, Z.; Liu, D.; Zhang, Z. The characteristic of cognitive dysfunction in remitted late life depression and amnestic mild cognitive impairment. *Psychiatry Res.* **2017**, *251*, 168–175. [CrossRef]
38. Chen, J.; Shu, H.; Wang, Z.; Zhan, Y.; Liu, D.; Liao, W.; Xu, L.; Liu, Y.; Zhang, Z. Convergent and divergent intranetwork and internetwork connectivity patterns in patients with remitted late-life depression and amnestic mild cognitive impairment. *Cortex* **2016**, *83*, 194–211. [CrossRef]
39. Li, W.; Wang, Y.; Ward, B.D.; Antuono, P.G.; Li, S.-J.; Goveas, J.S. Intrinsic inter-network brain dysfunction correlates with symptom dimensions in late-life depression. *J. Psychiatr. Res.* **2017**, *87*, 71–80. [CrossRef]
40. Yue, Y.; Jia, X.; Hou, Z.; Zang, Y.; Yuan, Y. Frequency-dependent amplitude alterations of resting-state spontaneous fluctuations in late-onset depression. *Biomed. Res. Int.* **2015**, *2015*, 1–9. [CrossRef]
41. Alexopoulos, G.S.; Hoptman, M.J.; Kanellopoulos, D.; Murphy, C.F.; Lim, K.O.; Gunning, F.M. Functional connectivity in the cognitive control network and the default mode network in late-life depression. *J. Affect. Disord.* **2012**, *139*, 56–65. [CrossRef]
42. Li, X.; Steffens, D.C.; Potter, G.G.; Guo, H.; Song, S.; Wang, L. Decreased between-hemisphere connectivity strength and network efficiency in geriatric depression. *Hum. Brain Mapp.* **2017**, *38*, 53–67. [CrossRef]
43. Ozer, S.; Young, J.; Champ, C.; Burke, M. A systematic review of the diagnostic test accuracy of brief cognitive tests to detect amnestic mild cognitive impairment. *Int. J. Geriatr. Psychiatry* **2016**, *31*, 1139–1150. [CrossRef] [PubMed]

44. Bai, F.; Shu, N.; Yuan, Y.; Shi, Y.; Yu, H.; Wu, D.; Wang, J.; Xia, M.; He, Y.; Zhang, Z. Topologically Convergent and Divergent Structural Connectivity Patterns between Patients with Remitted Geriatric Depression and Amnestic Mild Cognitive Impairment. *J. Neurosci.* **2012**, *32*, 4307–4318. [CrossRef] [PubMed]
45. Wang, Z.; Jia, X.; Liang, P.; Qi, Z.; Yang, Y.; Zhou, W.; Li, K. Changes in thalamus connectivity in mild cognitive impairment: Evidence from resting state fMRI. *Eur. J. Radiol.* **2012**, *81*, 277–285. [CrossRef] [PubMed]
46. Li, H.-J.; Hou, X.-H.; Liu, H.-H.; Yue, C.-L.; He, Y.; Zuo, X.-N. Toward systems neuroscience in mild cognitive impairment and Alzheimer's disease: A meta-analysis of 75 fMRI studies. *Hum. Brain Mapp.* **2015**, *36*, 1217–1232. [CrossRef] [PubMed]
47. Shimoda, K.; Kimura, M.; Yokota, M.; Okubo, Y. Comparison of regional gray matter volume abnormalities in Alzheimer's disease and late life depression with hippocampal atrophy using VSRAD analysis: A voxel-based morphometry study. *Psychiatry Res. Neuroimaging* **2015**, *232*, 71–75. [CrossRef]
48. Biswal, B.; Zerrin Yetkin, F.; Haughton, V.M.; Hyde, J.S. Functional connectivity in the motor cortex of resting human brain using echo-planar MRI. *Magn. Reson. Med.* **1995**, *34*, 537–541. [CrossRef]
49. Smitha, K.A.; Akhil Raja, K.; Arun, K.M.; Rajesh, P.G.; Thomas, B.; Kapilamoorthy, T.R.; Kesavadas, C. Resting state fMRI: A review on methods in resting state connectivity analysis and resting state networks. *Neuroradiol. J.* **2017**, *30*, 305–317. [CrossRef]
50. Rosenberg, M.D.; Finn, E.S.; Scheinost, D.; Papademetris, X.; Shen, X.; Constable, R.T.; Chun, M.M. A neuromarker of sustained attention from whole-brain functional connectivity. *Nat. Neurosci.* **2016**, *19*, 165–171. [CrossRef]
51. Hsu, W.-T.; Rosenberg, M.D.; Scheinost, D.; Constable, R.T.; Chun, M.M. Resting-state functional connectivity predicts neuroticism and extraversion in novel individuals. *Soc. Cogn. Affect. Neurosci.* **2018**, *13*, 224–232. [CrossRef]
52. Jiang, R.; Calhoun, V.D.; Zuo, N.; Lin, D.; Li, J.; Fan, L.; Qi, S.; Sun, H.; Fu, Z.; Song, M.; et al. Connectome-based individualized prediction of temperament trait scores. *Neuroimage* **2018**, *183*, 366–374. [CrossRef]
53. Beaty, R.E.; Kenett, Y.N.; Christensen, A.P.; Rosenberg, M.D.; Benedek, M.; Chen, Q.; Fink, A.; Qiu, J.; Kwapil, T.R.; Kane, M.J.; et al. Robust prediction of individual creative ability from brain functional connectivity. *Proc. Natl. Acad. Sci. USA* **2018**, *115*, 1087–1092. [CrossRef] [PubMed]
54. Siegel, J.S.; Ramsey, L.E.; Snyder, A.Z.; Metcalf, N.V.; Chacko, R.V.; Weinberger, K.; Baldassarre, A.; Hacker, C.D.; Shulman, G.L.; Corbetta, M. Disruptions of network connectivity predict impairment in multiple behavioral domains after stroke. *Proc. Natl. Acad. Sci. USA* **2016**, *113*, E4367–E4376. [CrossRef] [PubMed]
55. Jalbrzikowski, M.; Liu, F.; Foran, W.; Calabro, F.J.; Roeder, K.; Devlin, B.; Luna, B. Cognitive and default mode networks support developmental stability in functional connectome fingerprinting through adolescence. *bioRxiv* **2019**, 812719. [CrossRef]
56. Gratton, C.; Laumann, T.O.; Nielsen, A.N.; Greene, D.J.; Gordon, E.M.; Gilmore, A.W.; Nelson, S.M.; Coalson, R.S.; Snyder, A.Z.; Schlaggar, B.L.; et al. Functional Brain Networks Are Dominated by Stable Group and Individual Factors, Not Cognitive or Daily Variation. *Neuron* **2018**, *98*, 439–452.e5. [CrossRef] [PubMed]
57. Kühn, S.; Vanderhasselt, M.-A.; De Raedt, R.; Gallinat, J. Why ruminators won't stop: The structural and resting state correlates of rumination and its relation to depression. *J. Affect. Disord.* **2012**, *141*, 352–360. [CrossRef]
58. Brakowski, J.; Spinelli, S.; Dörig, N.; Bosch, O.G.; Manoliu, A.; Holtforth, M.G.; Seifritz, E. Resting state brain network function in major depression—Depression symptomatology, antidepressant treatment effects, future research. *J. Psychiatr. Res.* **2017**, *92*, 147–159. [CrossRef]
59. Takamura, T.; Hanakawa, T. Clinical utility of resting-state functional connectivity magnetic resonance imaging for mood and cognitive disorders. *J. Neural Transm.* **2017**, *124*, 821–839. [CrossRef]
60. Lee, M.H.; Smyser, C.D.; Shimony, J.S. Resting-state fMRI: A review of methods and clinical applications. *Am. J. Neuroradiol.* **2013**, *34*, 1866–1872. [CrossRef]
61. Zang, Y.; Jiang, T.; Lu, Y.; He, Y.; Tian, L. Regional homogeneity approach to fMRI data analysis. *Neuroimage* **2004**, *22*, 394–400. [CrossRef]
62. Mckeown, M.J.; Sejnowski, T.J. Independent Component Analysis of fMRI Data: Examining the Assumptions. *Hum. Brain Mapp.* **1998**, *6*, 368–372. [CrossRef]
63. Van De Ven, V.G.; Formisano, E.; Prvulovic, D.; Roeder, C.H.; Linden, D.E.J. Functional Connectivity as Revealed by Spatial Independent Component Analysis of fMRI Measurements During Rest. *Hum. Brain Mapp.* **2004**, *22*, 165–178. [CrossRef] [PubMed]
64. Bullmore, E.; Sporns, O. Complex brain networks: Graph theoretical analysis of structural and functional systems. *Nat. Rev. Neurosci.* **2009**, *10*, 186–198. [CrossRef] [PubMed]
65. Bassett, D.S.; Bullmore, E.T. Small-World Brain Networks Revisited. *Neuroscientist* **2016**, *23*, 499–516. [CrossRef]
66. Friston, K.J. Functional and effective connectivity in neuroimaging: A synthesis. *Hum. Brain Mapp.* **1994**, *2*, 56–78. [CrossRef]
67. Liang, P.; Li, Z.; Deshpande, G.; Wang, Z.; Hu, X.; Li, K. Altered causal connectivity of resting state brain networks in amnesic MCI. *PLoS ONE* **2014**, *9*, e88476. [CrossRef]
68. Yu-Feng, Z.; Yong, H.; Chao-Zhe, Z.; Qing-Jiu, C.; Man-Qiu, S.; Meng, L.; Li-Xia, T.; Tian-Zi, J.; Yu-Feng, W. Altered baseline brain activity in children with ADHD revealed by resting-state functional MRI. *Brain Dev.* **2007**, *29*, 83–91. [CrossRef]
69. Zou, Q.-H.; Zhu, C.-Z.; Yang, Y.; Zuo, X.-N.; Long, X.-Y.; Cao, Q.-J.; Wang, Y.-F.; Zang, Y.-F. An improved approach to detection of amplitude of low-frequency fluctuation (ALFF) for resting-state fMRI: Fractional ALFF. *J. Neurosci. Methods* **2008**, *172*, 137–141. [CrossRef]
70. Geng, J.; Yan, R.; Shi, J.; Chen, Y.; Mo, Z.; Shao, J.; Wang, X.; Yao, Z.; Lu, Q. Altered regional homogeneity in patients with somatic depression: A resting-state fMRI study. *J. Affect. Disord.* **2019**, *246*, 498–505. [CrossRef]

71. Peng, D.; Liddle, E.B.; Iwabuchi, S.J.; Zhang, C.; Wu, Z.; Liu, J.; Jiang, K.; Xu, L.; Liddle, P.F.; Palaniyappan, L.; et al. Dissociated large-scale functional connectivity networks of the precuneus in medication-naïve first-episode depression. *Psychiatry Res. Neuroimaging* **2015**, *232*, 250–256. [CrossRef]
72. Liu, F.; Hu, M.; Wang, S.; Guo, W.; Zhao, J.; Li, J.; Xun, G.; Long, Z.; Zhang, J.; Wang, Y.; et al. Abnormal regional spontaneous neural activity in first-episode, treatment-naive patients with late-life depression: A resting-state fMRI study. *Prog. Neuro-Psychopharmacol. Biol. Psychiatry* **2012**, *39*, 326–331. [CrossRef]
73. Gray, J.P.; Müller, V.I.; Eickhoff, S.B.; Fox, P.T. Multimodal Abnormalities of Brain Structure and Function in Major Depressive Disorder: A Meta-Analysis of Neuroimaging Studies. *Am. J. Psychiatry* **2020**, *177*, 422–434. [CrossRef] [PubMed]
74. Müller, V.I.; Cieslik, E.C.; Serbanescu, I.; Laird, A.R.; Fox, P.T.; Eickhoff, S.B. Altered Brain Activity in Unipolar Depression Revisited: Meta-analyses of Neuroimaging Studies. *JAMA Psychiatry* **2017**, *74*, 47–55. [CrossRef] [PubMed]
75. Marek, S.; Tervo-Clemmens, B.; Nielsen, A.N.; Wheelock, M.D.; Miller, R.L.; Laumann, T.O.; Earl, E.; Foran, W.W.; Cordova, M.; Doyle, O.; et al. Identifying reproducible individual differences in childhood functional brain networks: An ABCD study. *Dev. Cogn. Neurosci.* **2019**, *40*, 100706. [CrossRef] [PubMed]
76. Mulders, P.C.; van Eijndhoven, P.F.; Schene, A.H.; Beckmann, C.F.; Tendolkar, I. Resting-state functional connectivity in major depressive disorder: A review. *Neurosci. Biobehav. Rev.* **2015**, *56*, 330–344. [CrossRef]
77. Yuen, G.S.; Gunning-Dixon, F.M.; Hoptman, M.J.; AbdelMalak, B.; McGovern, A.R.; Seirup, J.K.; Alexopoulos, G.S. The salience network in the apathy of late-life depression. *Int. J. Geriatr. Psychiatry* **2014**, *29*, 1116–1124. [CrossRef]
78. Hohenfeld, C.; Werner, C.J.; Reetz, K. Resting-state connectivity in neurodegenerative disorders: Is there potential for an imaging biomarker? *NeuroImage Clin.* **2018**, *18*, 849–870. [CrossRef]
79. Greicius, M.D.; Ben, K.; Allan, L.R.; Vinod, M. Functional connectivity in the resting brain: A network analysis of the default mod hypothesis. *Proc. Natl. Acad. Sci. USA* **2003**, *100*, 253–258. [CrossRef]
80. Buckner, R.L.; Andrews-Hanna, J.R.; Schacter, D.L. The Brain's Default Network. *Ann. N. Y. Acad. Sci.* **2008**, *1124*, 1–38. [CrossRef]
81. Mohan, A.; Roberto, A.J.; Mohan, A.; Lorenzo, A.; Jones, K.; Carney, M.J.; Liogier-Weyback, L.; Hwang, S.; Lapidus, K.A.B. The Significance of the Default Mode Network (DMN) in Neurological and Neuropsychiatric Disorders: A Review. *Yale J. Biol. Med.* **2016**, *89*, 49–57.
82. Kyeong, S.; Kim, J.; Kim, J.; Kim, E.J.; Kim, H.E.; Kim, J.-J. Differences in the modulation of functional connectivity by self-talk tasks between people with low and high life satisfaction. *Neuroimage* **2020**, *217*, 116929. [CrossRef]
83. Spreng, R.N.; Mar, R.A.; Kim, A.S.N. The common neural basis of autobiographical memory, prospection, navigation, theory of mind, and the default mode: A quantitative meta-analysis. *J. Cogn. Neurosci.* **2009**, *21*, 489–510. [CrossRef] [PubMed]
84. Raichle, M.E. The Brain's Default Mode Network. *Annu. Rev. Neurosci.* **2015**, *38*, 433–447. [CrossRef] [PubMed]
85. Buckner, R.L.; Sepulcre, J.; Talukdar, T.; Krienen, F.M.; Liu, H.; Hedden, T.; Andrews-Hanna, J.R.; Sperling, R.A.; Johnson, K.A. Cortical Hubs Revealed by Intrinsic Functional Connectivity: Mapping, Assessment of Stability, and Relation to Alzheimer's Disease. *J. Neurosci.* **2009**, *29*, 1860–1873. [CrossRef] [PubMed]
86. Andrews-Hanna, J.R.; Reidler, J.S.; Sepulcre, J.; Poulin, R.; Buckner, R.L. Functional-Anatomic Fractionation of the Brain's Default Network. *Neuron* **2010**, *65*, 550–562. [CrossRef] [PubMed]
87. Andrews-Hanna, J.R.; Smallwood, J.; Spreng, R.N. The default network and self-generated thought: Component processes, dynamic control, and clinical relevance. *Ann. N. Y. Acad. Sci.* **2014**, *1316*, 29–52. [CrossRef] [PubMed]
88. Leech, R.; Sharp, D.J. The role of the posterior cingulate cortex in cognition and disease. *Brain* **2014**, *137*, 12–32. [CrossRef]
89. Menon, V. Large-scale brain networks and psychopathology: A unifying triple network model. *Trends Cogn. Sci.* **2011**, *15*, 483–506. [CrossRef]
90. Scalabrini, A.; Vai, B.; Poletti, S.; Damiani, S.; Mucci, C.; Colombo, C.; Zanardi, R.; Benedetti, F.; Northoff, G. All roads lead to the default-mode network—global source of DMN abnormalities in major depressive disorder. *Neuropsychopharmacology* **2020**, *45*, 2058–2069. [CrossRef]
91. Connolly, C.G.; Wu, J.; Ho, T.C.; Hoeft, F.; Wolkowitz, O.; Eisendrath, S.; Frank, G.; Hendren, R.; Max, J.E.; Paulus, M.P.; et al. Resting-State Functional Connectivity of Subgenual Anterior Cingulate Cortex in Depressed Adolescents. *Biol. Psychiatry* **2013**, *74*, 898–907. [CrossRef]
92. Yin, Y.; He, X.; Xu, M.; Hou, Z.; Song, X.; Sui, Y.; Liu, Z.; Jiang, W.; Yue, Y.; Zhang, Y.; et al. Structural and functional connectivity of default mode network underlying the cognitive impairment in late-onset depression. *Sci. Rep.* **2016**, *6*, 1–10. [CrossRef]
93. Posner, J.; Hellerstein, D.J.; Gat, I.; Mechling, A.; Klahr, K.; Wang, Z.; McGrath, P.J.; Stewart, J.W.; Peterson, B.S. Antidepressants Normalize the Default Mode Network in Patients with Dysthymia. *JAMA Psychiatry* **2013**, *70*, 373–382. [CrossRef] [PubMed]
94. Yuan, Y.; Zhang, Z.; Bai, F.; Yu, H.; Shi, Y.; Qian, Y.; Liu, W.; You, J.; Zhang, X.; Liu, Z. Abnormal neural activity in the patients with remitted geriatric depression: A resting-state functional magnetic resonance imaging study. *J. Affect. Disord.* **2008**, *111*, 145–152. [CrossRef] [PubMed]
95. Chen, J.; Liu, F.; Xun, G.; Chen, H.; Hu, M.; Guo, X.; Xiao, C.; Wooderson, S.C.; Guo, W.; Zhao, J. Early and late onset, first-episode, treatment-naive depression: Same clinical symptoms, different regional neural activities. *J. Affect. Disord.* **2012**, *143*, 56–63. [CrossRef] [PubMed]
96. Steffens, D.C.; Wang, L.; Manning, K.J.; Pearlson, G.D. Negative Affectivity, Aging, and Depression: Results from the Neurobiology of Late-Life Depression (NBOLD) Study. *Am. J. Geriatr. Psychiatry* **2017**, *25*, 1135–1149. [CrossRef]

97. Guo, W.; Liu, F.; Zhang, J.; Zhang, Z.; Yu, L.; Liu, J.; Chen, H.; Xiao, C. Abnormal default-mode network homogeneity in first-episode, drug-naive major depressive disorder. *PLoS ONE* **2014**, *9*, e91102. [CrossRef]
98. Zhu, X.; Wang, X.; Xiao, J.; Liao, J.; Zhong, M.; Wang, W.; Yao, S. Evidence of a Dissociation Pattern in Resting-State Default Mode Network Connectivity in First-Episode, Treatment-Naive Major Depression Patients. *Biol. Psychiatry* **2012**, *71*, 611–617. [CrossRef]
99. Li, B.; Liu, L.; Friston, K.J.; Shen, H.; Wang, L.; Zeng, L.-L.; Hu, D. A Treatment-Resistant Default Mode Subnetwork in Major Depression. *Biol. Psychiatry* **2013**, *74*, 48–54. [CrossRef]
100. Wu, M.; Andreescu, C.; Butters, M.A.; Tamburo, R.; Reynolds, C.F.; Aizenstein, H. Default-mode network connectivity and white matter burden in late-life depression. *Psychiatry Res. Neuroimaging* **2011**, *194*, 39–46. [CrossRef]
101. Andreescu, C.; Tudorascu, D.L.; Butters, M.A.; Tamburo, E.; Patel, M.; Price, J.; Karp, J.F.; Reynolds, C.F.; Aizenstein, H. Resting state functional connectivity and treatment response in late-life depression. *Psychiatry Res. Neuroimaging* **2013**, *214*, 313–321. [CrossRef]
102. Sheline, Y.I.; Price, J.L.; Yan, Z.; Mintun, M.A. Resting-state functional MRI in depression unmasks increased connectivity between networks via the dorsal nexus. *Proc. Natl. Acad. Sci. USA* **2010**, *107*, 11020–11025. [CrossRef]
103. Van Tol, M.J.; Li, M.; Metzger, C.D.; Hailla, N.; Horn, D.I.; Li, W.; Heinze, H.J.; Bogerts, B.; Steiner, J.; He, H.; et al. Local cortical thinning links to resting-state disconnectivity in major depressive disorder. *Psychol. Med.* **2014**, *44*, 2053–2065. [CrossRef] [PubMed]
104. Braak, H.; Braak, E.; Bohl, J. Staging of Alzheimer-Related Cortical Destruction. *Eur. Neurol.* **1993**, *33*, 403–408. [CrossRef] [PubMed]
105. Braak, H.; Braak, E. Neuropathological stageing of Alzheimer-related changes. *Acta Neuropathol.* **1991**, *82*, 239–259. [CrossRef] [PubMed]
106. Hanseeuw, B.J.; Schultz, A.P.; Betensky, R.A.; Sperling, R.A.; Johnson, K.A. Decreased hippocampal metabolism in high-amyloid mild cognitive impairment. *Alzheimer's Dement.* **2016**, *12*, 1288–1296. [CrossRef] [PubMed]
107. Serra, L.; Bozzali, M.; Fadda, L.; De Simone, M.S.; Bruschini, M.; Perri, R.; Caltagirone, C.; Carlesimo, G.A. The role of hippocampus in the retrieval of autobiographical memories in patients with amnestic Mild Cognitive Impairment due to Alzheimer's disease. *J. Neuropsychol.* **2018**, *14*, 46–68. [CrossRef] [PubMed]
108. Den Heijer, T.; van der Lijn, F.; Koudstaal, P.J.; Hofman, A.; van der Lugt, A.; Krestin, G.P.; Niessen, W.J.; Breteler, M.M.B. A 10-year follow-up of hippocampal volume on magnetic resonance imaging in early dementia and cognitive decline. *Brain* **2010**, *133*, 1163–1172. [CrossRef]
109. Steffens, D.C.; McQuoid, D.R.; Payne, M.E.; Potter, G.G. Change in Hippocampal Volume on Magnetic Resonance Imaging and Cognitive Decline Among Older Depressed and Nondepressed Subjects in the Neurocognitive Outcomes of Depression in the Elderly Study. *Am. J. Geriatr. Psychiatry* **2011**, *19*, 4–12. [CrossRef]
110. Allen, G.; Barnard, H.; McColl, R.; Hester, A.L.; Fields, J.A.; Weiner, M.F.; Ringe, W.K.; Lipton, A.M.; Brooker, M.; McDonald, E.; et al. Reduced Hippocampal Functional Connectivity in Alzheimer Disease. *Arch. Neurol.* **2007**, *64*, 1482–1487. [CrossRef]
111. Li, S.-J.; Li, Z.; Wu, G.; Zhang, M.-J.; Franczak, M.; Antuono, P.G. Alzheimer Disease: Evaluation of a Functional MR Imaging Index as a Marker. *Radiology* **2002**, *225*, 253–259. [CrossRef]
112. Wang, L.; Zang, Y.; He, Y.; Liang, M.; Zhang, X.; Tian, L.; Wu, T.; Jiang, T.; Li, K. Changes in hippocampal connectivity in the early stages of Alzheimer's disease: Evidence from resting state fMRI. *Neuroimage* **2006**, *31*, 496–504. [CrossRef]
113. Das, S.R.; Pluta, J.; Mancuso, L.; Kliot, D.; Yushkevich, P.A.; Wolk, D.A. Anterior and posterior MTL networks in aging and MCI. *Neurobiol. Aging* **2015**, *36*, S141–S150. [CrossRef] [PubMed]
114. Kenny, E.R.; Blamire, A.M.; Firbank, M.J.; O'Brien, J.T. Functional connectivity in cortical regions in dementia with Lewy bodies and Alzheimer's disease. *Brain* **2012**, *135*, 569–581. [CrossRef] [PubMed]
115. Sohn, W.S.; Yoo, K.; Na, D.L.; Jeong, Y. Progressive Changes in Hippocampal Resting-state Connectivity Across Cognitive Impairment: A Cross-sectional Study from Normal to Alzheimer Disease. *Alzheimer Dis. Assoc. Disord.* **2014**, *28*, 239–246. [CrossRef] [PubMed]
116. Tahmasian, M.; Pasquini, L.; Scherr, M.; Meng, C.; Förster, S.; Mulej Bratec, S.; Shi, K.; Yakushev, I.; Schwaiger, M.; Grimmer, T.; et al. The lower hippocampus global connectivity, the higher its local metabolism in Alzheimer disease. *Neurology* **2015**, *84*, 1956–1963. [CrossRef]
117. Sun, Y.; Wang, Y.; Lu, J.; Liu, R.; Schwarz, C.G.; Zhao, H.; Zhang, Y.; Xu, L.; Zhu, B.; Zhang, B.; et al. Disrupted functional connectivity between perirhinal and parahippocampal cortices with hippocampal subfields in patients with mild cognitive impairment and Alzheimer's disease. *Oncotarget* **2017**, *8*, 99112–99124. [CrossRef]
118. Agosta, F.; Pievani, M.; Geroldi, C.; Copetti, M.; Frisoni, G.B.; Filippi, M. Resting state fMRI in Alzheimer's disease: Beyond the default mode network. *Neurobiol. Aging* **2012**, *33*, 1564–1578. [CrossRef]
119. Hafkemeijer, A.; Möller, C.; Dopper, E.G.P.; Jiskoot, L.C.; Schouten, T.M.; van Swieten, J.C.; van der Flier, W.M.; Vrenken, H.; Pijnenburg, Y.A.L.; Barkhof, F.; et al. Resting state functional connectivity differences between behavioral variant frontotemporal dementia and Alzheimer's disease. *Front. Hum. Neurosci.* **2015**, *9*, 1–12. [CrossRef]
120. Damoiseaux, J.S.; Prater, K.E.; Miller, B.L.; Greicius, M.D. Functional connectivity tracks clinical deterioration in Alzheimer's disease. *Neurobiol. Aging* **2012**, *33*, 828.e19–828.e30. [CrossRef]
121. Filippi, M.; Agosta, F.; Scola, E.; Canu, E.; Magnani, G.; Marcone, A.; Valsasina, P.; Caso, F.; Copetti, M.; Comi, G.; et al. Functional network connectivity in the behavioral variant of frontotemporal dementia. *Cortex* **2013**, *49*, 2389–2401. [CrossRef]

122. Franciotti, R.; Falasca, N.W.; Bonanni, L.; Anzellotti, F.; Maruotti, V.; Comani, S.; Thomas, A.; Tartaro, A.; Taylor, J.-P.; Onofrj, M. Default network is not hypoactive in dementia with fluctuating cognition: An Alzheimer disease/dementia with Lewy bodies comparison. *Neurobiol. Aging* **2013**, *34*, 1148–1158. [CrossRef]
123. Gili, T.; Cercignani, M.; Serra, L.; Perri, R.; Giove, F.; Maraviglia, B.; Caltagirone, C.; Bozzali, M. Regional brain atrophy and functional disconnection across Alzheimer's disease evolution. *J. Neurol. Neurosurg. Psychiatry* **2011**, *82*, 58–66. [CrossRef] [PubMed]
124. Griffanti, L.; Dipasquale, O.; Laganà, M.M.; Nemni, R.; Clerici, M.; Smith, S.M.; Baselli, G.; Baglio, F. Effective artifact removal in resting state fMRI data improves detection of DMN functional connectivity alteration in Alzheimer's disease. *Front. Hum. Neurosci.* **2015**, *9*, 1–11. [CrossRef] [PubMed]
125. Schwindt, G.C.; Chaudhary, S.; Crane, D.; Ganda, A.; Masellis, M.; Grady, C.L.; Stefanovic, B.; Black, S.E. Modulation of the Default-Mode Network Between Rest and Task in Alzheimer's Disease. *Cereb. Cortex* **2013**, *23*, 1685–1694. [CrossRef] [PubMed]
126. Wang, Z.; Yan, C.; Zhao, C.; Qi, Z.; Zhou, W.; Lu, J.; He, Y.; Li, K. Spatial patterns of intrinsic brain activity in mild cognitive impairment and alzheimer's disease: A resting-state functional MRI study. *Hum. Brain Mapp.* **2011**, *32*, 1720–1740. [CrossRef] [PubMed]
127. Weiler, M.; Fukuda, A.; Massabki, L.; Lopes, T.; Franco, A.; Damasceno, B.; Cendes, F.; Balthazar, M. Default Mode, Executive Function, and Language Functional Connectivity Networks are Compromised in Mild Alzheimer's Disease. *Curr. Alzheimer Res.* **2014**, *11*, 274–282. [CrossRef]
128. Zhang, Z.; Liu, Y.; Jiang, T.; Zhou, B.; An, N.; Dai, H.; Wang, P.; Niu, Y.; Wang, L.; Zhang, X. Altered spontaneous activity in Alzheimer's disease and mild cognitive impairment revealed by Regional Homogeneity. *Neuroimage* **2012**, *59*, 1429–1440. [CrossRef]
129. Zhou, W.; Xia, Z.; Bi, Y.; Shu, H. Altered connectivity of the dorsal and ventral visual regions in dyslexic children: A resting-state fMRI study. *Front. Hum. Neurosci.* **2015**, *9*, 495–504. [CrossRef]
130. Balthazar, M.L.F.; Pereira, F.R.S.; Lopes, T.M.; da Silva, E.L.; Coan, A.C.; Campos, B.M.; Duncan, N.W.; Stella, F.; Northoff, G.; Damasceno, B.P.; et al. Neuropsychiatric symptoms in Alzheimer's disease are related to functional connectivity alterations in the salience network. *Hum. Brain Mapp.* **2014**, *35*, 1237–1246. [CrossRef]
131. Binnewijzend, M.A.A.; Schoonheim, M.M.; Sanz-Arigita, E.; Wink, A.M.; van der Flier, W.M.; Tolboom, N.; Adriaanse, S.M.; Damoiseaux, J.S.; Scheltens, P.; van Berckel, B.N.M.; et al. Resting-state fMRI changes in Alzheimer's disease and mild cognitive impairment. *Neurobiol. Aging* **2012**, *33*, 2018–2028. [CrossRef]
132. Brier, M.R.; Thomas, J.B.; Snyder, A.Z.; Benzinger, T.L.; Zhang, D.; Raichle, M.E.; Holtzman, D.M.; Morris, J.C.; Ances, B.M. Loss of Intranetwork and Internetwork Resting State Functional Connections with Alzheimer's Disease Progression. *J. Neurosci.* **2012**, *32*, 8890–8899. [CrossRef]
133. Badhwar, A.; Tam, A.; Dansereau, C.; Orban, P.; Hoffstaedter, F.; Bellec, P. Resting-state network dysfunction in Alzheimer's disease: A systematic review and meta-analysis. *Alzheimer's Dement. Diagn. Assess. Dis. Monit.* **2017**, *8*, 73–85. [CrossRef] [PubMed]
134. Koch, K.; Myers, N.E.; Göttler, J.; Pasquini, L.; Grimmer, T.; Förster, S.; Manoliu, A.; Neitzel, J.; Kurz, A.; Förstl, H.; et al. Disrupted Intrinsic Networks Link Amyloid-β Pathology and Impaired Cognition in Prodromal Alzheimer's Disease. *Cereb. Cortex* **2015**, *25*, 4678–4688. [CrossRef] [PubMed]
135. Jones, D.T.; Vemuri, P.; Murphy, M.C.; Gunter, J.L.; Senjem, M.L.; Machulda, M.M.; Przybelski, S.A.; Gregg, B.E.; Kantarci, K.; Knopman, D.S.; et al. Non-Stationarity in the "Resting Brain's" Modular Architecture. *PLoS ONE* **2012**, *7*, e39731. [CrossRef] [PubMed]
136. Song, J.; Qin, W.; Liu, Y.; Duan, Y.; Liu, J.; He, X.; Li, K.; Zhang, X.; Jiang, T.; Yu, C. Aberrant Functional Organization within and between Resting-State Networks in AD. *PLoS ONE* **2013**, *8*, e63727. [CrossRef] [PubMed]
137. Guo, Z.; Liu, X.; Hou, H.; Wei, F.; Liu, J.; Chen, X. Abnormal degree centrality in Alzheimer's disease patients with depression: A resting-state functional magnetic resonance imaging study. *Exp. Gerontol.* **2016**, *79*, 61–66. [CrossRef] [PubMed]
138. Brier, M.R.; Thomas, J.B.; Fagan, A.M.; Hassenstab, J.; Holtzman, D.M.; Benzinger, T.L.; Morris, J.C.; Ances, B.M. Functional connectivity and graph theory in preclinical Alzheimer's disease. *Neurobiol. Aging* **2014**, *35*, 757–768. [CrossRef] [PubMed]
139. Sun, Y.; Yin, Q.; Fang, R.; Yan, X.; Wang, Y.; Bezerianos, A. Disrupted Functional Brain Connectivity and Its Association to Structural Connectivity in Amnestic Mild Cognitive Impairment and Alzheimer's Disease. *PLoS ONE* **2014**, *9*, e96505. [CrossRef]
140. Toussaint, P.-J.; Maiz, S.; Coynel, D.; Doyon, J.; Messé, A.; de Souza, L.C.; Sarazin, M.; Perlbarg, V.; Habert, M.-O.; Benali, H. Characteristics of the default mode functional connectivity in normal ageing and Alzheimer's disease using resting state fMRI with a combined approach of entropy-based and graph theoretical measurements. *Neuroimage* **2014**, *101*, 778–786. [CrossRef]
141. Sanz-arigita, E.J.; Schoonheim, M.M.; Damoiseaux, J.S.; Rombouts, S.A.R.B. Loss of 'Small-World' Networks in Alzheimer's Disease: Graph Analysis of fMRI Resting-State Functional Connectivity. *PLoS ONE* **2010**, *5*, e13788. [CrossRef]
142. Wang, J.; Zuo, X.; Dai, Z.; Xia, M.; Zhao, Z.; Zhao, X.; Jia, J.; Han, Y. Disrupted Functional Brain Connectome in Individuals at Risk for Alzheimer's Disease. *Biol. Psychiatry* **2013**, *73*, 472–481. [CrossRef]
143. Zhao, X.; Liu, Y.; Wang, X.; Liu, B.; Xi, Q.; Guo, Q.; Jiang, H.; Jiang, T.; Wang, P. Disrupted Small-World Brain Networks in Moderate Alzheimer's Disease: A Resting-State fMRI Study. *PLoS ONE* **2012**, *7*, e33540. [CrossRef] [PubMed]
144. Wang, J.; Wang, X.; He, Y.; Yu, X.; Wang, H.; He, Y. Apolipoprotein E ε4 modulates functional brain connectome in Alzheimer's disease. *Hum. Brain Mapp.* **2015**, *36*, 1828–1846. [CrossRef] [PubMed]
145. Quiroz, Y.T.; Schultz, A.P.; Chen, K.; Protas, H.D.; Brickhouse, M.; Fleisher, A.S.; Langbaum, J.B.; Thiyyagura, P.; Fagan, A.M.; Shah, A.R.; et al. Brain Imaging and Blood Biomarker Abnormalities in Children with Autosomal Dominant Alzheimer Disease: A Cross-Sectional Study. *JAMA Neurol.* **2015**, *72*, 912–919. [CrossRef] [PubMed]

146. Chhatwal, J.P.; Schultz, A.P.; Johnson, K.; Benzinger, T.L.S.; Jack, C.; Ances, B.M.; Sullivan, C.A.; Salloway, S.P.; Ringman, J.M.; Koeppe, R.A.; et al. Impaired default network functional connectivity in autosomal dominant Alzheimer disease. *Neurology* **2013**, *81*, 736–744. [CrossRef] [PubMed]
147. Sala-Llonch, R.; Fortea, J.; Bartrés-Faz, D.; Bosch, B.; Lladó, A.; Peña-Gómez, C.; Antonell, A.; Castellanos-Pinedo, F.; Bargalló, N.; Molinuevo, J.L.; et al. Evolving Brain Functional Abnormalities in PSEN1 Mutation Carriers: A Resting and Visual Encoding fMRI Study. *J. Alzheimer's Dis.* **2013**, *36*, 165–175. [CrossRef] [PubMed]
148. Adriaanse, S.M.; Sanz-Arigita, E.J.; Binnewijzend, M.A.A.; Ossenkoppele, R.; Tolboom, N.; van Assema, D.M.E.; Wink, A.M.; Boellaard, R.; Yaqub, M.; Windhorst, A.D.; et al. Amyloid and its association with default network integrity in Alzheimer's disease. *Hum. Brain Mapp.* **2014**, *35*, 779–791. [CrossRef]
149. Thomas, J.B.; Brier, M.R.; Bateman, R.J.; Snyder, A.Z.; Benzinger, T.L.; Xiong, C.; Raichle, M.; Holtzman, D.M.; Sperling, R.A.; Mayeux, R.; et al. Functional Connectivity in Autosomal Dominant and Late-Onset Alzheimer Disease. *JAMA Neurol.* **2014**, *71*, 1111–1122. [CrossRef]
150. Li, X.; Westman, E.; Thordardottir, S.; Ståhlbom, A.K.; Almkvist, O.; Blennow, K.; Wahlund, L.-O.; Graff, C. The Effects of Gene Mutations on Default Mode Network in Familial & Alzheimer's Disease. *J. Alzheimer's Dis.* **2017**, *56*, 327–334. [CrossRef]
151. Matura, S.; Prvulovic, D.; Butz, M.; Hartmann, D.; Sepanski, B.; Linnemann, K.; Oertel-Knöchel, V.; Karakaya, T.; Fußer, F.; Pantel, J.; et al. Recognition memory is associated with altered resting-state functional connectivity in people at genetic risk for Alzheimer's disease. *Eur. J. Neurosci.* **2014**, *40*, 3128–3135. [CrossRef]
152. Sheline, Y.I.; Morris, J.C.; Snyder, A.Z.; Price, J.L.; Yan, Z.; D'Angelo, G.; Liu, C.; Dixit, S.; Benzinger, T.; Fagan, A.; et al. APOE4 Allele Disrupts Resting State fMRI Connectivity in the Absence of Amyloid Plaques or Decreased CSF Aβ42. *J. Neurosci.* **2010**, *30*, 17035–17040. [CrossRef]
153. Su, Y.Y.; Liang, X.; Schoepf, U.J.; Varga-Szemes, A.; West, H.C.; Qi, R.; Kong, X.; Chen, H.J.; Lu, G.M.; Zhang, L.J. APOE Polymorphism Affects Brain Default Mode Network in Healthy Young Adults: A STROBE Article. *Medicine* **2015**, *94*, e1734. [CrossRef] [PubMed]
154. Filippini, N.; MacIntosh, B.J.; Hough, M.G.; Goodwin, G.M.; Frisoni, G.B.; Smith, S.M.; Matthews, P.M.; Beckmann, C.F.; Mackay, C.E. Distinct patterns of brain activity in young carriers of the APOE-ε4 allele. *Proc. Natl. Acad. Sci. USA* **2009**, *106*, 7209–7214. [CrossRef] [PubMed]
155. Song, H.; Long, H.; Zuo, X.; Yu, C.; Liu, B.; Wang, Z.; Wang, Q.; Wang, F.; Han, Y.; Jia, J. APOE effects on default mode network in Chinese cognitive normal elderly: Relationship with clinical cognitive performance. *PLoS ONE* **2015**, *10*, 1–11. [CrossRef] [PubMed]
156. Goveas, J.S.; Xie, C.; Chen, G.; Li, W.; Ward, B.D.; Franczak, M.B.; Jones, J.L.; Antuono, P.G.; Li, S.J. Functional Network Endophenotypes Unravel the Effects of Apolipoprotein E Epsilon 4 in Middle-Aged Adults. *PLoS ONE* **2013**, *8*, 1–10. [CrossRef]
157. Westlye, E.T.; Lundervold, A.; Rootwelt, H.; Lundervold, A.J.; Westlye, L.T. Increased hippocampal default mode synchronization during rest in middle-aged and elderly APOE ε4 carriers: Relationships with memory performance. *J. Neurosci.* **2011**, *31*, 7775–7783. [CrossRef]
158. Zhang, H.-Y.; Wang, S.-J.; Xing, J.; Liu, B.; Ma, Z.-L.; Yang, M.; Zhang, Z.-J.; Teng, G.-J. Detection of PCC functional connectivity characteristics in resting-state fMRI in mild Alzheimer's disease. *Behav. Brain Res.* **2009**, *197*, 103–108. [CrossRef]
159. Han, S.D.; Arfanakis, K.; Fleischman, D.A.; Leurgans, S.E.; Tuminello, E.R.; Edmonds, E.C.; Bennett, D.A. Functional connectivity variations in mild cognitive impairment: Associations with cognitive function. *J. Int. Neuropsychol. Soc.* **2012**, *18*, 39–48. [CrossRef]
160. Bai, F.; Watson, D.R.; Yu, H.; Shi, Y.; Yuan, Y.; Zhang, Z. Abnormal resting-state functional connectivity of posterior cingulate cortex in amnestic type mild cognitive impairment. *Brain Res.* **2009**, *1302*, 167–174. [CrossRef]
161. Qureshi, M.N.I.; Ryu, S.; Song, J.; Lee, K.H.; Lee, B. Evaluation of Functional Decline in Alzheimer's Dementia Using 3D Deep Learning and Group ICA for rs-fMRI Measurements. *Front. Aging Neurosci.* **2019**, *11*, 8–16. [CrossRef]
162. Goveas, J.S.; Xie, C.; Ward, B.D.; Wu, Z.; Li, W.; Franczak, M.; Jones, J.L.; Antuono, P.G.; Li, S. Recovery of Hippocampal Network Connectivity Correlates with Cognitive Improvement in Mild Alzheimer's Disease Patients Treated with Donepezil Assessed by Resting-State fMRI. *J. Magn. Reson. Imaging* **2011**, *34*, 764–773. [CrossRef]
163. Li, W.; Antuono, P.G.; Xie, C.; Chen, G.; Jones, J.L.; Ward, B.D.; Franczak, M.; Goveas, J.S.; Li, S. NeuroImage Changes in regional cerebral blood flow and functional connectivity in the cholinergic pathway associated with cognitive performance in subjects with mild Alzheimer's disease after 12-week donepezil treatment. *Neuroimage* **2012**, *60*, 1083–1091. [CrossRef]
164. Ferreira, L.K.; Busatto, G.F. Resting-state functional connectivity in normal brain aging. *Neurosci. Biobehav. Rev.* **2013**, *37*, 384–400. [CrossRef] [PubMed]
165. Wang, L.; Brier, M.R.; Snyder, A.Z.; Thomas, J.B.; Fagan, A.M.; Xiong, C.; Benzinger, T.L.; Holtzman, D.M.; Morris, J.C.; Ances, B.M. Cerebrospinal Fluid Aβ42, Phosphorylated Tau181, and Resting-State Functional Connectivity. *JAMA Neurol.* **2013**, *70*, 1242–1248. [CrossRef] [PubMed]
166. Elman, J.A.; Madison, C.M.; Baker, S.L.; Vogel, J.W.; Marks, S.M.; Crowley, S.; O'Neil, J.P.; Jagust, W.J. Effects of Beta-Amyloid on Resting State Functional Connectivity Within and Between Networks Reflect Known Patterns of Regional Vulnerability. *Cereb. Cortex* **2016**, *26*, 695–707. [CrossRef]
167. Hafkemeijer, A.; Möller, C.; Dopper, E.G.P.; Jiskoot, L.C.; van den Berg-Huysmans, A.A.; van Swieten, J.C.; van der Flier, W.M.; Vrenken, H.; Pijnenburg, Y.A.L.; Barkhof, F.; et al. A Longitudinal Study on Resting State Functional Connectivity in Behavioral Variant Frontotemporal Dementia and Alzheimer's Disease. *J. Alzheimer's Dis.* **2017**, *55*, 521–537. [CrossRef] [PubMed]

168. Hart, B.; Cribben, I.; Fiecas, M. A longitudinal model for functional connectivity networks using resting-state fMRI. *Neuroimage* **2018**, *178*, 687–701. [CrossRef]
169. Lau, W.K.-W.; Leung, P.P.-Y.; Chung, C.L.-P. Effects of the Satir Model on Mental Health: A Randomized Controlled Trial. *Res. Soc. Work Pract.* **2018**, *29*, 775–785. [CrossRef]
170. Zhou, J.; Greicius, M.D.; Gennatas, E.D.; Growdon, M.E.; Jang, J.Y.; Rabinovici, G.D.; Kramer, J.H.; Weiner, M.; Miller, B.L.; Seeley, W.W. Divergent network connectivity changes in behavioural variant frontotemporal dementia and Alzheimer's disease. *Brain* **2010**, *133*, 1352–1367. [CrossRef]
171. Fox, M.D.; Corbetta, M.; Snyder, A.Z.; Vincent, J.L.; Raichle, M.E. Spontaneous neuronal activity distinguishes human dorsal and ventral attention systems. *Proc. Natl. Acad. Sci. USA* **2006**, *103*, 10046–10051. [CrossRef]
172. Dosenbach, N.U.F.; Fair, D.A.; Miezin, F.M.; Cohen, A.L.; Wenger, K.K.; Dosenbach, R.A.T.; Fox, M.D.; Snyder, A.Z.; Vincent, J.L.; Raichle, M.E.; et al. Distinct brain networks for adaptive and stable task control in humans. *Proc. Natl. Acad. Sci. USA* **2007**, *104*, 11073–11078. [CrossRef]
173. Sylvester, C.M.; Shulman, G.L.; Jack, A.I.; Corbetta, M. Anticipatory and Stimulus-Evoked Blood Oxygenation Level-Dependent Modulations Related to Spatial Attention Reflect a Common Additive Signal. *J. Neurosci.* **2009**, *29*, 10671–10682. [CrossRef] [PubMed]
174. Challis, E.; Hurley, P.; Serra, L.; Bozzali, M.; Oliver, S.; Cercignani, M. Gaussian process classification of Alzheimer's disease and mild cognitive impairment from resting-state fMRI. *Neuroimage* **2015**, *112*, 232–243. [CrossRef] [PubMed]
175. Khazaee, A.; Ebrahimzadeh, A.; Babajani-Feremi, A. Identifying patients with Alzheimer's disease using resting-state fMRI and graph theory. *Clin. Neurophysiol.* **2015**, *126*, 2132–2141. [CrossRef] [PubMed]
176. Shen, K.; Welton, T.; Lyon, M.; McCorkindale, A.N.; Sutherland, G.T.; Burnham, S.; Fripp, J.; Martins, R.; Grieve, S.M. Structural core of the executive control network: A high angular resolution diffusion MRI study. *Hum. Brain Mapp.* **2020**, *41*, 1226–1236. [CrossRef]
177. Niendam, T.A.; Laird, A.R.; Ray, K.L.; Dean, Y.M.; Glahn, D.C.; Carter, C.S. Meta-analytic evidence for a superordinate cognitive control network subserving diverse executive functions. *Cogn. Affect. Behav. Neurosci.* **2012**, *12*, 241–268. [CrossRef]
178. Reineberg, A.E.; Banich, M.T. Functional connectivity at rest is sensitive to individual differences in executive function: A network analysis. *Hum. Brain Mapp.* **2016**, *37*, 2959–2975. [CrossRef]
179. Zhu, Z.; Johnson, N.F.; Kim, C.; Gold, B.T. Reduced frontal cortex efficiency is associated with lower white matter integrity in aging. *Cereb. Cortex* **2015**, *25*, 138–146. [CrossRef]
180. Rosenberg-Katz, K.; Herman, T.; Jacob, Y.; Mirelman, A.; Giladi, N.; Hendler, T.; Hausdorff, J.M. Fall risk is associated with amplified functional connectivity of the central executive network in patients with Parkinson's disease. *J. Neurol.* **2015**, *262*, 2448–2456. [CrossRef]
181. Cai, S.; Peng, Y.; Chong, T.; Zhang, Y.; von Deneen, K.M.; Huang, L. Differentiated Effective Connectivity Patterns of the Executive Control Network in Progressive MCI: A Potential Biomarker for Predicting AD. *Curr. Alzheimer Res.* **2017**, *14*. [CrossRef]
182. Zhao, Q.; Lu, H.; Metmer, H.; Li, W.X.Y.; Lu, J. Evaluating functional connectivity of executive control network and frontoparietal network in Alzheimer's disease. *Brain Res.* **2018**, *1678*, 262–272. [CrossRef]
183. Cieri, F.; Esposito, R.; Cera, N.; Pieramico, V.; Tartaro, A.; Di Giannantonio, M. Late-life depression: Modifications of brain resting state activity. *J. Geriatr. Psychiatry Neurol.* **2017**, *30*, 140–150. [CrossRef] [PubMed]
184. Respino, M.; Hoptman, M.J.; Victoria, L.W.; Alexopoulos, G.S.; Solomonov, N.; Stein, A.T.; Coluccio, M.; Morimoto, S.S.; Blau, C.J.; Abreu, L.; et al. Cognitive Control, Network Homogeneity and Executive Functions in Late-Life Depression. *Biol. Psychiatry Cogn. Neurosci. Neuroimaging* **2020**, *5*, 213–221. [CrossRef] [PubMed]
185. Manning, K.; Wang, L.; Steffens, D. Recent advances in the use of imaging in psychiatry: Functional magnetic resonance imaging of large-scale brain networks in late-life depression. *F1000Research* **2019**, *8*, 1–9. [CrossRef]
186. Alalade, E.; Denny, K.; Potter, G.; Steffens, D.; Wang, L. Altered Cerebellar-Cerebral Functional Connectivity in Geriatric Depression. *PLoS ONE* **2011**, *6*, e20035. [CrossRef] [PubMed]
187. Yin, Y.; Hou, Z.; Wang, X.; Sui, Y.; Yuan, Y. Association between altered resting-state cortico-cerebellar functional connectivity networks and mood/cognition dysfunction in late-onset depression. *J. Neural Transm.* **2015**, *122*, 887–896. [CrossRef]
188. Yue, Y.; Yuan, Y.; Hou, Z.; Jiang, W.; Bai, F.; Zhang, Z. Abnormal Functional Connectivity of Amygdala in Late-Onset Depression Was Associated with Cognitive Deficits. *PLoS ONE* **2013**, *8*, e75058. [CrossRef] [PubMed]
189. Wang, Z.; Yuan, Y.; Bai, F.; Shu, H.; You, J.; Li, L.; Zhang, Z. Altered functional connectivity networks of hippocampal subregions in remitted late-onset depression: A longitudinal resting-state study. *Neurosci. Bull.* **2015**, *31*, 13–21. [CrossRef]
190. Lockwood, K.A.; Alexopoulos, G.S.; van Gorp, W.G. Executive dysfunction in geriatric depression. *Am. J. Psychiatry* **2002**, *159*, 1119–1126. [CrossRef]
191. Manning, K.J.; Alexopoulos, G.S.; Mcgovern, A.R.; Morimoto, S.S.; Yuen, G.; Kanellopoulos, T.; Gunning, F.M. Executive functioning in late-life depression. *Psychiatr. Ann.* **2014**, *44*, 143–146. [CrossRef]
192. Gandelman, J.A.; Albert, K.; Boyd, B.D.; Park, J.W.; Riddle, M.; Woodward, N.D.; Kang, H.; Landman, B.A.; Taylor, W.D. Intrinsic Functional Network Connectivity Is Associated with Clinical Symptoms and Cognition in Late-Life Depression. *Biol. Psychiatry Cogn. Neurosci. Neuroimaging* **2019**, *4*, 160–170. [CrossRef]
193. Alexopoulos, G.S.; Kiosses, D.N.; Klimstra, S.; Kalayam, B.; Bruce, M.L. Clinical Presentation of the "Depression–Executive Dysfunction Syndrome" of Late Life. *Am. J. Geriatr. Psychiatry* **2002**, *10*, 98–106. [CrossRef] [PubMed]
194. Alexopoulos, G.S.; Kiosses, D.N.; Heo, M.; Murphy, C.F.; Shanmugham, B.; Gunning-Dixon, F. Executive Dysfunction and the Course of Geriatric Depression. *Biol. Psychiatry* **2005**, *58*, 204–210. [CrossRef] [PubMed]

195. Manning, K.J.; Alexopoulos, G.S.; Banerjee, S.; Morimoto, S.S.; Seirup, J.K.; Klimstra, S.A.; Yuen, G.; Kanellopoulos, T.; Gunning-Dixon, F. Executive functioning complaints and escitalopram treatment response in late-life depression. *Am. J. Geriatr. Psychiatry* **2015**, *23*, 440–445. [CrossRef] [PubMed]
196. Morimoto, S.S.; Kanellopoulos, D.; Manning, K.J.; Alexopoulos, G.S. Diagnosis and treatment of depression and cognitive impairment in late life. *Ann. N. Y. Acad. Sci.* **2015**, *1345*, 36–46. [CrossRef] [PubMed]
197. Castellazzi, G.; Palesi, F.; Casali, S.; Vitali, P.; Sinforiani, E.; Wheeler-Kingshott, C.A.M.; D'Angelo, E. A comprehensive assessment of resting state networks: Bidirectional modification of functional integrity in cerebro-cerebellar networks in dementia. *Front. Neurosci.* **2014**, *8*, 223–250. [CrossRef] [PubMed]
198. Gour, N.; Ranjeva, J.-P.; Ceccaldi, M.; Confort-Gouny, S.; Barbeau, E.; Soulier, E.; Guye, M.; Didic, M.; Felician, O. Basal functional connectivity within the anterior temporal network is associated with performance on declarative memory tasks. *Neuroimage* **2011**, *58*, 687–697. [CrossRef] [PubMed]
199. Firbank, M.; Kobeleva, X.; Cherry, G.; Killen, A.; Gallagher, P.; Burn, D.J.; Thomas, A.J.; O'Brien, J.T.; Taylor, J.P. Neural correlates of attention-executive dysfunction in lewy body dementia and Alzheimer's disease. *Hum. Brain Mapp.* **2016**, *37*, 1254–1270. [CrossRef]
200. Levine, M.E.; Lu, A.T.; Bennett, D.A.; Horvath, S. Epigenetic age of the pre-frontal cortex is associated with neuritic plaques, amyloid load, and Alzheimer's disease related cognitive functioning. *Aging* **2015**, *7*, 1198–1211. [CrossRef]
201. Liu, Y.; Yu, J.T.; Wang, H.F.; Han, P.R.; Tan, C.C.; Wang, C.; Meng, X.F.; Risacher, S.L.; Saykin, A.J.; Tan, L. APOE genotype and neuroimaging markers of Alzheimer's disease: Systematic review and meta-analysis. *J. Neurol. Neurosurg. Psychiatry* **2015**, *86*, 127–134. [CrossRef]
202. Menon, V.; Uddin, L.Q. Saliency, switching, attention and control: A network model of insula function. *Brain Struct. Funct.* **2010**, *214*, 655–667. [CrossRef]
203. Seeley, X.W.W. The Salience Network: A Neural System for Perceiving and Responding to Homeostatic Demands. *J. Neurosci.* **2019**, *39*, 9878–9882. [CrossRef] [PubMed]
204. Downar, J.; Crawley, A.P.; Mikulis, D.J.; Davis, K.D. A multimodal cortical network for the detection of changes in the sensory environment. *Nat. Neurosci.* **2000**, *3*, 277–283. [CrossRef] [PubMed]
205. Touroutoglou, A.; Hollenbeck, M.; Dickerson, B.C.; Feldman Barrett, L. Dissociable large-scale networks anchored in the right anterior insula subserve affective experience and attention. *Neuroimage* **2012**, *60*, 1947–1958. [CrossRef] [PubMed]
206. Seeley, W.W.; Menon, V.; Schatzberg, A.F.; Keller, J.; Glover, G.H.; Kenna, H.; Reiss, A.L.; Greicius, M.D. Dissociable Intrinsic Connectivity Networks for Salience Processing and Executive Control. *J. Neurosci.* **2007**, *27*, 2349–2356. [CrossRef] [PubMed]
207. Chand, G.B.; Wu, J.; Hajjar, I.; Qiu, D. Interactions of the Salience Network and Its Subsystems with the Default-Mode and the Central-Executive. *Brain Connect.* **2017**, *7*, 401–412. [CrossRef] [PubMed]
208. Elton, A.; Gao, W. Divergent task-dependent functional connectivity of executive control and salience networks. *Cortex* **2014**, *51*, 56–66. [CrossRef]
209. Bonnelle, V.; Ham, T.E.; Leech, R.; Kinnunen, K.M.; Mehta, M.A.; Greenwood, R.J.; Sharp, D.J. Salience network integrity predicts default mode network function after traumatic brain injury. *Proc. Natl. Acad. Sci. USA* **2012**, *109*, 4690–4695. [CrossRef]
210. Dai, L.; Zhou, H.; Xu, X.; Zuo, Z. Brain structural and functional changes in patients with major depressive disorder: A literature review. *PeerJ* **2019**, *7*, e8170. [CrossRef]
211. Cullen, K.R.; Westlund, M.K.; Klimes-Dougan, B.; Mueller, B.A.; Houri, A.; Eberly, L.E.; Lim, K.O. Abnormal Amygdala Resting-State Functional Connectivity in Adolescent Depression. *JAMA Psychiatry* **2014**, *71*, 1138–1147. [CrossRef]
212. Luking, K.R.; Repovs, G.; Belden, A.C.; Gaffrey, M.S.; Botteron, K.N.; Luby, J.L.; Barch, D.M. Functional Connectivity of the Amygdala in Early-Childhood-Onset Depression. *J. Am. Acad. Child Adolesc. Psychiatry* **2011**, *50*, 1027–1041.e3. [CrossRef]
213. Davey, C.G.; Whittle, S.; Harrison, B.J.; Simmons, J.G.; Byrne, M.L.; Schwartz, O.S.; Allen, N.B. Functional brain-imaging correlates of negative affectivity and the onset of first-episode depression. *Psychol. Med.* **2015**, *45*, 1001–1009. [CrossRef] [PubMed]
214. Zhang, H.; Li, L.; Wu, M.; Chen, Z.; Hu, X.; Chen, Y.; Zhu, H.; Jia, Z.; Gong, Q. Brain gray matter alterations in first episodes of depression: A meta-analysis of whole-brain studies. *Neurosci. Biobehav. Rev.* **2016**, *60*, 43–50. [CrossRef] [PubMed]
215. Wang, L.; Chou, Y.H.; Potter, G.G.; Steffens, D.C. Altered synchronizations among neural networks in geriatric depression. *Biomed. Res. Int.* **2015**, *2015*. [CrossRef]
216. Steffens, D.C.; Wang, L.; Pearlson, G.D. Functional connectivity predictors of acute depression treatment outcome. *Int. Psychogeriatr.* **2019**, *31*, 1831–1835. [CrossRef] [PubMed]
217. Fredericks, C.A.; Sturm, V.E.; Brown, J.A.; Hua, A.Y.; Bilgel, M.; Wong, D.F.; Resnick, S.M.; Seeley, W.W. Early affective changes and increased connectivity in preclinical Alzheimer's disease. *Alzheimer's Dement.* **2018**, *10*, 471–479. [CrossRef]
218. Machulda, M.M.; Jones, D.T.; Vemuri, P.; McDade, E.; Avula, R.; Przybelski, S.; Boeve, B.F.; Knopman, D.S.; Petersen, R.C.; Jack, C.R., Jr. Effect of APOE ε4 status on intrinsic network connectivity in cognitively normal elderly subjects. *Arch. Neurol.* **2011**, *68*, 1131–1136. [CrossRef]
219. He, X.; Qin, W.; Liu, Y.; Zhang, X.; Duan, Y.; Song, J.; Li, K.; Jiang, T.; Yu, C. Abnormal salience network in normal aging and in amnestic mild cognitive impairment and Alzheimer's disease. *Hum. Brain Mapp.* **2014**, *35*, 3446–3464. [CrossRef]
220. Rami, L.; Sala-Llonch, R.; Solé-Padullés, C.; Fortea, J.; Olives, J.; Lladó, A.; Peña-Gómez, C.; Balasa, M.; Bosch, B.; Antonell, A.; et al. Distinct Functional Activity of the Precuneus and Posterior Cingulate Cortex During Encoding in the Preclinical Stage of Alzheimer's Disease. *J. Alzheimer's Dis.* **2012**, *31*, 517–526. [CrossRef]

221. Scheff, S.W.; Price, D.A.; Ansari, M.A.; Roberts, K.N.; Schmitt, F.A.; Ikonomovic, M.D.; Mufson, E.J. Synaptic Change in the Posterior Cingulate Gyrus in the Progression of Alzheimer's Disease. *J. Alzheimer's Dis.* **2015**, *43*, 1073–1090. [CrossRef]
222. Mutlu, J.; Landeau, B.; Tomadesso, C.; de Flores, R.; Mézenge, F.; de La Sayette, V.; Eustache, F.; Chételat, G. Connectivity Disruption, Atrophy, and Hypometabolism within Posterior Cingulate Networks in Alzheimer's Disease. *Front. Neurosci.* **2016**, *10*, 582–591. [CrossRef]
223. Jamieson, A.; Goodwill, A.M.; Termine, M.; Campbell, S.; Szoeke, C. Depression related cerebral pathology and its relationship with cognitive functioning: A systematic review. *J. Affect. Disord.* **2019**, *250*, 410–418. [CrossRef] [PubMed]
224. Dong, X.; Yan, L.; Huang, L.; Guan, X.; Dong, C.; Tao, H.; Wang, T.; Qin, X.; Wan, Q. Repetitive transcranial magnetic stimulation for the treatment of Alzheimer's disease: A systematic review and meta-analysis of randomized controlled trials. *PLoS ONE* **2018**, *13*, 1–13. [CrossRef] [PubMed]
225. Crossley, N.A.; Mechelli, A.; Scott, J.; Carletti, F.; Fox, P.T.; McGuire, P.; Bullmore, E.T. The hubs of the human connectome are generally implicated in the anatomy of brain disorders. *Brain* **2014**, *137*, 2382–2395. [CrossRef] [PubMed]
226. Sepulcre, J.; Schultz, A.P.; Sabuncu, M.; Gomez-Isla, T.; Chhatwal, J.; Becker, A.; Sperling, R.; Johnson, K.A. In Vivo Tau, Amyloid, and Gray Matter Profiles in the Aging Brain. *J. Neurosci.* **2016**, *36*, 7364–7374. [CrossRef]
227. Curado, M.; Escolano, F.; Lozano, M.A.; Hancock, E.R. Early Detection of Alzheimer's Disease: Detecting Asymmetries with a Return Random Walk Link Predictor. *Entropy* **2020**, *22*, 465. [CrossRef]
228. Dachena, C.; Casu, S.; Fanti, A.; Lodi, M.B.; Mazzarella, G. Combined Use of MRI, fMRI and Cognitive Data for Alzheimer's Disease: Preliminary Results. *Appl. Sci.* **2019**, *9*, 3156. [CrossRef]

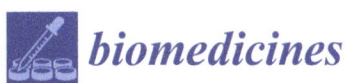

Article

Sex-Dependent End-of-Life Mental and Vascular Scenarios for Compensatory Mechanisms in Mice with Normal and AD-Neurodegenerative Aging

Aida Muntsant [1,2,†], Francesc Jiménez-Altayó [2,3,*,†], Lidia Puertas-Umbert [3], Elena Jiménez-Xarrie [4], Elisabet Vila [3] and Lydia Giménez-Llort [1,2,*]

1. Department of Psychiatry and Forensic Medicine, School of Medicine, Universitat Autònoma de Barcelona, 08193 Barcelona, Spain; aida.muntsant@uab.cat
2. Institut de Neurociències, Universitat Autònoma de Barcelona, 08193 Barcelona, Spain
3. Department of Pharmacology, Toxicology and Therapeutics, School of Medicine, Universitat Autònoma de Barcelona, 08193 Barcelona, Spain; lidiapu28@gmail.com (L.P.-U.); elisabet.vila@uab.cat (E.V.)
4. Stroke Unit, Department of Neurology, Institut d'Investigació Biomèdica (IIB)-Sant Pau, 08041 Barcelona, Spain; ejimenezx@santpau.cat
* Correspondence: francesc.jimenez@uab.cat (F.J.-A.); lidia.gimenez@uab.cat (L.G.-L.); Tel.: +34-93-581-1952 (F.J.-A.); +34-93-581-2378 (L.G.-L.); Fax: +34-93-581-1953 (F.J.-A.); +34-93-581-1435 (L.G.-L.)
† These authors contributed equally to this work.

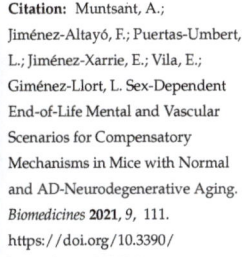

Citation: Muntsant, A.; Jiménez-Altayó, F.; Puertas-Umbert, L.; Jiménez-Xarrie, E.; Vila, E.; Giménez-Llort, L. Sex-Dependent End-of-Life Mental and Vascular Scenarios for Compensatory Mechanisms in Mice with Normal and AD-Neurodegenerative Aging. *Biomedicines* 2021, 9, 111. https://doi.org/10.3390/biomedicines9020111

Academic Editor: Masaru Tanaka
Received: 26 October 2020
Accepted: 20 January 2021
Published: 24 January 2021

Publisher's Note: MDPI stays neutral with regard to jurisdictional claims in published maps and institutional affiliations.

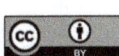

Copyright: © 2021 by the authors. Licensee MDPI, Basel, Switzerland. This article is an open access article distributed under the terms and conditions of the Creative Commons Attribution (CC BY) license (https://creativecommons.org/licenses/by/4.0/).

Abstract: Life expectancy decreases with aging, with cardiovascular, mental health, and neurodegenerative disorders strongly contributing to the total disability-adjusted life years. Interestingly, the morbidity/mortality paradox points to females having a worse healthy life expectancy. Since bidirectional interactions between cardiovascular and Alzheimer's diseases (AD) have been reported, the study of this emerging field is promising. In the present work, we further explored the cardiovascular–brain interactions in mice survivors of two cohorts of non-transgenic and 3xTg-AD mice, including both sexes, to investigate the frailty/survival through their life span. Survival, monitored from birth, showed exceptionally worse mortality rates in females than males, independently of the genotype. This mortality selection provided a "survivors" cohort that could unveil brain–cardiovascular interaction mechanisms relevant for normal and neurodegenerative aging processes restricted to long-lived animals. The results show sex-dependent distinct physical (worse in 3xTg-AD males), neuropsychiatric-like and cognitive phenotypes (worse in 3xTg-AD females), and hypothalamic–pituitary–adrenal (HPA) axis activation (higher in females), with higher cerebral blood flow and improved cardiovascular phenotype in 3xTg-AD female mice survivors. The present study provides an experimental scenario to study the suggested potential compensatory hemodynamic mechanisms in end-of-life dementia, which is sex-dependent and can be a target for pharmacological and non-pharmacological interventions.

Keywords: healthy life expectancy (HALE); morbidity/mortality paradox; anxiety; cognition; systolic blood pressure; cerebral blood flow; arterial properties; angiogenesis; gender medicine; neurodegenerative disorders

1. Introduction

In a life expectancy that decreases with the aging process, cardiovascular, mental health, and neurodegenerative disorders strongly contribute to the total disability-adjusted life years (DALYs) with significant sex differences observed [1,2]. On the other hand, the morbidity/mortality paradox points to females having greater longevity but worse healthy life expectancy (HALE) than males [3]. Neurodegenerative disorders such as dementia are associated with increased mortality compared to aged control populations [4–6]. Besides, in recent years, the high degree of heterogeneity in the clinical and temporal patterns of advanced stages of Alzheimer's disease (AD) in the elderly population evidences the existence of several subgroups of patients and demands clinical prognosticators of end-of-life dementia [7]. At the translational level, the shorter life span of animal models provides a particular scenario for studying and long-term monitoring of the factors relevant for health/disease and those factors involved in its fine-tuning modulation, from genetic and epigenetic to morphological, structural, and functional levels.

Among the animal models of AD, we have proposed long-term survivors of the widely used 3xTg-AD mice as a model for mortality selection bias and heterogeneity in end-of-life dementia [8]. This model, homozygous for the familial AD mutations PS1/M146V and APPSwe, also harboring the tauP301L human transgene, progressively develops temporal- and regional-specific neuropathological patterns and other hallmarks of the human disease [9–11]. The mortality rates of 3xTg-AD mice at 15 months of age, an advanced stage of amyloid and tau neuropathology, are higher than in the non-transgenic (NTg) counterparts [12]. Thus, survivors could be used to investigate the frailty/survival paradigm in normal and pathological aging, since a small number of animals overcome advanced neuropathological stages of the disease. Across the literature, most experimental research of our and other laboratories has shown higher mortality rates in homozygous [12,13] and heterozygous [14] male 3xTg-AD mice, despite female 3xTg-AD mice exhibiting worse neuropathological status than males [15].

Peripheral cardiovascular dysfunction as a risk factor in AD is among the promising emerging fields, since bidirectional interactions have been reported in these patients. Thus, amyloid pathology affects patients' hearts [16], and the impact of cerebrovascular dysfunction independently of cerebral amyloid angiopathy has also been demonstrated [17]. The arterial function is crucial to regulate blood pressure and flow through the body by the contraction and relaxation of the vascular smooth muscle cells. Increasing evidence obtained in different mouse models suggests that AD is associated with vascular dysfunction affecting different circulation arterial beds [18–21]. Angiogenesis, or growth of new blood vessels from pre-existent vessels, is a fundamental process, such as during development, wound healing, and restoring blood flow from hypoxic regions. Previous studies support a role of angiogenesis as a compensatory response to impaired cerebral blood flow (CBF) in AD [22]. However, extensive angiogenesis can lead to increased vascular permeability and subsequent hypervascularization and brain damage in AD [23,24]. Overall, although the "vascular hypothesis" of AD is increasingly being understood, the influence of sex on the vascular features present in AD has been a neglected topic.

Cardiovascular disease resulting from oxidative stress inflammation can exacerbate Alzheimer's disease. We recently reported the first evidence of sex-dependent worse physiologically relevant structural (increased passive external and internal diameters, cross sectional area) and functional (increased active internal diameters) properties in small peripheral mesenteric resistance arteries (MRA) in 15-month-old 3xTg-AD mice (advanced stages of disease) compared to age-matched mice with normal aging [21]. Thus, at both physiological and high intraluminal pressures, vascular alterations of female 3xTg-AD mice were found more pronounced than those found in age-matched male 3xTg-AD mice. Besides, a correlation between MRA properties and anxiety-like behavioral profile was found in both 3xTg-AD mice and age-matched non-transgenic counterparts with normal aging, pointing at the relevant interaction between vascular and mental health in the aging process.

The present work aimed to further explore the cardiovascular–brain interactions in normal and AD-neurodegenerative aging models using a life span paradigm. For that purpose, we studied two cohorts of NTg and 3xTg-AD mice, including both sexes, until the end of life. Survival, monitored from birth, showed exceptional worse mortality rates in females than males, independently of the genotype. This mortality selection provided a "survivors" sample that could unveil brain–cardiovascular interaction mechanisms relevant for normal and neurodegenerative aging processes in long-lived animals. The results show sex-dependent distinct physical (worse in 3xTg-AD males), neuropsychiatric-like and cognitive phenotypes (worse in 3xTg-AD females), and hypothalamic–pituitary–adrenal (HPA) axis activation (higher in females), with higher cerebral blood flow and improved cardiovascular phenotype in 3xTg-AD female mice survivors. The present study suggests a potential compensatory hemodynamic mechanism in end-of-life dementia, which is sex-dependent and can be a target for pharmacological and non-pharmacological interventions.

2. Materials and Methods

2.1. Animals

Homozygous triple-transgenic 3xTg-AD mice harboring human $PS1_{M146V}$, APP_{Swe}, and tau_{P301L} transgenes were genetically engineered at the University of California Irvine, as previously described [9]. Briefly, two independent transgenes (encoding human APP_{Swe} and human tauP301L, both under control of the mouse Thy1.2 regulatory element) were co-injected into single-cell embryos harvested from homozygous mutant PS1M146V knock-in (PS1KI) mice. The PS1 knock-in mice were originally generated after embryonic transfer into pure C57BL/6.

A total of thirty-six 14-month-old homozygous male and female mice from the Spanish colonies of 3xTg-AD ($n = 19$, 10 males, 9 females) and C57BL/6 ($n = 17$, 10 males and 7 females) wild-type mice (from now, referred as non-transgenic mice, NTg) from litters of a breeding program established after embryonic transfer to C57BL/6 strain background were used in this study. All the animals were housed three to four per cage and maintained (Makrolon, $35 \times 35 \times 25$ cm ^{3}) under standard laboratory conditions (12 h light/dark, cycle starting at 8:00 h, food and water available ad libitum, $22 \pm 2\ °C$, 50–60% humidity) at the Universitat Autònoma de Barcelona. Behavioral tests were performed from 9:00 h to 13:00 h. Assessments were performed blind to the experiment in a counterbalanced manner.

All procedures were in accordance with Spanish legislation on "Protection of Animals Used for Experimental and Other Scientific Purposes" and the EU Council directive (2010/63/EU) on this subject. The protocol CEEAH 3588/DMAH 9452 was approved the 8th of March 2019 by Departament de Medi Ambient i Habitatge, Generalitat de Catalunya. The study complies with the ARRIVE guidelines developed by the NC3Rs and aims to reduce the number of animals used [25].

2.2. Experimental Design

A longitudinal study divided into successive phases was performed, starting at 14 months of age, with the characterization of their physical and mental health status (behavioral phenotype and physical condition (weight, Mouse Clinical Frailty Index Assessment, and Survival) 441.7 ± 1.55 days (14.52 months). Thereafter, different physiological variables were evaluated: systolic blood pressure 470.9 ± 1.41 days (15.48 months); relative cerebral blood flow 477.9 ± 1.49 days (15.71 months); aortic function and angiogenesis 499.6 ± 2.14 days (16.43 month). Survival was continuously monitored, and glucocorticoid levels, as an indicator of HPA axis function, were analyzed from blood samples collected during the euthanasia.

2.3. Behavioral

At 14 months of age, a comprehensive screening of physical, emotional, and cognitive functions was successively performed. A battery of 7 tests was used, based on three main behavioral dimensions [12] that can be described as follows:

2.3.1. Neuropsychiatric-Like Behaviors

Changes in emotionality increased neophobia, and other signs of anxiety-like responses, all of them BPSD-like behaviors modeled in 3xTg-AD mice [10], were measured in classical unconditioned tests. The test evaluates locomotion/exploration, anxiety-like behaviors, and emotionality under three different anxiogenic conditions: mild neophobia in a new home-cage (corner test), direct exposure to an illuminated field (open-field test), a choice between a dark and a lit chamber (dark–light box test), black corridors of a maze resembling burrows (T-maze test), and interaction with small objects (marble burying test).

2.3.2. Corner Test (CT) and Open-Field Test (OF)

Neophobia was assessed in the corner test for 30 s. Animals were individually placed in the center of a clean standard home cage, filled with wood save bedding. The number of corners visited were recorded during 30 s [26]. Latency to realize the first rearing and the number of rearings were also registered [10]. Immediately after the CT, mice were placed in the center of an open field (metalwork, white box, $42 \times 38 \times 15$ cm^3) and observed for 5 min [27]. The ethogram, described by the temporal profile of the following sequence of behavioral events, was recorded: duration of freezing behavior, latency to leave the central square, and that of entering the peripheral ring and latency and total duration of self-grooming behavior. Horizontal (crossings of 10×10 cm^2 squares) and vertical (rearings with wall support) locomotor activities were also measured. During the tests, defecation boli and urination were also recorded. The repeated test, 24 h later, was used to evaluate the long-term memory of these experiences [28].

2.3.3. Dark–Light Box Test (DLB)

Anxiety and risk assessment were measured for 5 min after introducing the animals into the dark compartment of the DLB (Panlab, S.L., Barcelona, Spain). The apparatus consisted of two compartments (black, $27 \times 18 \times 27$ cm^3, white, $27 \times 27 \times 27$ cm^3 illuminated by a red 20 W bulb) connected by an opening (7×7 cm^3). The experimental room was kept in darkness (without illumination). Latency to enter, time spent, and the number of entries into the lit compartment were recorded. The number of stretch attendances and self-grooming were also recorded.

2.3.4. Marble Burying Test (MB)

Mice were placed individually in a standard home cage containing nine glass marbles (dimensions $1 \times 1 \times 1$ cm^3) evenly spaced making a square (three rows of three marbles per row only in the left area of the cage) on a 5 cm thick layer of sawdust. The mice were left in the cage with marbles for a 30 min period after which the test was terminated by removing the mice and counting the number of marbles: intact (untouched), rotated (90 or 180°), half-buried (at least $\frac{1}{2}$ buried by sawdust), and buried (completely hidden).

2.3.5. T-maze Test (TM)

Two different paradigms were carried out in a T-shaped maze (woodwork; two short arms of 30×10 cm^2 and a long arm of 50×10 cm^2). Copying with stress strategies, risk assessment, and working memory were assessed in a spontaneous alternation task [29]. Animals were placed inside the maze's long arm with its head facing the end wall, and it was allowed to explore the maze during a maximum of 5 min. The latencies to each one of the goals in this task, namely, to move and turn (freezing behavior), then to reach the intersection, the time elapsed until the animal crossed (4 paws criteria) the intersection of the three arms, and the total time invested in exploring the three arms of the maze (test completion criteria) were recorded. The entry of an already visited arm in the trial before completing the test was considered an error. Defecation boli and urination were also noted.

The working memory paradigm was studied 24 h later and consisted of two consecutive trials: one forced choice followed, 60 s later, by one free choice (recall trial). In this case, mice were placed inside the short arm of the maze and the latencies to each one of the goals in this task, namely, to move and turn, then to reach the intersection, the time elapsed until the animal crossed (4 paws criteria) the intersection of the three arms and the time elapsed until the mice completed 20 s in the forced arm were recorded (time to reach the criteria). Sixty seconds later, the animals that completed the forced trial in less than the cut-off time (10 min) were allowed to explore the maze in a free choice trial where both arms were accessible for 5 min. The arm chosen by the mice and the time spent to reach the correct arm during the free choice were recorded (exploration criteria). The choice of the already visited arm in the previous trial was considered as an error, and the total number was calculated. Finally, defecation boli and urination were also recorded.

2.3.6. Morris Water Maze Test (MWM)

Animals were tested for spatial learning and memory in the MWM test consisting of 1 day of cue learning and 2 days of place learning for spatial reference memory. We used this short protocol, adapted from the 2 day water maze protocol [30], as more suitable in studies where the repeated swimming or the water maze situation—which is stressful for mice but not for rats—can have an impact on other variables, such as cardiovascular system or blood pressure. Mice were trained to locate a hidden platform (7 cm diameter, 1 cm below the water surface) in a circular pool for mice (120 cm in diameter and 60 cm deep, 25 °C opaque water). Mice that failed to find the platform within 60 s were placed on it for 10 s, the same period as was allowed for the successful animals.

Cue learning with a visible platform: On the first day, the animals were tested for the cue learning of a visual platform consisting of four trials in 1 day. In each trial, the mouse was gently released (facing the wall) from one randomly selected starting point (W-S-E-N) and allowed to swim until it escaped onto the platform, elevated 1 cm above the water level in the NE position and indicated by a visible striped flag ($5.3 \times 8.3 \times 15$ cm^3). Extra maze cues were absent in the black walls of the room.

Place learning with a hidden platform: On the following day, the place learning task consisted of four trial sessions per day for 2 days with trials spaced 30 min apart. The mouse was gently released (facing the wall) from one randomly selected starting point (N-E-W-S; E-N-S-W) and allowed to swim until escaped onto the hidden platform, which was now located in the middle of the SW quadrant (reversal). Different geometric figures hung on each wall of the room were used as external visual clues.

Variables of time (escape latency), distance covered, and swimming speed were analyzed in all the tasks' trials. The escape latency was readily measured with a stopwatch by an observer unaware of the animal's genotype and confirmed during the subsequent video-tracking analysis (ANY-Maze v. 5.14, Stoelting, Dublin, Ireland).

2.4. Body Weight, Mouse Clinical Frailty Index Assessment, and Survival

After the behavioral assessment, the body weight was recorded. Frailty was assessed using an adaptation of the MCFI [31], including 30 "clinically" assessed non-invasive items. For 29 of these items, mice were given a score 0 if not presented, 0.5 if there was a mild deficit, and 1 for severe deficit. Weight was scored based on the number of standard deviations from a reference mean. The clinical evaluation included the integument, the physical/musculoskeletal system, the vestibulocochlear/auditory systems, the ocular and nasal systems, the digestive system, the urogenital system, the respiratory system, signs of discomfort, and body weight. Survival was recorded continuously with a daily cadence.

2.5. Systolic Blood Pressure

Measurement of systolic blood pressure was performed in conscious NTg and 3xTg-AD mice using the tail-cuff method (NIPREM 645; Cibertec, Madrid, Spain). The average systolic blood pressure of each mouse was determined from six consecutive measurements after habituation, as described [32].

2.6. MRI-ASL—Relative Cerebral Blood Flow

MRI was carried out at the joint nuclear magnetic resonance facility of the Universitat Autònoma de Barcelona and Centro de Investigación Biomédica en Red—Bioingeniería, Biomateriales y Nanomedicina (CIBER-BBN) (Cerdanyola del Vallès, Spain) in a 7-Tesla horizontal magnet (BioSpec 70/30, Bruker BioSpin, Ettlingen Germany), equipped with actively shielded gradients (B-GA12 gradient coil inserted into a B-GA20S gradient system). For signal reception, a mouse brain surface coil was used actively decoupled from a 72 mm inner diameter volume resonator. Animals were anaesthetized using an average 2.5% isoflurane in O2, and both animal respiration and temperature were constantly monitored with a preclinical monitoring and gating system (SA Instruments, New York, USA). High-resolution T2-weighted images (T2w) were acquired for anatomical references using rapid acquisition with relaxation enhancement sequence with double echoes. The acquisition parameters were the following: orientation = axial plane, echo train length or rare factor = 8, field of view (FOV) = 1.92 × 1.92 cm^2, matrix size (MTX) = 256 × 256 (75 × 75 µm/pixel), number of slices = 11, slice thickness = 1 mm, interslice distance = 1 mm, repetition time (TR)/ effective echo time (TEeff) = 5000/36 ms, number of averages = 1, and total acquisition time (TAT) = 2 min. Perfusion-weighted imaging was obtained using the MRI arterial spin labelling (MRI-ASL) technique without contrast. Two consecutive axial slices were placed in two different sections (Bregma −1.5 mm, −2.5 mm) according to the mouse brain atlas by Paxinos and Franklin [33] using a T2w sagital plane image as anatomic reference. The vendor provided ASL protocol using a flow-sensitive alternating inversion-recovery rapid acquisition with relaxation enhancement (FAIR-RARE) sequence. The parameters were the following: echo train length = 72, TR/TEeff = 16,000/ 50 ms, slice thickness = 1 mm, thickness of the selective inversion slice = 4 mm, FOV = 1.92 × 1.92 cm^2 (150 × 150 µm/ pixel), MTX = 128 × 128, inversion recovery time (TIR) = 30 ms, increment of TIR = 100 ms, number of TIR = 22, and TAT = 13 min. The obtained ASL images were analyzed using the workstation software Paravision 5.1 (Bruker Española S.A., Madrid, Spain) to generate rCBF images. rCBF values were measured using a region of interest (ROI) created corresponding to cortex (Bregma −1.5 mm, −2.5 mm), striatum (Bregma −1.5 mm, −2.5 mm), caudate putamen (Bregma −1.5 mm), basolateral amygdala (−1.5 mm), and hippocampus (−2.5 mm) in both hemispheres (Figure 5). Bilateral ROIs from the same mouse were analyzed together as a mean value and separately to evaluated left-right rCBF asymmetries between hemispheres. For correlations, asymmetry index (AI) defined as (right-left)/(right + left) * 100 was used.

2.7. Angiogenesis

Segments of MCA and the descending thoracic aorta were dissected in ice-cold physiological salt solution (PSS; composition in mM: NaCl 112.0; KCl 4.7; $CaCl_2$ 2.5; KH_2PO_4 1.1; $MgSO_4$ 1.2; $NaHCO_3$ 25.0 and glucose 11.1) supplemented with amphotericin B (15 mg/l) (Biowhittaker ®, Lonza, Basel, Switzer- land) and gentamicine (30mg/l) (Genta-gobens ®, Laboratorios Normon SA, Tres Cantos, Madrid, Spain) and gassed with 95% O_2 and 5% CO_2. Afterwards, vessels were immersed into Matrigel® (50 µL; BD Bioscience, San Jose, CA, USA) following the protocol previously described [34,35]. Angiogenic growth was measured using an inverted microscope equipped with a camera (10× objective; TE2000 Nikon Eclipse-S, Nikon España, Madrid, Spain) at day 4, 5, 6, and 6 after seeding. The longest vessel sprouting from the artery's outer surface (starting point) determined the angiogenic growth [34,35], and at least three fields per arterial segment were measured.

2.8. Aortic Function

Segments (2 mm) of the descending thoracic aorta were dissected free of fat and connective tissue in ice-cold PSS gassed with 95% O_2 and 5% CO_2 and set up on an isometric wire myograph (model 410 A; Danish Myo Technology, Aarhus, Denmark) filled with PSS (37 °C; 95% O_2 and 5% CO_2), as described [36]. The vessels were stretched to 6 mN and allowed to equilibrate for 45 min. Afterwards, aortas were contracted twice with 100 mM KCl, and after washing, vessels were left to equilibrate (30 min) before starting the experiments. Endothelial-dependent vasodilatations to acetylcholine (ACh; 10^{-9} to 10^{-4} M) and endothelial-independent vasodilatations to sodium nitroprusside (10^{-10} to 10^{-3} M) were performed in phenylephrine (Phe)-precontracted (70–100% of 100 mM KCl contraction) vessels. Contractile responses to the α_1-adrenoceptors agonist Phe (10^{-9} to 3×10^{-4} M) were also studied.

2.9. HPA Axis Endocrine Status

Blood samples were collected; plasma was obtained by centrifugation and stored at −80 °C until corticosterone analysis. Corticosterone content (ng/mL) was analyzed using a commercial kit (Corticosterone EIA Immunodiagnostic Systems Ltd., Boldon, UK) and read at 450 nm of absorbance with Varioskan LUX ESW 1.00.38 (Thermo Fisher Scientific, Massachusetts, MA, USA)

2.10. Statistics

Results are expressed as mean ± SEM. SPSS 15.0 (SPSS Inc., Chicago, IL, USA) and GraphPad Prism 5.0 (GraphPad Software Inc., San Diego, CA, USA) software were used. A 2 × 2 factorial design with multivariate general lineal model analysis evaluated genotype (G) and sex (S) effects. Two independent groups were compared with Student's t-test, while comparisons for related samples were made with the paired t-test. The survival curve was analyzed with the Kaplan–Meier test. Relaxations to ACh and sodium nitroprusside were expressed as the percentage change from the Phe precontracted level. Contractions to Phe are expressed as a percentage of the tone generated by 100 mM KCl. The area under the curve was individually calculated from each concentration–response curve to ACh, sodium nitroprusside, and Phe and was expressed as arbitrary units. Differences between concentration–response curves were assessed by two-way repeated measures ANOVA with Tukey's post-test. The correlations between the different variables studied were evaluated with Pearson's correlation. In all the tests, $p < 0.05$ was considered statistically significant.

3. Results

3.1. Survival

Survival, from birth to 16 months of age, of an initial sample of fifty-nine mice (29 NTg, 17 males, 12 females; 30 3xTg-AD, 16 males; 14 females) is illustrated in Figure 1A. Log-rank analyses show an overall difference in survival curves over the four groups ($\chi 2(3) = 10.634$, $p = 0.014$). There was no significant difference between the curves for NTg male and female mice, but female 3xTg-AD mice had a shorter lifespan than male 3xTg-AD mice ($\chi 2(1) = 5.168$, $p = 0.023$). Pairwise comparisons in the survival curve confirmed the effect of sex factor with females' worse survival, independently of the genotype ($\chi 2(1) = 8.224$, $p = 0.004$). Both groups of females exhibited an early 10% mortality rate before young adulthood (2 months of age), and their mean life expectancy was achieved at late adulthood (459 days or 15.1 months in NTg females, 493 days or 16.2 months in 3xTg-AD females). However, they differed in the temporal course of mortality, with a young adulthood and late adulthood mortality pattern in NTg and 3xTg-AD mice, respectively. In this cohort, the drop of survival for male NTg mice was at middle age (12 months), and at the end of the experiment (16 months), their survival rate was 62%. In contrast, the survival of male 3xTg-AD mice was 92%. Rates of censored data for each group ranged from 93.8 to 50%. Thirty-six animals started the experimental design, 17 NTg (10 males, seven females) mice, and 19 3xTg-AD (10 males, nine females). During the experimental research, three NTg males, two NTg females, and four 3xTg-AD females died.

3.2. HPA Axis Endocrine Status

A sex effect was observed with increased levels of corticosterone in the plasma of females (Sex (S), Factorial analysis (F) (1,27) = 30.015, $p < 0.001$) as compared to respective male counterparts (post hoc test, $p < 0.006$). This effect was more notorious in the NTg groups, leading to an overall genotype difference as well (Figure 1B) (G, F (1,27) = 4.634, $p = 0.042$).

SURVIVAL, FRAILTY STATUS AND HPA AXIS

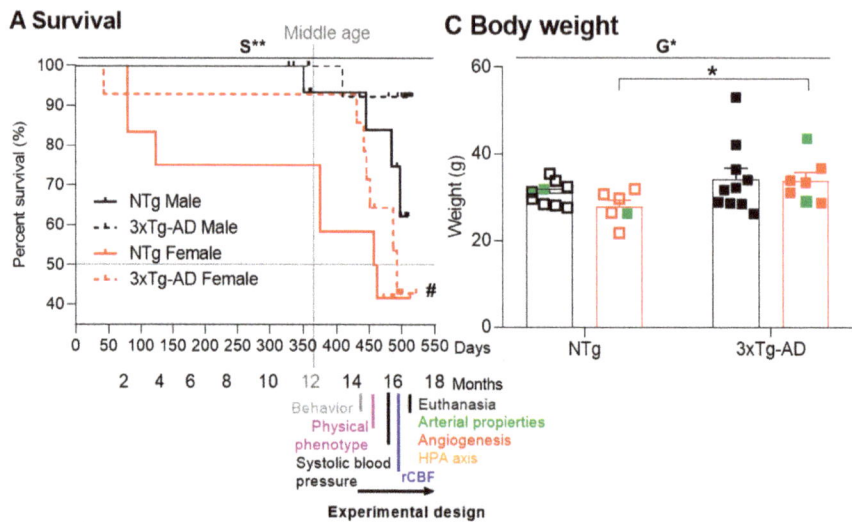

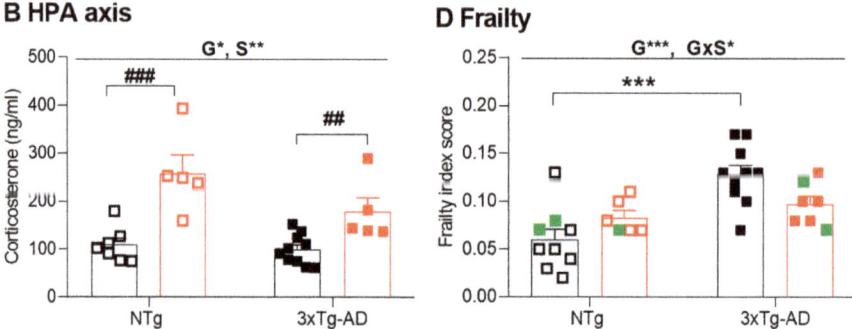

Figure 1. Survival, hypothalamic–pituitary–adrenal (HPA) axis endocrine status and physical health. (**A**) Survival; (**B**) corticosterone levels; physical health: (**C**) body weight, and (**D**) frailty scores of 14-month-old mice. Results are expressed as the mean ± SEM. Initial sample size: NTg, male n = 10, female n = 7; 3xTg-AD, male n = 10, female n = 9. Bars illustrate the genotype groups, as indicated in the abscissae. Symbols are used to illustrate individual values of males (black, left panel) and females (red, right panel). In green: the no-survivors. Statistics: 2 × 2 factorial ANOVA analysis design: genotype (G), sex (S) and genotype × sex (G×S) interaction effects, * p < 0.05, ** p < 0.01, *** p < 0.001 (above line). Student t-test comparisons: * p < 0.05, ** p < 0.01, *** p < 0.001 vs. the corresponding NTg group; ## p < 0.01, ### p < 0.001 vs. the corresponding male group.

3.3. Behavioral Assessment for Physical, Emotional, and Cognitive Phenotypes

At 14 months of age, a comprehensive screening of three main behavioral dimensions and functions, namely, physical, emotional, and cognitive, was performed using a battery of seven tests as previously described [37].

3.3.1. Physical Phenotype

Genotype differences were found in body weight (Figure 1C), which was increased in 3xTg-AD mice (Genotype (G), $F(1,32)$ = 5.204; p = 0.030), an effect that was more clearly observed among females (post hoc test, p < 0.05).

Frailty score (Figure 1D) was increased in 3xTg-AD mice (G, $F(1,32) = 12.052$, $p = 0.002$) with a statistically significant two-fold increase in male mice as compared to NTg counterparts (post hoc test, $p = 0.001$), while NTg and 3xTg-AD females exhibited similar frailty scores (GxS; $F(1,32) = 6.136$; $p = 0.020$).

3.3.2. Neuropsychiatric symptoms (NPS)-like phenotype and cognitive impairment under different anxiogenic conditions

In the corner test (CT) for neophobia (Figure 2A), NTg females exhibited increased behavior, as measured by a higher number of visited corners and faster onset of rearing than NTg males (Student t-test, $p < 0.05$). In the 3xTg-AD mice, the behavior was slightly increased compared to male NTg response but did not reach statistical significance. Overall, the sex difference was shown in the visited corners (S, $F(1,36) = 8.032$, $p = 0.008$). Genotype per sex interaction effects in the variables for vertical exploratory behavior indicated the consistent results between male and female 3xTg-AD mice in this regard, while in the NTg mice, sex differences were shown (GxS, $F(1,36) = 4.267$, $p = 0.047$).

In the open-field (OF) test (Figure 2B), male and female NTg mice behaved quite similarly, as shown by the time course and total counts of their horizontal and vertical activities. In contrast, male 3xTg-AD mice exhibited sustained horizontal activity during the test and higher total counts than their NTg counterparts (OF1, repeated measures ANOVA (RMA); crossings: time × genotype × sex, $F(1,36) < 0.001$, $p = 0.003$). Female 3xTg-AD behaved like NTg mice, with a drop of activity from the first to the second minute of the test. These patterns resulted in statistically significant genotype x sex interaction effects (OF1 min 5, $F(1,36) = 17.187$, $p = 0.001$). When central and peripheral activity were distinguished, male 3xTg-AD mice showed an increased number of peripheral crossings in the third, fourth, and fifth minutes of the test (not shown) and, as a result, also on the total number, as compared to NTg animals and 3xTg-AD females.

In the repeated corner test (24 h later), all the groups showed lower levels of activity (paired t-test, $p < 0.05$). The genotype × sex factors interaction effects shown on the first day were also found here.

In the repeated open-field test (24 h later), the time course of horizontal and vertical activity was also dependent on the genotype and sex or both (OF2, RMA crossings: TxG, TxS and RMA rearing: TxG, TxS, TxGxS, all Fs $(1,36) > 4.251.000$, $p < 0.047$). NTg mice performed similar total activity levels than the precedent day. During the first minute of the repeated open-field test, performance did not differ from that shown in their first experience in the test (OF21 vs. OF11, n.s. in all the groups). Here, genotype effects on the number of crossings and rearing in the first minute of the test ($F(1,36) > 4.584$, $p < 0.05$) indicated higher performances in 3xTg-AD mice than NTg mice. Still, male 3xTg-AD reduced their total activity to control levels.

A GxS effect was observed when we calculated the difference between the crossings performed in the first minute of the test on day2 (OF21) and those in the last minute of day 1 (OF15) ($F(1,36) = 10.889$, $p = 0.002$), with only female 3xTg-AD mice differing from their NTg counterparts ($p < 0.05$).

In the dark–light box (DLB) test (Figure 2C), 3xTg-AD mice exhibited a disinhibitory behavior, as shown by the increased number of crossings in the lit area (data not shown, G, $F(1,35) = 5.186$, $p = 0.03$) and increased total time spent into it (G, $F(1,35) = 4.387$, $p = 0.044$), as compared to the NTg genotype. Emotionality in 3xTg-AD mice was also increased, as they spent more time grooming (G, $F(1,35) > 4.919$, $p = 0.034$).

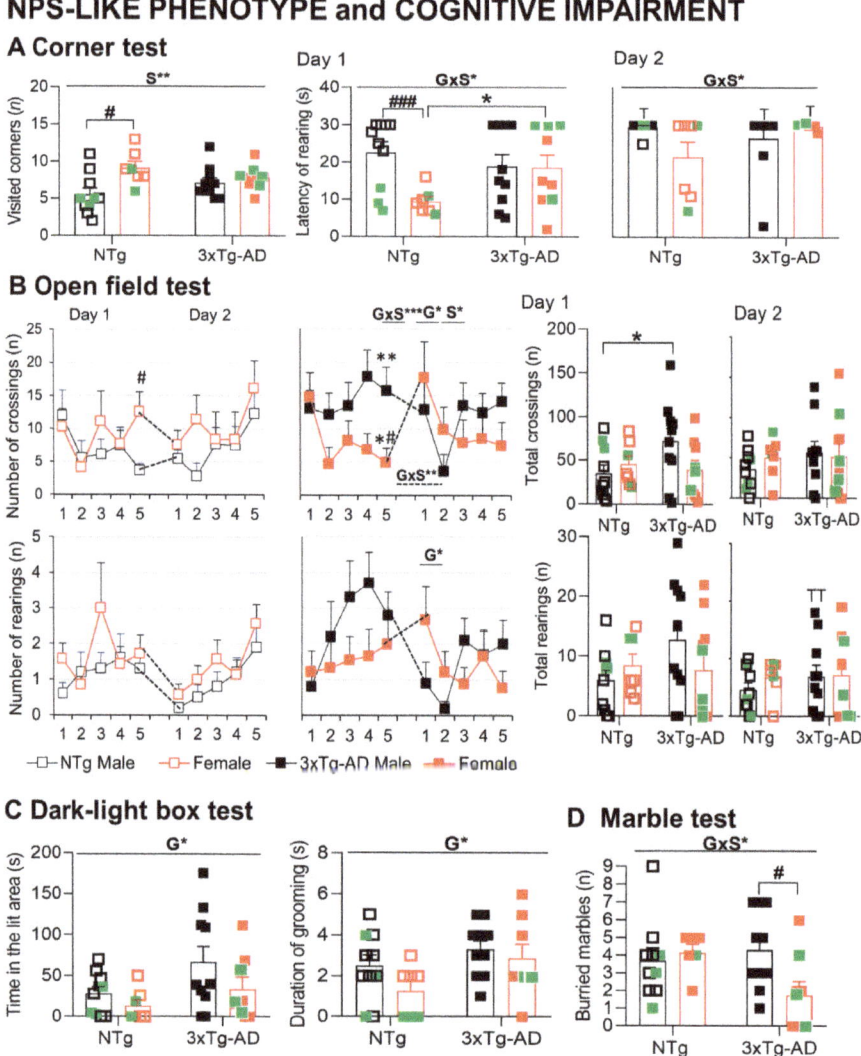

Figure 2. Mental health: Neuropsychiatric-like phenotype and cognitive impairment under different anxiogenic conditions. (**A**) Two-day corner test, (**B**) two-day open-field test, (**C**) dark–light box, (**D**) marble test. Results are the mean ± SEM. Bars illustrate the genotype groups, as indicated in the abscissae. Symbols are used to illustrate individual values of males (black, left panel) and females (red, right panel). In green: the no-survivors. Genotype (G) and sex (S) effects and GxS interaction were analyzed by 2 × 2 factorial ANOVA analysis, * $p < 0.05$, ** $p < 0.01$, *** $p < 0.001$ (above line). Time (T) factor (day-by-day) was analyzed by repeated measures ANOVA, $^T p < 0.05$, $^{TT} p < 0.01$, vs. the corresponding day 1 results. Student t-test comparisons: * $p < 0.05$, ** $p < 0.01$, *** $p < 0.001$ vs. the corresponding NTg group; # $p < 0.05$, ### $p < 0.001$ vs. the corresponding male group.

In the marble (MB) test (Figure 2D), 44.4% (4/9) of the marbles were buried on average by the groups except in the group of 3xTg-AD females that buried only 22.2% (2/9), resulting in a sex difference not found in NTg genotype (GxS, F (1,34) = 4.254, $p = 0.048$). A sex effect was also observed when we measured the marbles left intact (not shown, S, F (1,34) = 4.501, $p = 0.042$).

Two different paradigms were carried out in a T-shaped maze, as depicted in Figure 3A; all the groups included animals that failed to complete the T-maze spontaneous alternation test (latency, 300 s) and the forced memory test (latency, 600 s). On average, all the groups showed similar latencies in the ethogram of behaviors exhibited in the T-maze spontaneous alternation (TMSA) test (turning, reaching the intersection, crossing the intersection with four paw criteria, completing the test) (G, S, all Fs (1,34) < 0.231; p > 0.05). The most representative of these latencies—that of achieving "test completion criteria"—is illustrated. The number of spatial working memory errors (revisiting an explored area) were recorded in those animals able to initiate the task. No statistically significant differences were observed between groups in spatial alternation.

In the second paradigm for working memory in the T-maze (TM) test (Figure 3B), all the groups needed the same time to reach the acquisition criteria in the forced trial (G, S, all Fs(1,33) < 0.708; p > 0.05). In the recall trial, considering the animals that completed the test (n = 25; nine NTg males; four NTg females; seven 3xTg-AD males and five 3xTg-AD females), sex differences, clearer among NTg, were found (S, F (1,25) = 10.063, p = 0.005), with males investing shorter times than females to reach the exploration criteria. Despite the small number of animals, an increased number of errors in working memory (revisiting an explored area) was noted in females (S, F (1,19) = 34.135, p < 0.001).

In the Morris water maze (MWM) (Figure 3C), genotype differences were found in the navigation speed, reaching statistically significant differences in the cue learning paradigm. Thus, 3xTg-AD mice were swimming slower than NTg counterparts (CUE: G, F (1,32) = 4.437, p = 0.044), an effect that was more clearly shown in females (p < 0.05). Therefore, the distance covered to reach the platform was used to illustrate all the paradigms' performances. Genotype x sex interaction effects in the cue and the place tasks (PT) indicate that males' and females' performances were dependent on the genotype. Here, sex differences in the cue learning were shown in NTg mice, but not 3xTg-AD mice. Female NTg covered more distance than NTg males, whereas both sexes performed equally in the 3xTg-AD genotype. At the end of the four trial sessions of the cue learning task, all the groups could reach the platform in 20 s and cover 2 to 3 m.

In the two daily sessions of the place learning task, where the platform was hidden and located in a reversed position, animals exhibited a genotype effect in the distance covered to find the new location of the platform (PT11: G, F(1,32) = 6.228, p = 0.019). NTg mice were faster (shorter latency, not shown) and covered less distance to find the hidden platform. After that, the performances between NTg and 3xTg-AD mice differed in some trials. Genotype effect was also observed in the last trial of the second day; in this case, as in the mean distance of place task, two 3xTg-AD male mice performed less distance to arrive at the platform (PT24: G, F (1,32) = 4.964, p = 0.034; meanPT2, G, F(1,32) = 5.926, p = 0.022). The sex effect was observed in PT23, with females covering more distance to find the platform (PT23: S, F(1,32) = 4.716, p = 0.039).

In summary, different survival and behavioral signatures were found in these cohorts. Namely, (1) physical: An early mortality window of the female sex found enhanced in the AD-genotype and increased frailty only in male 3xTg-AD mice. (2) Neuropsychiatric-like: increased and persistent neophobia in female 3xTg-AD mice, a hyperactive pattern of male 3xTg-AD mice, and disinhibitory behavior in male and female 3xTg-AD mice. (3) Worse long-term memory of female 3xTg-AD in the open-field test; overall bad performances of all the animals in the mazes, with worse performance and working memory of female 3xTg-AD mice, a slower swimming speed of female 3xTg-AD mice, and paradoxical performances of male 3xg-AD mice, probably related to emotional and physical comorbidities. As discussed in previous work, these sex-dependent effects point at the relevance of the sex-specific analysis of AD disease. The results also illustrate the relevance of controlling for frailty and mortality rates to discriminate against the confounding factors (synopsis; Table 1).

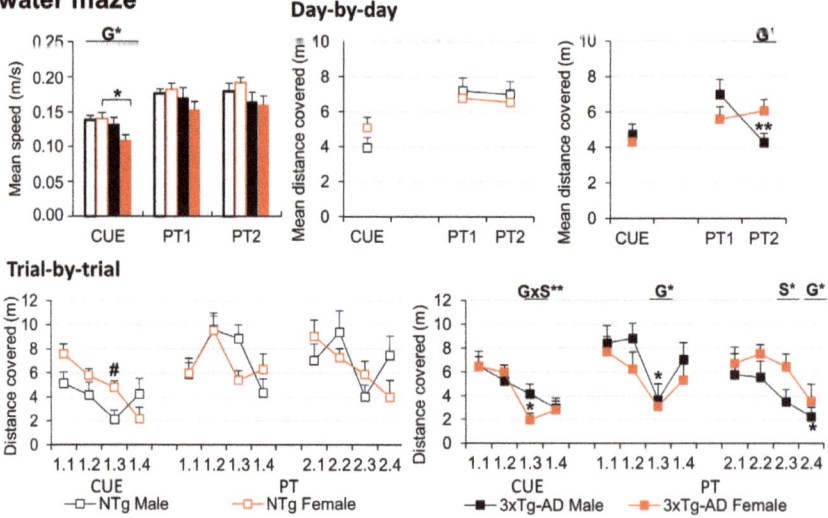

Figure 3. Mental health: cognitive impairment (**A**) Spontaneous alternation T-maze, (**B**) T-maze, (**C**) Morris water maze. Results are the mean ± SEM. Bars illustrate the genotype groups, as indicated in the abscissae. Symbols are used to illustrate individual values of males (black, left panel) and females (red, right panel). In green: the no-survivors. Genotype (G) and sex (S) effects and GxS interaction were analyzed by 2 × 2 factorial ANOVA analysis, * $p < 0.05$, ** $p < 0.01$, *** $p < 0.001$ (above line). Student *t*-test comparisons: * $p < 0.05$, ** $p < 0.01$, *** $p < 0.001$ vs. the corresponding NTg group; # $p < 0.05$, ### $p < 0.001$ vs. the corresponding male group.

Table 1. Synopsys of main genotype and sex effects in the physical condition and behavioral phenotype.

Domains	Tests	Effect	Between Groups Differences	Figure
		Physical Condition		
Survival	Survival curve	Sex **	3xTg-AD females vs. males	Figure 1A
Frailty	Frailty index	Genotype ***	3xTg-AD males vs. NTg males	Figure 1D
Weight	Body weight	Genotype *	3xTg-AD females vs. NTg females	Figure 1B
HPA axis	Corticosterone	Genotype*; Sex**	Females vs. males	Figure 1C
		Behavioral Phenotype Neuropsychiatric-Like Domain		
Neophobia	CT,OF	Sex *		Figure 2A,B
Hyperactivity	OF	Genotype *	3xTg-AD males vs. NTg males	Figure 2B
Disinhibition	DLB	Genotype *		Figure 2C
		Cognitive Domain		
Long-term memory	OF2	Genotype *		Figure 2B
Working memory	TM	Sex ***	Females vs. males	Figure 3B
Swimming speed	MWM	Genotype *	3xTg-AD females vs. NTg females	Figure 3C
Paradoxical performance	MWM	Genotype *	3xTg-AD males vs. NTg males	Figure 3C

Domains studied, tests used (CT, corner test; OF, open-field test; OF2, open-field test day 2; DLB, dark–light box test and MWM, Morris water maze). Statistics: genotype and sex effect; between groups differences; * $p < 0.05$; ** $p < 0.01$; *** $p < 0.001$ and related figures.

3.4. Systolic Blood Pressure

Figure 4 illustrates the systolic blood pressure. Two transgenic animals could not be assessed because of a lack of vasodilation (1 animal) and overweight (1 animal). The sex effect was observed, with males presenting an increased systolic blood pressure compared to females (S, $F (1,30) = 8.163$, $p = 0.008$). These differences were especially observed between 3xTg-AD mice (Student t-test, $p = 0.022$).

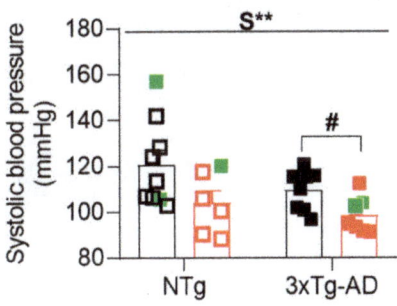

Figure 4. Systolic blood pressure. Results are the mean ± SEM. Bars illustrate the genotype groups, as indicated in the abscissae. Symbols are used to illustrate individual values of males (black, left panel) and females (red, right panel). In green: the no-survivors. Genotype (G) and sex (S) effects and GxS interaction were analyzed by 2 × 2 factorial ANOVA analysis, ** $p < 0.01$ (above line). Student t-test comparisons: ** $p < 0.01$, vs. the corresponding NTg group; # $p < 0.05$ vs. the corresponding male group.

3.5. MRI Relative Cerebral Blood Flow

Representative relative cerebral blood flow (rCBF) images in five regions of interest: cortex, striatum, hippocampus (HC), caudate-putamen (CPu), and basolateral amygdala (BLA) from two 1mm consecutive slices (approximately, Bregma −1.5 mm and −2.5 mm) are presented in Figure 5. No statistically significant differences in rCBF were observed (Figure 6A). However, 3xTg-AD female mice survivors had increased rCBF in the cortex and hippocampus compared with their NTg counterparts (Student t-test $p < 0.05$). In particular, genotype per sex interaction effects were observed in cortical rCBF (GxS, $F(1,27) = 4.545$, $p = 0.044$).

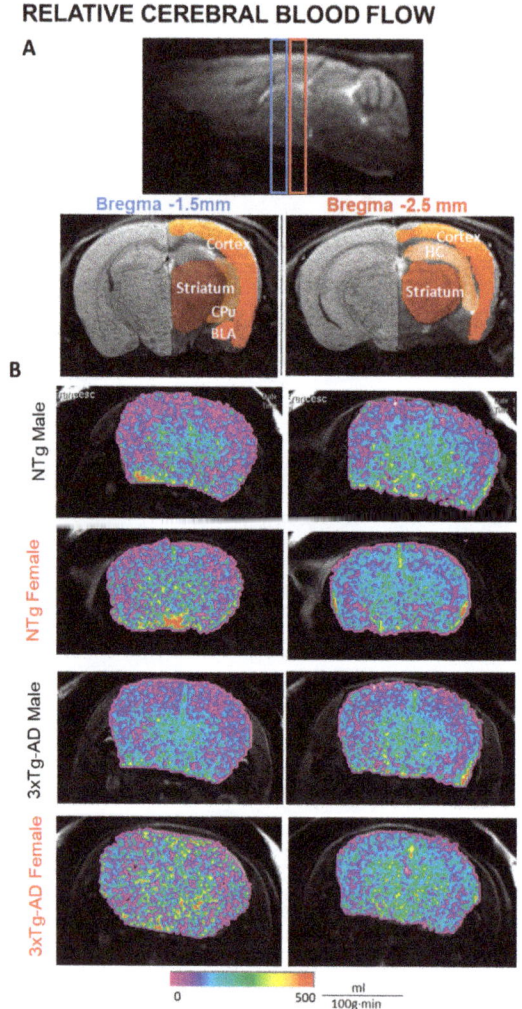

Figure 5. MRI arterial spin labeling (ASL)—relative cerebral blood flow in regions of interest. (**A**) Global cerebral blood flow and five regions of interest were examined in the present study from two different sections (Bregma −1.5 mm, −2.5 mm). Cortex; striatum; caudate putamen (CPu); basolateral amygdala (BLA); hippocampus (HC). (**B**) Representative images from rCBF maps superimposed to T2w-image from NTg male, NTg female, 3xTg-AD male, and 3xTg-AD female.

RELATIVE CEREBRAL BLOOD FLOW

A Mean rCBF

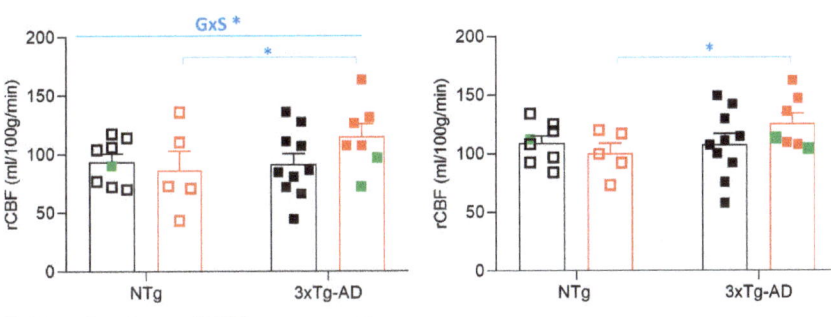

B Hemisphere CBF asymmetry

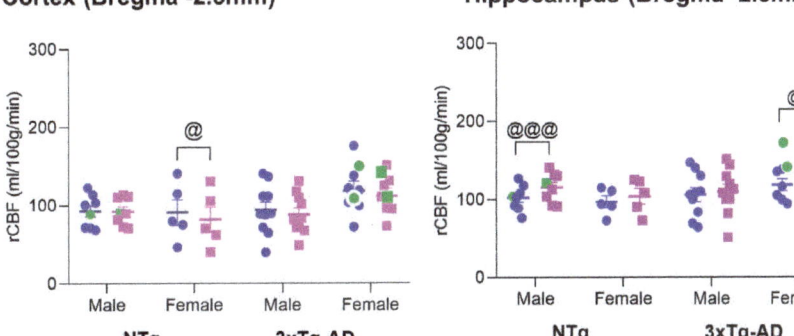

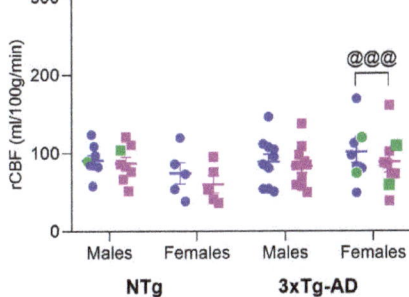

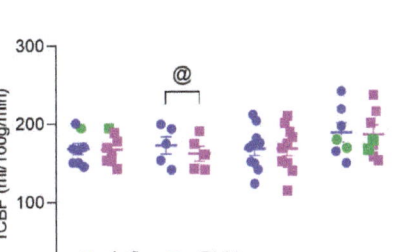

Figure 6. MRI-ASL—relative cerebral blood flow. (**A**) Mean relative blood flow in cortex and hippocampus. (**B**) Hemisphere relative cerebral blood flow asymmetry. Results are the mean ± SEM. Bars illustrate the genotype groups, as indicated in the abscissae. Symbols are used to illustrate individual values of males (black, left panel) and females (red, right panel). Left hemisphere: blue; right hemisphere: purple. In green: the no-survivors. Genotype (G) and sex (S) effects and GxS interaction were analyzed by 2x2 factorial ANOVA analysis, * $p < 0.05$ (above line). Student *t*-test comparisons: * $p < 0.05$ vs. the corresponding NTg group; Paired *t*-test in asymmetry between right/left hemispheres: @ $p < 0.05$, @@@ $p < 0.001$.

For each group, the asymmetries in the rCBF of the left and right hemispheres are illustrated in Figure 6 B. In the cortex, rCBF asymmetries were found in females. The asymmetry between left–right hemispheres was also observed in the hippocampus of NTg males and 3xTg females and the striatum of NTg females (paired t-test, $p < 0.05$).

3.6. Angiogenesis

The middle cerebral artery (MCA) (Figure 7A,B) and the aorta (Figure 7C,D) was longitudinally measured at day 4, 5, 6, 7 after seeding in growth medium containing Matrigel. Sex did not modify MCA angiogenic growth either in NTg or 3xTg-AD mice, though female 3xTg-AD mice showed an enhanced ($p < 0.01$) growth from day 4 to 6 compared to female NTg. In the aorta, although NTg females showed an initially lower angiogenic growth than males, growth was significantly increased ($p < 0.05$) in 3xTg-AD females compared to 3xTg-AD males (Figure 7D) and NTg females (Figure 7C vs. 7D).

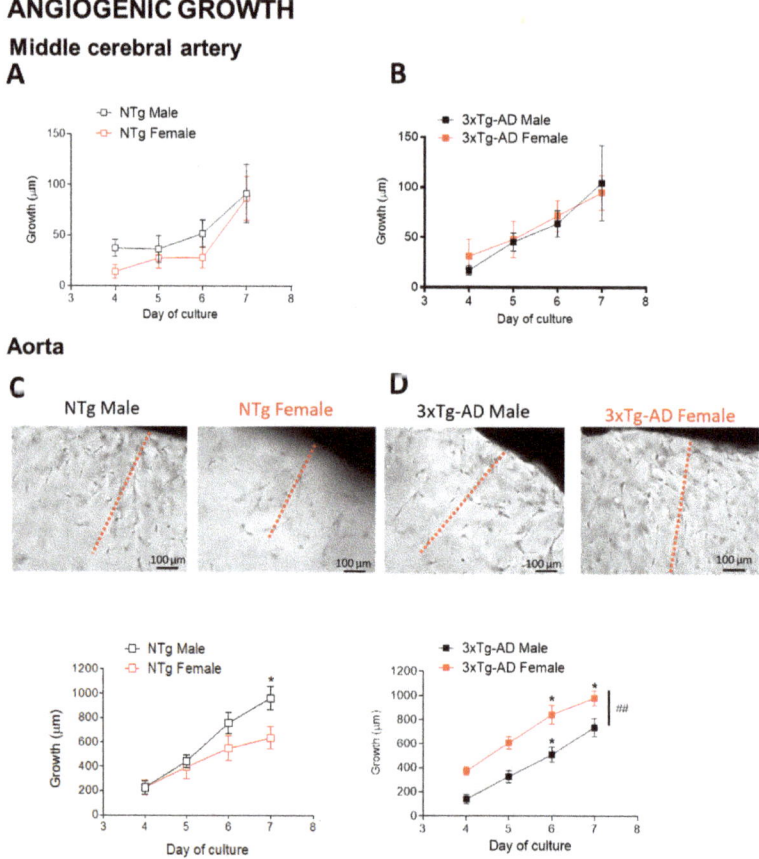

Figure 7. Influence of sex and genotype on the MCA and aortic angiogenic response. Analysis of neovessel growth progression in MCA from NTg (**A**) and 3xTg-AD (**B**) male and female mice. Representative images of neovessel sprouting (above) at day 7 (left) or 6 (right) and analysis of neovessel growth (below) in aorta from NTg (**C**) and 3xTg-AD (**D**) male and female mice. Red dotted lines represent the length of the longest vessel sprouting from the artery's outer surface (starting point). Results are the mean ± SEM from NTg, male $n = 6$–7, female $n = 4$–5; 3xTg-AD, male $n = 10$, female $n = 5$. Data were analyzed by two-way repeated measures ANOVA with Tukey post-test. * $p < 0.05$, ## $p < 0.01$.

3.7. Arterial Properties

Endothelium-dependent ACh-induced vasodilatation in the aorta of female NTg mice was slightly higher than NTg males, whereas no sex-dependent differences were found in 3xTg-AD mice (Figure 8A). Sodium nitroprusside relaxations were not affected by sex, either in NTg or 3xTg-AD mice (Figure 8B). However, these relaxations were impaired ($p < 0.05$) in 3xTg-AD compared to NTg males. These results suggest an impairment of smooth muscle relaxing responses in 3xTg-AD males. We subsequently measured contractile responses to KCl (100 mM) (Figure 8C) and Phe (Figure 8D). Responses to KCl were significantly higher ($p < 0.01$) in the 3xTg-AD genotype in males but not females, an effect that culminated in greater ($p < 0.05$) contractions in 3xTg-AD males than females (Figure 8C). Nevertheless, concentration-dependent contractions to Phe were not affected either by sex or genotype (Figure 8D).

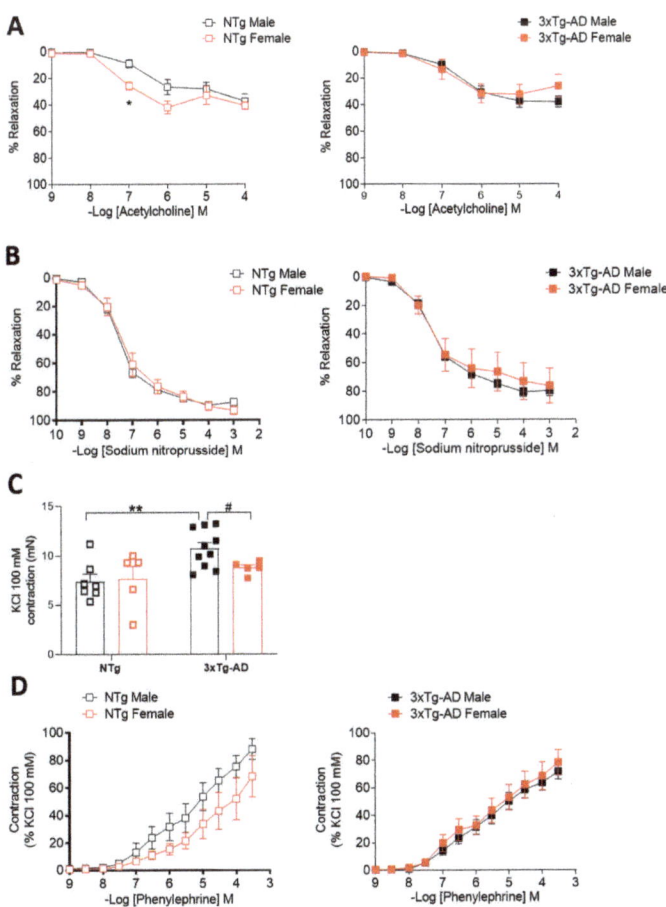

Figure 8. Influence of sex and genotype on aortic function. Concentration-dependent relaxations to acetylcholine (**A**) and sodium nitroprusside (**B**) in thoracic aortas from NTg and 3xTg-AD male and female mice. Contractions to KCL 100 mM (**C**) and concentration-dependent contractions to phenylephrine (**D**). Results are the mean ± SEM from NTg, male $n = 7$, female $n = 5$; 3xTg-AD, male $n = 10$, female $n = 5$. Data were analyzed by ×-way repeated measures (**A,B,D**) or regular (**C**) two-way ANOVA with Tukey post-test. * $p < 0.05$, ** $p < 0.01$, # $p < 0.05$.

3.8. Mental Health and Cardiovascular Function Correlates

Behavioral correlates with cardiovascular function and HPA axis activation were analyzed. The most statistically significant correlations found when considering the whole sample of animals are illustrated in Figure 9. Amygdala CBF was positively correlated with body weight (Figure 9A, $p = 0.001$), and corticosterone levels with the number of intact marbles (Figure 9B, $p = 0.002$) and errors in the T-maze (Figure 9C, $p < 0.001$). Systolic blood pressure was positively correlated with the number of half-buried marbles (Figure 9D, $p = 0.009$) and negatively correlated with latency to arrive to T-intersection with four paws in the TMSA test (Figure 9E, $p = 0.007$) and TM test (Figure 9F, $p = 0.005$). Sodium nitroprusside relaxations (area under the curve), a measure of endothelium-independent relaxations, were negatively correlated with the total horizontal activity in the first open-field test (Figure 9G) and vertical activity in the two open-fields (Figure 9H, $p = 0.007$, and 9I, $p = 0.006$). Asymmetry of several brain regions was also correlated with behavior. Cortical areas were positively correlated with risk assessment behavior (Figure 9J, $p = 0.003$), neophobia in the corner test (Figure 9K, $p = 0.004$), and errors in the T-maze (Figure 9L, $p = 0.008$). Hippocampal's asymmetry index (AI), defined as (right-left)/(right + left) * 100 was negatively correlated with neophobia in the corner test (Figure 9M, $p = 0.009$), while amygdala's asymmetry index was positively correlated with neophobia in the second open-field test (Figure 9N, $p = 0.005$).

The functional correlates of the behavioral signatures were also analyzed for the corresponding group and are presented as supplementary data (supplementary material). Briefly, the increased and persistent neophobia in female 3xTg-AD mice, confirmed also in the open-field test, was correlated with Phe %KCL- pEC50 ($r > -0.983$, $p < 0.003$), area under the curve (AUC) ($r = -0.983$, $p = 0.001$), PEC50 ($r = -0.983$, $p = 0.007$), and KCL ($r > -0.965$, $p < 0.008$). The hyperactive pattern of male 3xTg-AD mice in the open-field test was correlated with the striatum (Bregma -1.5 mm) asymmetry index (AI) ($r = 0.790$, $p = 0.006$), systolic blood pressure ($r = -0.910$, $p = 0.002$), PEC50 Acetylcholine (% Phe) ($r = -0.842$, $p = 0.002$), and amygdala (Bregma -1.5 mm) AI ($r > 0.776$, $p < 0.009$). The disinhibitory behavior in male and female 3xTg-AD mice in the dark–light box was correlated with acetylcholine (% Phe)- area under curve ($r = 0.707$, $+$, $p = 0.003$); cortex (Bregma -2.5 mm) AI ($r = 0.612$, $+$, $p = 0.009$), acetylcholine (% Phe)- maximum effect ($r = -0.679$, $+$, $p = 0.005$); the frailty index FI ($r = 0.616$, $+$, $p = 0.009$) and global cerebral blood flow in the selected slices ($r = 0.660$, $+$, $p = 0.004$), striatum ($r = 0.709$, $+$, $p = 0.001$), caudate putamen ($r = 0.671$, $+$, $p = 0.003$), amygdala ($r = 0.622$, $+$, $p = 0.009$); striatum (Bregma -2.5 mm) AI ($r = -0.766$, $p < 0.001$). The slower speed of female 3xTg-AD mice in the water maze was correlated with the cerebral blood flow of whole brain ($r = -0.878$, $p = 0.009$), striatum ($r = -0.893$, $+$, $p = 0.007$), caudate putamen ($r = -0.916$, $+$, $p = 0.004$), and hippocampus ($r = -0.906$, $p = 0.005$). Finally, paradoxal performances in male 3xg-AD mice probably related to their emotional and physical comorbid conditions to cognitive function were found correlated with acetylcholine (% Phe)- PEC50 ($r = 0.774$, $+$, $p = 0.009$), sodium nitroprusside (% Phe)- PEC50 ($r = 0.784$, $+$, $p = 0.007$), cerebral blood flow of whole brain ($r = 0.778$, $+$, $p = 0.008$), striatum ($r = 0.795$, $+$, $p = 0.006$), caudate putamen ($r = 0.807$, $+$, $p = 0.005$), and cortex (Bregma -1.5 mm) AI ($r = 0.844$, $+$, $p = 0.002$).

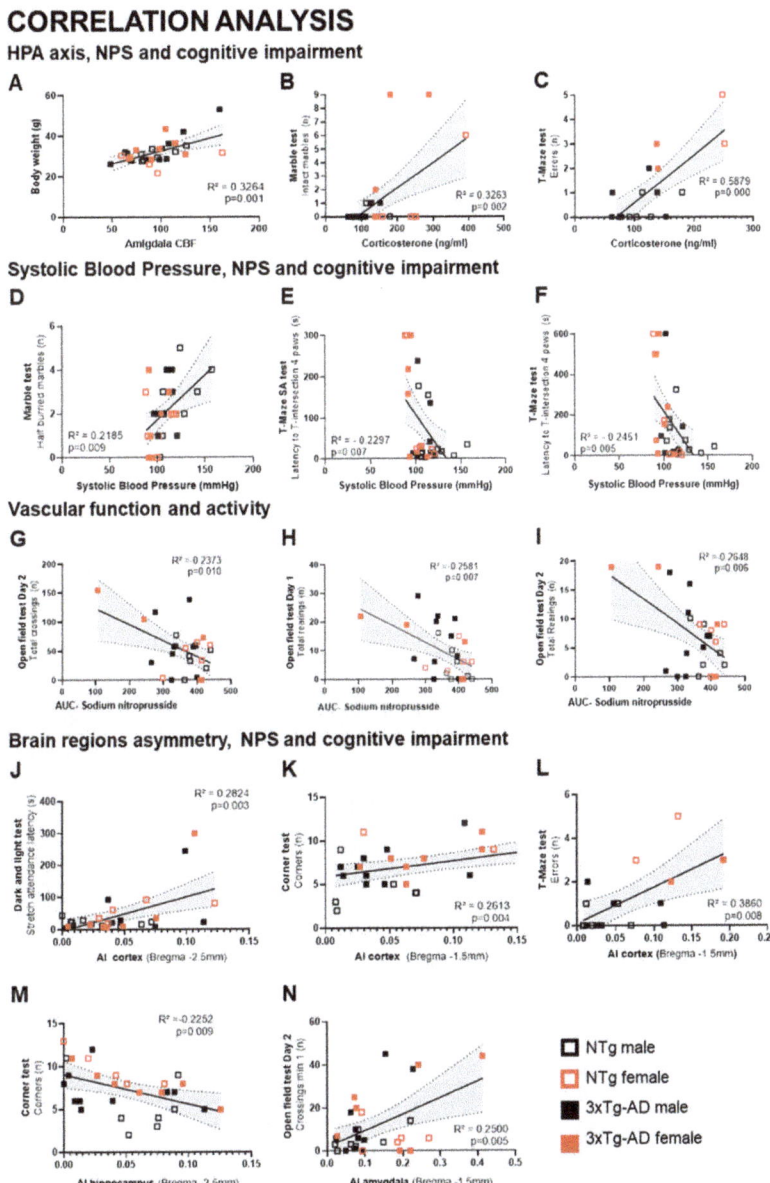

Figure 9. Mental health—cardiovascular function correlation analysis. Meaningful significant Pearson r correlations between behavior and cardiovascular function and HPA axis. (**A**) Amygdala CBF with body weight (**B**) corticosterone levels with the number of intact marbles, and (**C**) errors in the T-maze. (**D**) Systolic blood pressure with the number of half-buried marbles and (**E**) with the latency to arrive to T-intersection with 4 paws in TMSA test and (**F**) TM test. (**G**) Vascular function, as measured by the area under the curve (AUC) of sodium nitroprusside and the total horizontal activity in the first open-field test and (**H**,**I**) vertical activity in the two open fields. (**J**) Cortical asymmetry index (AI) and risk assessment behavior, (**K**) neophobia in the corner test, and (**L**) errors in the T-maze. (**M**) Hippocampal's asymmetry index and neophobia in the corner test, (**N**) amygdala's asymmetry index and neophobia in the second open-field test.

4. Discussion

The present work investigated the interaction between mental health and cardiovascular disease under a translational gender-medicine perspective. We used two strains of mice modeling normal (NTg) and neurodegenerative (3xTg-AD) aging, where first evidence of compromised small peripheral mesenteric resistance artery (MRA) properties was recently shown [21]. Worse physiologically relevant MRA structural and functional alterations of 3xTg-AD females suggested sex-dependent dysfunctions. We hypothesize that those findings would also extend to other cardiovascular health measures. Since the aging process is very heterogeneous [7], here, we studied two cohorts where females exhibited worse mortality rates than males since birth. We were interested in exploring brain–cardiovascular interaction mechanisms relevant for long-lived animals. Eight functional aspects were successively studied from middle age to natural death or euthanasia at 16 months. First, we determined the physical (including frailty) and behavioral (neuropsychiatric-like and cognitive) phenotypes of animals. Once the "mental health" of each animal was characterized, we determined their "cardiovascular phenotype" through systolic blood pressure, rCBF, angiogenesis, and arterial function. Survival was continuously monitored. Glucocorticoid levels, an indicator of HPA axis function, were analyzed from blood samples collected during the euthanasia. In the results, the analysis includes the sample size at each time point; so that the results of a certain functional analysis are those taking into account the highest sample available. The results agreed with those from the analysis performed only using the final sample size of survivors (censored data).

4.1. Sex- and Genotype-Dependent Mortality/Morbidity Paradox

People with AD show worse survival than the general old population, and deranged neuro-immuno-endocrine system in males could explain their worse survival than females despite their less bad neuropathological status [4,6]. At the translational level, we have consistently reported increased vulnerability of 3xTg-AD mice concurrent with impairment of the neuro-immuno-endocrine system and in agreement with this sex-dependent profile [11,12,38]. However, we found cohorts that offered a distinct survival scenario, with pairwise comparisons in the survival curves confirming an effect of sex factor with worse survival of females, independently of the genotype. 3xTg-AD mice females had a shorter lifespan than males, and sex differences were less pronounced in NTg mice. The retrospective analysis of survival indicated that both groups of females exhibited an early mortality window, starting as soon as 2–3 months of age. While the male sex has worse cardiovascular mortality rates than females, the burden of cardiovascular disease in the female sex is widely reported [39]. Less is known in this regard in Alzheimer's disease. Therefore, the present cohorts offer an interesting experimental setting to study the morbidity/mortality paradox in surviving females. In this scenario, we were interested in studying the relationship between frailty, mental health, and cardiovascular phenotype.

Heterogeneity is found in the aging process, and prognostic tools to identify end-of-life dementia stages are difficult [7]. In NTg and 3xTg-AD mice, we described heterogeneity as part of the complexity of age-related scenarios [8,40,41]. The frailty index, a common tool to measure health status that seems to be sensitive to predict mortality [5], is a valuable tool in longevity and aging studies in mice [31]. In the general population, women usually present higher frailty scores and a reduced risk of mortality than men [42]. In contrast, higher frailty scores are recorded in men with AD [43]. In agreement, the Mouse Clinical Frailty Index, a translational adaptation of the frailty index data in humans [31], was increased in male 3xTg-AD mice compared to NTg counterparts, while females exhibited similar frailty scores. A worse sensorimotor function was also previously reported [8,10,12]. Using the same frailty index, other researchers also noticed that 3xTg-AD males show higher scores, with sex differences in health span predicting lifespan in the 3xTg-AD mouse model of AD [44].

4.2. Down-Regulation of HPA Axis Endocrine Status in Female 3xTg-AD Mice

At the endocrine level, mild hypercortisolemia is observed in AD patients [45], and the stimulation of the HPA can result in peripheral immune depression [46]. In the present work, the HPA axis exhibited sexual dimorphism, with higher levels of plasma corticosterone in females than males. The AD–genotype effect reduced plasmatic corticosterone levels in 3xTg-AD females, attenuating the sexual dimorphism in one degree of magnitude. These data agree with our first report in 15-month NTg and 3xTg-AD [12]. In all groups, the corticosterone levels were higher than those reported at 15 months, which could be due to the animals' increased stress response to the experimental design, especially observed in females [47]. These corticosterone levels were similar to those observed in NTg and 3xTg-AD mice after chronic treatment with caffeine and vehicle [48].

4.3. Different Behavioral Signatures for Physical, Emotional, and Cognitive Phenotypes

The patterns of innate neophobia (fear of novelty) response shown by NTg mice were found broken in the 3xTg-AD genotype, and it is most prominently observable in the mutants with female sex, as consistently described since our first work [10] and confirmed afterwards [21,37,49]. We proposed increased neophobia, as delayed and reduced rearing, an early behavioral marker of the onset of behavioral and psychological symptoms of dementia (BPSD)-like symptoms since premorbid disease stages [28]. Here, the corner test was sensitive to old 3xTg-AD females' genotype, where neophobia is enhanced. For the first time, we describe these patterns as also observable on the repeated test.

In the open-field test, no sex differences were found in normal aging. In contrast, the frail male 3xTg-AD exhibited sustained activity, mostly as a thigmotaxis response and slower habituation pattern. A hyperactive pattern in frail 3xTg-AD males is also observed after social isolation [50]. The repetition of the test elicited reduced activity, in all the groups. In agreement with previous reports showing a 24 h long-term memory deficit in male 3xTg-AD mice at 2, 4, and 6 months of age [28], the behavioral response did not benefit from previous experience. Here, we show that these genotype effects in the immediate re-confrontation with the test are extensive to 14 months of age and mostly observed in females.

As shown by increased crossings and time in the lit area and grooming, disinhibitory behavior in the dark–light box confirmed a consistent BPSD-like phenotype in male and female 3xTg-AD mice. These disinhibitory patterns were first described at 4 months of age as part of the profile mimicking AD's prodromal stage [51]. The marble test, assessing anxiety-like behaviors and screen drugs for obsessive-compulsive disorders and psychotic symptoms [52], also showed a specific pattern for females 3xTg-AD mice.

In the paradigms for learning and memory in mazes [37], the number of animals failing to complete the T-maze indicates their aged status and/or poor motivation [8]. The latency to achieve the first goal of the test (crossing the intersection) has been related to immunosenescence and reduced survival [53]. This ceiling effect resulted in a sample of "successful animals" that equally performed the spontaneous alternation task. However, these animals committed errors attributed to working memory (revisiting explored areas) when assessed in a more complex task (the forced-choice paradigm) in a sex-specific manner. Here, females of both genotypes spent more time choosing the right choice and committed more errors.

The water maze's performance was strongly determined by genotype differences in the swimming speed (slower in 3xTg-AD mice) mostly found among females. Motor features can be discarded (the frail animals were males), but the swimming performance can reflect their emotional status in an aquatic environment known to be anxiogenic for mice [54]. To control this factor, the distance covered was used instead of the latency. Two learning and memory tasks differing on the level of complexity and involving short (15 min) and long-term (24 h) memory were used. The day-by-day and trial-by-trial analysis showed a notorious aged profile compared to previous reports in young [10,11,28,37,49,51,55] or old animals [8,38,48,56]. Worse performance of female NTg mice was observed on the visual perceptual learning task. Long-term spatial reference learning and memory deficits were shown by all the groups in their first day of place learning task where the hidden platform, located in a reversed location, had to be found. Finally, the two-day place task indicated paradoxical better performances in male 3xTg-AD mice, which could be explained by the strong need that a frail animal may have to find and remember a safe place.

4.4. Increased MRI-ASL Regional Cerebral Blood Flow in 3xTg-AD Survivor Females

In the present study, we evaluated CBF in five different brain regions, namely, hippocampus, cortex, striatum, caudate putamen, and amygdala using arterial spin labeling (ASL), a magnetic resonance imaging (MRI) technique for non-invasive measurements of cerebral blood blow. The results indicated sex- and brain-region-associated changes in CBF. Among all, 3xTg-AD female mice survivors had increased CBF in the cortex and hippocampus as compared with their wild-type counterparts.

Although CBF alteration seems to be involved in AD pathogenesis, the perfusion patterns remain unclear, since both hypoperfusion and hyperperfusion have been described in different brain areas and involved in different brain functions [57].

Oxidative stress, inflammation, and cerebrovascular disease have been suggested to be involved in AD. In one of our recent collaborative studies in 3xTg-AD mice, we have reported that the number of β-amyloid (Aβ) plaques in the hippocampus and entorhinal cortex at advanced stages of the disease was higher in females than in males [58]. Interestingly, co-localization of hypoxic areas and Aβ plaques in the hippocampus and entorhinal cortex were observed only in females. In the present study, the increased CBF in the cortex and hippocampus in female survivors suggests a potential compensatory hemodynamic mechanism in end-of-life dementia, which is sex- and brain-region-dependent. This is interesting to note, since recent work in APP/PS1 transgenic mice at the early stages of AD has shown longitudinal changes in regional CBF, indicating age- and brain-region-dependent alterations of cerebral blood flow [59]. At the clinical level, an increased CBF has also been observed in patients at preclinical stages of AD when cognitive performance is still preserved, suggesting a compensatory response to the accumulation of Aβ pathology [60]. Moreover, the reduction in CBF seems to be an important factor contributing to the cognitive dysfunction associated with dementia. One study performed with APP/PS1 mice in the late stages of the disease reported that a treatment that consists of the increase in the cerebral blood flow improves cognition [61].

4.5. Sex- and Brain-Region-Dependent Asymmetry in the MRI-ASL Regional Cerebral Blood Flow

Brain structural and functional asymmetry in health/disease is an emerging field. The neurodegeneration of subcortical structures is not symmetric, with neuroimaging studies reporting volumetric regional, hemispheric asymmetries. Thus, asymmetric hippocampal atrophy has been recently reported in normal aging, mild cognitive impairment, and AD [62]. A whole-brain analysis revealed increased neuroanatomical asymmetries in dementia for the hippocampus and amygdala and is proposed as a powerful imaging biomarker [63]. At the translational level, hippocampal asymmetry was important in rodents for acquiring spatial reference memory, retaining working memory [64], and some features of non-spatial learning [65]. At the neurochemical and molecular levels, left–right hippocampal asymmetry has been demonstrated for the glutamatergic system [65]. We have just provided the first evidence of brain atrophy asymmetry in male 3xTg-AD mice, thus modeling that found in human patients with AD [50]. However, little is known about the alterations in CBF hemisphere asymmetries. In the present work, the MRI-ASL rCBF results unveiled, for the first time, the asymmetry between left–right hemispheres in the female's cortex, in the hippocampus of control males, and 3xTg-AD females, as well as in the striatum of control females. Therefore, the present results show asymmetry between left–right hemispheres in the 3xTg-AD model and aging mice, in both sexes (but mostly in females) and in cortical and subcortical structures. Moreover, to ensure that these detected asymmetries in rCBF measurements were not affected by differences in mice's head positioning (rotation respect to the sagittal plane) or differences in signal-to-noise ratio (SNR) or contrast-to-noise ratio (CNR) between hemispheres, a SNR/CNR quality check analysis was performed that showed no statistically significant differences among the experimental groups (data not shown). This modeling will be useful for the translational development and assessment of the preventive/ therapeutic interventions and those of the risk factors and hazards and monitoring disease progression.

4.6. Improved Vascular Profile in 3xTg-AD Survivor Females

Hypertension is a risk factor to develop cognitive impairment and dementia [66] and is associated with the pathological manifestations of Alzheimer's disease [67]. Although it is more prevalent in men, a recent study demonstrated that midlife hypertension increases the risk of dementia in women but not in males [68]. Arterial pressure increases in a sex- and age-specific manner similar to humans, showing sex differences until 14 months [69]. In agreement with this, the sex effect was observed in this study, with males presenting an increased systolic blood pressure. Although our results did not demonstrate a higher systolic blood pressure in 3xTg-AD mice than NTg mice, as it has been observed in AβPP/PS1 mice [70], a correlation between higher levels of systolic blood pressure and decreased regional cerebral blood flow was observed in 3xTg-AD mice.

AD is associated with cerebral and peripheral artery dysfunction, a process that can lead to altered blood flow to the brain, which in turn can increase the risk of developing AD or impair AD pathology [71,72]. In mice models of AD disease, both peripheral large [18–20] and small [21] artery dysfunction have been reported. A previous study showed decreased ACh- and sodium-nitroprusside-dependent relaxations in conjunction with increased endothelin-1 contractions in aortas from 11-month-old male 3xTg-AD mice [18]. Consistently, in the 16-month-old male 3xTg-AD compared to NTg mice of the present study, similar low levels of ACh-induced relaxations, impairments of sodium nitroprusside responses, and enhanced contractions to KCl 100 mM were observed. Notably, 3xTg-AD female mice survivors had an improved vascular profile.

On the one hand, although 3xTg-AD females showed similar low levels of ACh relaxation than males, relaxations to sodium nitroprusside and contractions to KCl were unaltered compared to NTg mice. On the other hand, the angiogenic growth capacity of the MCA and aorta was higher in 3xTg-AD compared to NTg females, and 3xTg-AD females showed greater aortic angiogenesis than 3xTg-AD males. In a precedent work, the anxious-like behavioral profile correlated with vascular alterations in small mesenteric arteries from 15-month-old 3xTg-AD female mice [21]. Altogether, we suggest that the vascular profile is tightly linked to the overall health status, especially in female 3xTg-AD mice.

The increased angiogenic response correlated with increased CBF in the cortex and hippocampus in 3xTg-AD compared to NTg females, an effect that is consistent with the concept that angiogenesis, would be a compensatory response to impaired CBF in AD [22]. These findings agree with previous studies that found increased angiogenesis in the hippocampus, midfrontal cortex, substantia nigra, pars compacta, and locus ceruleus of post mortem human AD brains [73]. It is worth noting that increased angiogenesis, which has been associated with the presence of Aβ [24,74–76], could be linked to increased vascular permeability, especially under pro-oxidant and pro-inflammatory environments, such as in AD [23,24]. A non-invasive method was used to measure blood pressure due to the old age of mice. However, a high-fidelity blood pressure phenotyping method (e.g., radiotelemetry) would be necessary to confirm blood pressure data. Besides, we used the thoracic aorta (i.e., a large conductance artery) as a model for generic peripheral artery function. Therefore, the present study is limited by the lack of information on vascular function in peripheral resistance arteries, which might reflect better what happens at the level of cerebral vasculature.

4.7. Behavioral Correlates Mental Health and Cardiovascular Measurements

Correlation analysis through all the components suggests functional interactions between NPS and cognitive impairment with amygdala and HPA axis. The vascular function correlated with activity, while the left and right hemispheres' asymmetry of rCBF with NPS and cognitive impairments. Increased activation of the amygdala in 3xTg-AD mice [55] could explain the specific correlation between amygdala CBF and body weight. Corticosterone level correlations agree with our first report on the increase in glucocorticoid levels concomitantly to increased anxiety and peripheral immune dysfunction [12] and recent work of other laboratories [77]. Systolic blood pressure correlated positively with the number of half-buried marbles and negatively correlated with latency to cross the T-intersection and TM test, which are indicators of a worse neuro-immunoendocrine function, accelerated aging, and premature death in mice [53]. These correlates agree with mice chronically subjected to high blood pressure being more active in the open-field and faster in a spontaneous alternation test [78]. Recently, we demonstrated the correlation between peripheral small vessel properties and anxiety in both NTg and 3xTg-AD mice, mostly in females [21]. Here, we show that the animals with lower endothelial-independent vasodilatations to sodium nitroprusside (i.e., lower muscle relaxation capacity) were the most active in the open-field test, in both non-goal- (horizontal activity) and goal-directed (rearing) behaviors [79,80]. The correlation was consistent, as also observed in the repeated test. Regarding relative cerebral blood flow and neuropsychiatric and cognitive impairment, the cortex was the better area correlated with behavior. Cortex hemisphere asymmetry correlated with risk assessment (stretch attendance), neophobia in the corner test, and worse memory performance in the T-maze test. Correlation between asymmetry and neophobia was also observed in the hippocampus and amygdala. Since testing the pairwise correlations between dozens of variables without multiple comparison correction may involve a high risk of type-1 error, only those which are meaningful, obtained a maximum statistical significance ($p < 0.001$), and could be verified with close-related variables were considered. Despite our aim to highlight and explore the sex-based differences, the statistical power of the sample size per sex did not allow to compare whether the correlations between these variables were different between male and female mice and thus modulated by the sex. Overall, this correlation analysis allows for finding meaningful functional correlations between behavioral responses related to the levels of anxiety, cognition and locomotor activity, and cardiovascular measurements. Especially, the present work provides pieces of evidence of the brain regions' asymmetry of both males and females with normal and AD-neurodegenerative aging correlation with neuropsychiatric symptoms and cognitive deficits.

4.8. Future Research Directions

The present study suggests a potential compensatory hemodynamic mechanism in end-of-life dementia, which is sex-dependent. Those vascular adaptations observed in 3xTg-AD female mice survivors might provide clues to understand potential vascular targets for pharmacological and non-pharmacological interventions.

Supplementary Materials: Supplementary materials can be found at https://www.mdpi.com/2227-9059/9/2/111/s1. Supplementary data: Mental health and cardiovascular function correlates.

Author Contributions: Conceptualization, L.G.-L. and F.J.-A.; methodology: behavior, asymmetry quantifications, and correlation analysis, A.M.; systolic blood pressure, E.V.; MRI-ASL-rCBF, E.J.-X.; angiogenesis, L.P.-U. and F.J.-A.; aortic function, F.J.-A.; writing—original draft: L.G.-L., F.J.-A. and A.M.; writing—manuscript: all the authors. Funding acquisition, L.G.-L. and F.J.-A. All authors have read and agreed to the published version of the manuscript.

Funding: This work was funded by UAB-GE-260408 to L.G.-L and SAF2014-56111 to F.J.-A. The colony of 3xTg-AD mice is sustained by European Union's Horizon 2020 research and innovation program under grant agreement No 737390 to L.G.-L.

Institutional Review Board Statement: The study was conducted according to the guidelines of the Declaration of Helsinki, and approved by the Ethics Committee of Departament de Medi Ambient i Habitatge, Generalitat de Catalunya (CEEAH 3588/DMAH 9452) the 8th of March 2019.

Informed Consent Statement: Not applicable.

Data Availability Statement: Not applicable.

Acknowledgments: We thank Frank M. LaFerla, Institute for Memory Impairments and Neurological Disorders, University of California Irvine, CA, USA for kindly providing the progenitors of the Spanish colonies of homozygous 3xTg-AD and NTg mice. Thanks to Javier Carrasco, The INc Molecular Biology Unit for corticosterone determination. The joint nuclear magnetic resonance facility of the UAB and Centro de Investigación Biomédica en Red-Bioingeniería, Biomateriales y Nanomedicina (CIBER-BBN) (Cerdanyola del Vallès, Spain), Unit 25 of NANBIOSIS.

Conflicts of Interest: The authors declare no conflict of interest. The funders had no role in the design of the study; in the collection, analyses, or interpretation of data; in the writing of the manuscript, or in the decision to publish the results.

Abbreviations

3xTg-AD	Triple transgenic mice
AD	Alzheimer's disease
AI	Asymmetry index
ASL	Arterial spin labeling
AUC	Area under the curve
BLA	Basolateral amygdala
BPSD	Behavioral and psychological symptoms of dementia
CBF	Cerebral blood flow
CPu	Caudate putamen
CNR	Contrast-to-noise ratio
CT1	Corner test—Day 1
CT2	Corner test—Day 2
DALYs	Disability-adjusted life years
DLB	Dark–light box test
G	Genotype
HC	Hippocampus
HALE	Healthy life expectancy
HPA	Hypothalamic–pituitary–adrenal
MB	Marble test
MCA	Middle cerebral artery
MCFI	Mouse Clinical Frailty Index
MRA	Mesenteric resistance arteries
MRI	Magnetic resonance imaging
MWM	Morris water maze
NPS	Neuropsychiatric symptoms
NTg	Non transgenic mice
OF1	Open-field test—Day 1
OF1n	Open-field test—Day 1, minute n of the test
OF2	Open-field test—Day 2
OF2n	Open-field test—Day 2, minute n of the test
PT n n	Place task—Day, trial n of the test
RMA	Repeated measures ANOVA
ROI	Region of interest
S	Sex
SNR	Signal-to-noise ratio
T	Time
TM	T-maze
TMSA	T-maze spontaneous alternation

References

1. Kyu, H.H.; Abate, D.; Abate, K.H.; Abay, S.M.; Abbafati, C.; Abbasi, N.; Abbastabar, H.; Abd-Allah, F.; Abdela, J.; Abdelalim, A.; et al. Global, Regional, and National Disability-Adjusted Life-Years (dalys) for 359 Diseases and Injuries and Healthy Life Expectancy (HALE) for 195 Countries and Territories, 1990–2017: A Systematic Analysis for the Global Burden of Disease Study 2017. *Lancet* **2018**, *392*, 1859–1922. [CrossRef]
2. Mattiuzzi, C.; Lippi, G. Worldwide Disease Epidemiology in the Older Persons. *Eur. Geriatr. Med.* **2020**, *11*, 147–153. [CrossRef] [PubMed]
3. Alberts, S.C.; Archie, E.A.; Gesquiere, L.R.; Altmann, J.; Vaupel, J.W.; Christensen, K. The Male-Female Health-Survival Paradox: A Comparative Perspective on Sex Differences in Aging and Mortality. In *Sociality, Hierarchy, Health: Comparative Biodemography: A Collection of Papers.*; Maxine Weinstein, M.A.L., Ed.; National Academies Press (US): Washington, DC, USA, 2014; pp. 339–363. ISBN 978-0-309-30661-4.
4. Mitchell, S.L.; Miller, S.C.; Teno, J.M.; Kiely, D.K.; Davis, R.B.; Shaffer, M.L. Prediction of 6-Month Survival of Nursing Home Residents with Advanced Dementia Using ADEPT vs Hospice Eligibility Guidelines. *JAMA* **2010**, *304*, 1929–1935. [CrossRef] [PubMed]
5. Zeng, A.; Song, X.; Dong, J.; Mitnitski, A.; Liu, J.; Guo, Z.; Rockwood, K. Mortality in Relation to Frailty in Patients Admitted to a Specialized Geriatric Intensive Care Unit. *J. Gerontol. Ser. A Biol. Sci. Med. Sci.* **2015**, *70*, 1586–1594. [CrossRef] [PubMed]
6. van Dijk, P.T.; Dippel, D.W.; Habbema, J.D.F. Survival of Patients with Dementia. *J. Am. Geriatr. Soc.* **1991**, *39*, 603–610. [CrossRef]
7. Komarova, N.L.; Thalhauser, C.J. High Degree of Heterogeneity in Alzheimer's Disease Progression Patterns. *PLoS Comput. Biol.* **2011**, *7*, e1002251. [CrossRef]
8. Torres-Lista, V.; De la Fuente, M.; Giménez-Llort, L. Survival Curves and Behavioral Profiles of Female 3xTg-AD Mice Surviving to 18-Months of Age as Compared to Mice with Normal Aging. *J. Alzheimer's Dis. Rep.* **2017**, *1*, 47–57. [CrossRef]
9. Oddo, S.; Caccamo, A.; Shepherd, J.D.; Murphy, M.P.; Golde, T.E.; Kayed, R.; Metherate, R.; Mattson, M.P.; Akbari, Y.; LaFerla, F.M. Triple-Transgenic Model of Alzheimer's Disease with Plaques and Tangles: Intracellular Abeta and Synaptic Dysfunction. *Neuron* **2003**, *39*, 409–421. [CrossRef]
10. Giménez-Llort, L.; Blázquez, G.; Cañete, T.; Johansson, B.; Oddo, S.; Tobeña, A.; LaFerla, F.M.; Fernández-Teruel, A. Modeling Behavioral and Neuronal Symptoms of Alzheimer's Disease in Mice: A Role for Intraneuronal Amyloid. *Neurosci. Biobehav. Rev.* **2007**, *31*, 125–147. [CrossRef]
11. Blázquez, G.; Cañete, T.; Tobeña, A.; Giménez-Llort, L.; Fernández-Teruel, A. Cognitive and Emotional Profiles of Aged Alzheimer's Disease (3×TgAD) Mice: Effects of Environmental Enrichment and Sexual Dimorphism. *Behav. Brain Res.* **2014**, *268*, 185–201. [CrossRef]
12. Giménez-Llort, L.; Arranz, L.; Maté, I.; De La Fuente, M. Gender-Specific Neuroimmunoendocrine Aging in a Triple-Transgenic 3×Tg-AD Mouse Model for Alzheimer's Disease and Its Relation with Longevity. *Neuroimmunomodulation* **2008**, *15*, 331–343. [CrossRef] [PubMed]
13. Garcia-Mesa, Y.; Colie, S.; Corpas, R.; Cristòfol, R.; Comellas, F.; Nebreda, A.R.; Giménez-Llort, L.; Sanfeliu, C. Oxidative Stress Is a Central Target for Physical Exercise Neuroprotection Against Pathological Brain Aging. *J. Gerontol. Ser. A Biol. Sci. Med. Sci.* **2015**, *71*, 40–49. [CrossRef] [PubMed]
14. Rae, E.A.; Brown, R.E. The Problem of Genotype and Sex Differences in Life Expectancy in Transgenic AD Mice. *Neurosci. Biobehav. Rev.* **2015**, *57*, 238–251. [CrossRef] [PubMed]
15. Hirata-Fukae, C.; Li, H.F.; Hoe, H.S.; Gray, A.J.; Minami, S.S.; Hamada, K.; Niikura, T.; Hua, F.; Tsukagoshi-Nagai, H.; Horikoshi-Sakuraba, Y.; et al. Females Exhibit More Extensive Amyloid, but Not Tau, Pathology in an Alzheimer Transgenic Model. *Brain Res.* **2008**, *1216*, 92–103. [CrossRef]
16. Jefferson, A.L. Cardiac Output as a Potential Risk Factor for Abnormal Brain Aging. *J. Alzheimer's Dis.* **2010**, *20*, 813–821. [CrossRef] [PubMed]
17. Troncone, L.; Luciani, M.; Coggins, M.; Wilker, E.H.; Ho, C.Y.; Codispoti, K.E.; Frosch, M.P.; Kayed, R.; del Monte, F. Aβ Amyloid Pathology Affects the Hearts of Patients with Alzheimer's Disease: Mind the Heart. *J. Am. Coll. Cardiol.* **2016**, *68*, 2395–2407. [CrossRef]
18. Sena, C.M.; Pereira, A.M.; Carvalho, C.; Fernandes, R.; Seiça, R.M.; Oliveira, C.R.; Moreira, P.I. Type 2 Diabetes Aggravates Alzheimer's Disease-Associated Vascular Alterations of the Aorta in Mice. *J. Alzheimer's Dis.* **2015**, *45*, 127–138. [CrossRef]
19. Navarro-Dorado, J.; Villalba, N.; Prieto, D.; Brera, B.; Martín-Moreno, A.M.; Tejerina, T.; de Ceballos, M.L. Vascular Dysfunction in a Transgenic Model of Alzheimer's Disease: Effects of CB1R and CB2R Cannabinoid Agonists. *Front. Neurosci.* **2016**, *10*, 422. [CrossRef]
20. Merlini, M.; Shi, Y.; Keller, S.; Savarese, G.; Akhmedov, A.; Derungs, R.; Spescha, R.D.; Kulic, L.; Nitsch, R.M.; Lüscher, T.F.; et al. Reduced Nitric Oxide Bioavailability Mediates Cerebroarterial Dysfunction Independent of Cerebral Amyloid Angiopathy in a Mouse Model of Alzheimer's Disease. *Am. J. Physiol. Heart Circ. Physiol.* **2017**, *312*, H232–H238. [CrossRef]
21. Jiménez-Altayó, F.; Sánchez-Ventura, J.; Vila, E.; Giménez-Llort, L. Crosstalk between Peripheral Small Vessel Properties and Anxious-like Profiles: Sex, Genotype, and Interaction Effects in Mice with Normal Aging and 3×Tg-AD Mice at Advanced Stages of Disease. *J. Alzheimer's Dis.* **2018**, *62*, 1531–1538. [CrossRef]
22. Vagnucci, A.H.; Li, W.W. Alzheimer's Disease and Angiogenesis. *Lancet* **2003**, *361*, 605–608. [CrossRef]

23. Jefferies, W.A.; Price, K.A.; Biron, K.E.; Fenninger, F.; Pfeifer, C.G.; Dickstein, D.L. Adjusting the Compass: New Insights into the Role of Angiogenesis in Alzheimer's Disease. *Alzheimer's Res. Ther.* **2013**, *5*, 64. [CrossRef] [PubMed]
24. Biron, K.E.; Dickstein, D.L.; Gopaul, R.; Jefferies, W.A. Amyloid Triggers Extensive Cerebral Angiogenesis Causing Blood Brain Barrier Permeability and Hypervascularity in Alzheimer's Disease. *PLoS ONE* **2011**, *6*, e23789. [CrossRef] [PubMed]
25. Kilkenny, C.; Browne, W.J.; Cuthill, I.C.; Emerson, M.; Altman, D.G. Improving Bioscience Research Reporting: The ARRIVE Guidelines for Reporting Animal Research. *PLoS Biol.* **2010**, *8*, e1000412. [CrossRef] [PubMed]
26. Belzung, C.; Le Pape, G. Comparison of Different Behavioral Test Situations Used in Psychopharmacology for Measurement of Anxiety. *Physiol. Behav.* **1994**, *56*, 623–628. [CrossRef]
27. Hall, C.; Ballachey, E.L. A Study of the Rat's Behavior in a Field. A Contribution to Method in Comparative Psychology. *Univ. Calif. Publ. Psychol.* **1932**, *6*, 1–12.
28. Torres-Lista, V.; Parrado-Fernández, C.; Alvarez-Montón, I.; Frontiñán-Rubio, J.; Durán-Prado, M.; Peinado, J.R.; Johansson, B.; Alcaín, F.J.; Giménez-Llort, L. Neophobia, NQO1 and SIRT1 as Premorbid and Prodromal Indicators of AD in 3xTg-AD Mice. *Behav. Brain Res.* **2014**, *271*, 140–146. [CrossRef]
29. Douglas, R.J. Cues for Spontaneous Alternation. *J. Comp. Physiol. Psychol.* **1966**, *62*, 171–183. [CrossRef]
30. Gulinello, M.; Gertner, M.; Mendoza, G.; Schoenfeld, B.P.; Oddo, S.; LaFerla, F.; Choi, C.H.; McBride, S.M.J.; Faber, D.S. Validation of a 2-Day Water Maze Protocol in Mice. *Behav. Brain Res.* **2009**, *196*, 220–227. [CrossRef]
31. Whitehead, J.C.; Hildebrand, B.A.; Sun, M.; Rockwood, M.R.; Rose, R.A.; Rockwood, K.; Howlett, S.E. A Clinical Frailty Index in Aging Mice: Comparisons with Frailty Index Data in Humans. *J. Gerontol. Ser. A Biomed. Sci. Med. Sci.* **2014**, *69*, 621–632. [CrossRef]
32. Orejudo, M.; García-Redondo, A.B.; Rodrigues-Diez, R.R.; Rodrigues-Díez, R.; Santos-Sanchez, L.; Tejera-Muñoz, A.; Egido, J.; Selgas, R.; Salaices, M.; Briones, A.M.; et al. Interleukin-17A Induces Vascular Remodeling of Small Arteries and Blood Pressure Elevation. *Clin. Sci. (Lond)* **2020**, *134*, 513–527. [CrossRef] [PubMed]
33. Franklin, K.; Paxinos, G. *The Mouse Brain in Stereotaxic Coordinates*, 3rd ed.; Elsevier Science: San Diego, CA, USA, 2008; ISBN 9780123742445.
34. Vicente, D.; Hernández, B.; Segura, V.; Pascual, D.; Fornaciari, G.; Monto, F.; Mirabet, V.; Montesinos, M.C.; D'Ocon, P. Methodological Approach to Use Fresh and Cryopreserved Vessels as Tools to Analyze Pharmacological Modulation of the Angiogenic Growth. *J. Cardiovasc. Pharmacol.* **2016**, *68*, 230–240. [CrossRef] [PubMed]
35. Vila, E.; Solé, M.; Masip, N.; Puertas-Umbert, L.; Amaro, S.; Dantas, A.P.; Unzeta, M.; D'Ocon, P.; Planas, A.M.; Chamorro, Á.; et al. Uric Acid Treatment after Stroke Modulates the Krüppel-like Factor 2-VEGF-A Axis to Protect Brain Endothelial Cell Functions: Impact of Hypertension. *Biochem. Pharmacol.* **2019**, *164*, 115–128. [CrossRef] [PubMed]
36. Jiménez-Altayó, F.; Siegert, A.-M.; Bonorino, F.; Meirelles, T.; Barberà, L.; Dantas, A.P.; Vila, E.; Egea, G. Differences in the Thoracic Aorta by Region and Sex in a Murine Model of Marfan Syndrome. *Front. Physiol.* **2017**, *8*, 933. [CrossRef] [PubMed]
37. Giménez-Llort, L.; García, Y.; Buccieri, K.; Revilla, S.; Suñol, C.; Cristofol, R.; Sanfeliu, C. Gender-Specific Neuroimmunoendocrine Response to Treadmill Exercise in 3xTg-AD Mice. *Int. J. Alzheimers. Dis.* **2010**, *2010*, 128354. [CrossRef] [PubMed]
38. Torres-Lista, V.; López-Pousa, S.; Giménez-Llort, L. Impact of Chronic Risperidone Use on Behavior and Survival of 3xTg-AD Mice Model of Alzheimer's Disease and Mice with Normal Aging. *Front. Pharmacol.* **2019**, *10*, 1061. [CrossRef] [PubMed]
39. Maas, A.H.E.M.; Appelman, Y.E.A. Gender Differences in Coronary Heart Disease. *Neth. Heart J.* **2010**, *18*, 598–603. [CrossRef]
40. Giménez-Llort, L.; Ratia, M.; Pérez, B.; Camps, P.; Muñoz-Torrero, D.; Badia, A.; Clos, M.V. AVCRI104P3, a Novel Multitarget Compound with Cognition-Enhancing and Anxiolytic Activities: Studies in Cognitively Poor Middle-Aged Mice. *Behav. Brain Res.* **2015**, *286*, 97–103. [CrossRef]
41. Giménez-Llort, L.; Ramírez-Boix, P.; de la Fuente, M. Mortality of Septic Old and Adult Male Mice Correlates with Individual Differences in Premorbid Behavioral Phenotype and Acute-Phase Sickness Behavior. *Exp. Gerontol.* **2019**, *127*, 110717. [CrossRef]
42. Gordon, E.H.; Peel, N.M.; Samanta, M.; Theou, O.; Howlett, S.E.; Hubbard, R.E. Sex Differences in Frailty: A Systematic Review and Meta-Analysis. *Exp. Gerontol.* **2017**, *89*, 30–40. [CrossRef]
43. Trebbastoni, A.; Canevelli, M.; D'Antonio, F.; Imbriano, L.; Podda, L.; Rendace, L.; Campanelli, A.; Celano, V.; Bruno, G.; de Lena, C. The Impact of Frailty on the Risk of Conversion from Mild Cognitive Impairment to Alzheimer's Disease: Evidences from a 5-Year Observational Study. *Front. Med.* **2017**, *4*, 178. [CrossRef] [PubMed]
44. Kane, A.E.; Shin, S.; Wong, A.A.; Fertan, E.; Faustova, N.S.; Howlett, S.E.; Brown, R.E. Sex Differences in Healthspan Predict Lifespan in the 3xTg-AD Mouse Model of Alzheimer's Disease. *Front. Aging Neurosci.* **2018**, *10*, 172. [CrossRef] [PubMed]
45. Hartmann, A.; Veldhuis, J.D.; Deuschle, M.; Standhardt, H.; Heuser, I. Twenty-Four Hour Cortisol Release Profiles in Patients with Alzheimer's and Parkinson's Disease Compared to Normal Controls: Ultradian Secretory Pulsatility and Diurnal Variation. *Neurobiol. Aging* **1997**, *18*, 285–289. [CrossRef]
46. Woiciechowsky, C.; Schöning, B.; Lanksch, W.R.; Volk, H.D.; Döcke, W.D. Mechanisms of Brain-Mediated Systemic Anti-Inflammatory Syndrome Causing Immunodepression. *J. Mol. Med.* **1999**, *77*, 769–780. [CrossRef] [PubMed]
47. Drude, S.; Geißler, A.; Olfe, J.; Starke, A.; Domanska, G.; Schuett, C.; Kiank-Nussbaum, C. Side Effects of Control Treatment Can Conceal Experimental Data When Studying Stress Responses to Injection and Psychological Stress in Mice. *Lab Anim. (NY)* **2011**, *40*, 119–128. [CrossRef] [PubMed]
48. Baeta-Corral, R.; Johansson, B.; Giménez-Llort, L. Long-Term Treatment with Low-Dose Caffeine Worsens BPSD-Like Profile in 3xTg-AD Mice Model of Alzheimer'S Disease and Affects Mice with Normal Aging. *Front. Pharmacol.* **2018**, *9*, 79. [CrossRef]

49. García-Mesa, Y.; López-Ramos, J.C.; Giménez-Llort, L.; Revilla, S.; Guerra, R.; Gruart, A.; Laferla, F.M.; Cristòfol, R.; Delgado-García, J.M.; Sanfeliu, C. Physical Exercise Protects against Alzheimer's Disease in 3xTg-AD Mice. *J. Alzheimer's Dis.* **2011**, *24*, 421–454. [CrossRef]
50. Muntsant, A.; Giménez-Llort, L. Impact of Social Isolation on the Behavioral, Functional Profiles, and Hippocampal Atrophy Asymmetry in Dementia in Times of Coronavirus Pandemic (COVID-19): A Translational Neuroscience Approach. *Front. Psychiatry* **2020**, *11*, 572583. [CrossRef]
51. Cañete, T.; Blázquez, G.; Tobeña, A.; Giménez-Llort, L.; Fernández-Teruel, A. Cognitive and Emotional Alterations in Young Alzheimer's Disease (3xTgAD) Mice: Effects of Neonatal Handling Stimulation and Sexual Dimorphism. *Behav. Brain Res.* **2015**, *281*, 156–171. [CrossRef]
52. Torres-Lista, V.; López-Pousa, S.; Giménez-Llort, L. Marble-Burying Is Enhanced in 3xTg-AD Mice, Can Be Reversed by Risperidone and It Is Modulable by Handling. *Behav. Process.* **2015**, *116*, 69–74. [CrossRef]
53. Guayerbas, N.; Puerto, M.; Ferrández, M.D.; De La Fuente, M. A Diet Supplemented with Thiolic Anti-Oxidants Improves Leucocyte Function in Two Strains of Prematurely Ageing Mice. *Clin. Exp. Pharmacol. Physiol.* **2002**, *29*, 1009–1014. [CrossRef] [PubMed]
54. D'Hooge, R.; De Deyn, P.P. Applications of the Morris Water Maze in the Study of Learning and Memory. *Brain Res. Rev.* **2001**, *36*, 60–90. [CrossRef]
55. España, J.; Giménez-Llort, L.; Valero, J.; Miñano, A.; Rábano, A.; Rodriguez-Alvarez, J.; LaFerla, F.M.; Saura, C.A. Intraneuronal β-Amyloid Accumulation in the Amygdala Enhances Fear and Anxiety in Alzheimer's Disease Transgenic Mice. *Biol. Psychiatry* **2010**, *67*, 513–521. [CrossRef] [PubMed]
56. Giménez-Llort, L.; Ratia, M.; Pérez, B.; Camps, P.; Muñoz-Torrero, D.; Badia, A.; Clos, M.V. Behavioural Effects of Novel Multitarget Anticholinesterasic Derivatives in Alzheimer's Disease. *Behav. Pharmacol.* **2017**, *28*, 124–131. [CrossRef] [PubMed]
57. Sierra-Marcos, A. Regional Cerebral Blood Flow in Mild Cognitive Impairment and Alzheimer's Disease Measured with Arterial Spin Labeling Magnetic Resonance Imaging. *Int. J. Alzheimers Dis.* **2017**, *2017*, 5479597. [CrossRef]
58. Frontiñán-Rubio, J.; Sancho-Bielsa, F.J.; Peinado, J.R.; LaFerla, F.M.; Giménez-Llort, L.; Durán-Prado, M.; Alcain, F.J. Sex-Dependent Co-Occurrence of Hypoxia and β-Amyloid Plaques in Hippocampus and Entorhinal Cortex Is Reversed by Long-Term Treatment with Ubiquinol and Ascorbic Acid in the 3xTg-AD Mouse Model of Alzheimer's Disease. *Mol. Cell. Neurosci.* **2018**, *92*, 67–81. [CrossRef]
59. Guo, Y.; Li, X.; Zhang, M.; Chen, N.; Wu, S.; Lei, J.; Wang, Z.; Wang, R.; Wang, J.; Liu, H. Age- and Brain Region-associated Alterations of Cerebral Blood Flow in Early Alzheimer's Disease Assessed in AβPP SWE /PS1 ΔE9 Transgenic Mice Using Arterial Spin Labeling. *Mol. Med. Rep.* **2019**, *19*, 3045–3052. [CrossRef]
60. Fazlollahi, A.; Calamante, F.; Liang, X.; Bourgeat, P.; Raniga, P.; Dore, V.; Fripp, J.; Ames, D.; Masters, C.L.; Rowe, C.C.; et al. Increased Cerebral Blood Flow with Increased Amyloid Burden in the Preclinical Phase of Alzheimer's Disease. *J. Magn. Reson. Imaging* **2020**, *51*, 505–513. [CrossRef]
61. Bracko, O.; Njiru, B.N.; Swallow, M.; Ali, M.; Haft-Javaherian, M.; Schaffer, C.B. Increasing Cerebral Blood Flow Improves Cognition into Late Stages in Alzheimer's Disease Mice. *J. Cereb. Blood Flow Metab.* **2020**, *40*, 1441–1452. [CrossRef]
62. Ardekani, B.A.; Hadid, S.A.; Blessing, E.; Bachman, A.H. Sexual Dimorphism and Hemispheric Asymmetry of Hippocampal Volumetric Integrity in Normal Aging and Alzheimer Disease. *Am. J. Neuroradiol.* **2019**, *40*, 276–282. [CrossRef]
63. Wachinger, C.; Salat, D.H.; Weiner, M.; Reuter, M. Whole-Brain Analysis Reveals Increased Neuroanatomical Asymmetries in Dementia for Hippocampus and Amygdala. *Brain* **2016**, *139*, 3253–3266. [CrossRef] [PubMed]
64. Goto, K.; Kurashima, R.; Gokan, H.; Inoue, N.; Ito, I.; Watanabe, S. Left-right Asymmetry Defect in the Hippocampal Circuitry Impairs Spatial Learning and Working Memory in IV Mice. *PLoS ONE* **2010**, *5*, e15468. [CrossRef] [PubMed]
65. Shimbo, A.; Kosaki, Y.; Ito, I.; Watanabe, S. Mice Lacking Hippocampal Left-Right Asymmetry Show Non-Spatial Learning Deficits. *Behav. Brain Res.* **2018**, *336*, 156–165. [CrossRef] [PubMed]
66. Tadic, M.; Cuspidi, C.; Hering, D. Hypertension and Cognitive Dysfunction in Elderly: Blood Pressure Management for This Global Burden. *BMC Cardiovasc. Disord.* **2016**, *16*, 208. [CrossRef] [PubMed]
67. Skoog, I.; Gustafson, D. Update on Hypertension and Alzheimer's Disease. *Neurol. Res.* **2006**, *28*, 605–611. [CrossRef] [PubMed]
68. Gilsanz, P.; Mayeda, E.R.; Glymour, M.M.; Quesenberry, C.P.; Mungas, D.M.; DeCarli, C.; Dean, A.; Whitmer, R.A. Female Sex, Early-Onset Hypertension, and Risk of Dementia. *Neurology* **2017**, *89*, 1886–1893. [CrossRef]
69. Barsha, G.; Denton, K.M.; Mirabito Colafella, K.M. Sex- and Age-Related Differences in Arterial Pressure and Albuminuria in Mice. *Biol. Sex Differ.* **2016**, *7*, 1–15. [CrossRef]
70. Wiesmann, M.; Zerbi, V.; Jansen, D.; Lütjohann, D.; Veltien, A.; Heerschap, A.; Kiliaan, A.J. Hypertension, Cerebrovascular Impairment, and Cognitive Decline in Aged AβPP/PS1 Mice. *Theranostics* **2017**, *7*, 1277–1289. [CrossRef]
71. Dede, D.S.; Yavuz, B.; Yavuz, B.B.; Cankurtaran, M.; Halil, M.; Ulger, Z.; Cankurtaran, E.S.; Aytemir, K.; Kabakci, G.; Ariogul, S. Assessment of Endothelial Function in Alzheimer's Disease: Is Alzheimer's Disease a Vascular Disease? *J. Am. Geriatr. Soc.* **2007**, *55*, 1613–1617. [CrossRef]
72. Dickstein, D.L.; Walsh, J.; Brautigam, H.; Stockton, S.D.; Gandy, S.; Hof, P.R. Role of Vascular Risk Factors and Vascular Dysfunction in Alzheimer's Disease. *Mt. Sinai J. Med.* **2010**, *77*, 82–102. [CrossRef]
73. Desai, B.S.; Schneider, J.A.; Li, J.L.; Carvey, P.M.; Hendey, B. Evidence of Angiogenic Vessels in Alzheimer's Disease. *J. Neural. Transm.* **2009**, *116*, 587–597. [CrossRef] [PubMed]

74. Ethell, D.W. An Amyloid-Notch Hypothesis for Alzheimer's Disease. *Neuroscientist* **2010**, *16*, 614–617. [CrossRef] [PubMed]
75. Cameron, D.J.; Galvin, C.; Alkam, T.; Sidhu, H.; Ellison, J.; Luna, S.; Ethell, D.W. Alzheimer's-Related Peptide Amyloid-β Plays a Conserved Role in Angiogenesis. *PLoS ONE* **2012**, *7*, e39598. [CrossRef] [PubMed]
76. Koike, M.A.; Lin, A.J.; Pham, J.; Nguyen, E.; Yeh, J.J.; Rahimian, R.; Tromberg, B.J.; Choi, B.; Green, K.N.; LaFerla, F.M. APP Knockout Mice Experience Acute Mortality as the Result of Ischemia. *PLoS ONE* **2012**, *7*, e42665. [CrossRef] [PubMed]
77. Gaelle, D.; Nadia, H.; Thomas, P.; Vincent, D.; Jean-Louis, G.; Catherine, B.; Nicole, M.; Daniel, B. Sustained Corticosterone Rise in the Prefrontal Cortex Is a Key Factor for Chronic Stress-Induced Working Memory Deficits in Mice. *Neurobiol. Stress* **2019**, *10*, 100161. [CrossRef]
78. Thifault, S.; Lalonde, R.; Joyal, C.C.; Hamet, P. Neurobehavioral Evaluation of High Blood Pressure and Low Blood Pressure Mice. *Psychobiology* **1999**, *27*, 415–425. [CrossRef]
79. Giménez-Llort, L.; Martínez, E.; Ferré, S. Different Effects of Dopamine Antagonists on Spontaneous and NMDA-Induced Motor Activity in Mice. *Pharmacol. Biochem. Behav.* **1997**, *56*, 549–553. [CrossRef]
80. Colorado, R.A.; Shumake, J.; Conejo, N.M.; Gonzalez-Pardo, H.; Gonzalez-Lima, F. Effects of Maternal Separation, Early Handling, and Standard Facility Rearing on Orienting and Impulsive Behavior of Adolescent Rats. *Behav. Process.* **2006**, *71*, 51–58. [CrossRef]

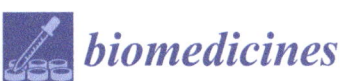

Article

Kisspeptin-8 Induces Anxiety-Like Behavior and Hypolocomotion by Activating the HPA Axis and Increasing GABA Release in the Nucleus Accumbens in Rats

Katalin Eszter Ibos [1,*], Éva Bodnár [1], Zsolt Bagosi [1], Zsolt Bozsó [2], Gábor Tóth [2], Gyula Szabó [3] and Krisztina Csabafi [1]

1. Department of Pathophysiology, Faculty of Medicine, University of Szeged, H-6720 Szeged, Hungary; dobo.eva@med.u-szeged.hu (É.B.); bagosi.zsolt@med.u-szeged.hu (Z.B.); csabafi.krisztina@med.u-szeged.hu (K.C.)
2. Department of Medical Chemistry, Faculty of Medicine, University of Szeged, H-6720 Szeged, Hungary; bozso.zsolt@med.u-szeged.hu (Z.B.); toth.gabor@med.u-szeged.hu (G.T.)
3. Office of International Affairs, Budapest Campus, McDaniel College, H-1071 Budapest, Hungary; gyula.szabo.prf@mcdaniel.hu
* Correspondence: ibos.katalin.eszter@med.u-szeged.hu

Abstract: Kisspeptins (Kp) are RF-amide neuropeptide regulators of the reproductive axis that also influence anxiety, locomotion, and metabolism. We aimed to investigate the effects of intracerebroventricular Kp-8 (an N-terminally truncated octapeptide) treatment in Wistar rats. Elevated plus maze (EPM), computerized open field (OF), and marble burying (MB) tests were performed for the assessment of behavior. Serum LH and corticosterone levels were determined to assess kisspeptin1 receptor (Kiss1r) activation and hypothalamic-pituitary-adrenal axis (HPA) stimulation, respectively. GABA release from the nucleus accumbens (NAc) and dopamine release from the ventral tegmental area (VTA) and NAc were measured via ex vivo superfusion. Kp-8 decreased open arm time and entries in EPM, and also raised corticosterone concentration, pointing to an anxiogenic effect. Moreover, the decrease in arm entries in EPM, the delayed increase in immobility accompanied by reduced ambulatory activity in OF, and the reduction in interactions with marbles show that Kp-8 suppressed exploratory and spontaneous locomotion. The increase in GABA release from the NAc might be in the background of hypolocomotion by inhibiting the VTA-NAc dopaminergic circuitry. As Kp-8 raised LH concentration, it could activate Kiss1r and stimulate the reproductive axis. As Kiss1r is associated with hyperlocomotion, it is more likely that neuropeptide FF receptor activation is involved in the suppression of locomotor activity.

Keywords: kisspeptin; anxiety; locomotion; Kiss1 receptor; HPA axis; HPG axis; nucleus accumbens

1. Introduction

The *KISS1* gene was discovered as a novel metastasis-suppressor in human melanoma cells in 1996 in Hershey, named after the famous chocolate of the city, Hershey's Kisses [1].

KISS1 encodes a 145-amino-acid propeptide, from which kisspeptin-54 (Kp-54) is cleaved. The proteolytical cleavage of this 54-amino-acid peptide results in shorter biologically active products, designated kisspeptin-14 (Kp-14), kisspeptin-13 (Kp-13) and kisspeptin-10 (Kp-10) [2]. Mammalian kisspeptins belong to the family of RF-amide peptides, as they carry the characteristic, conserved carboxyl-terminal Arg–Phe–NH$_2$ sequence [3].

The canonical receptor of kisspeptins is a G protein-coupled receptor, Gpr54, that is fully activated by all biologically active products of the *Kiss1* gene [4]. Although Gpr54 was initially described in 1999 as an orphan receptor similar to galanin receptors [5], after being deorphanized in 2001, it was designated kisspeptin-1 receptor (Kiss1r) [6].

Upon activation of the $G\alpha_{q/11}$-coupled Kiss1r, phospholipase C (PLC) is activated, leading to inositol 1,4,5-trisphosphate (IP3)-mediated intracellular Ca^{2+} mobilization. Moreover, the activation of protein kinase C (PKC) and the $G\alpha_q$-independent recruitment of β-arrestins result in the phosphorylation of several mitogen-activated protein kinases (MAPKs), including extracellular signal-regulated kinases 1/2 (ERK1/2) and p38 [4]. MAPKs in turn regulate gene expression and induce long-term alterations in a wide range of biological processes [7], including progesterone secretion [8], trophoblast adhesion [9], and glucose-induced insulin secretion [10].

Kisspeptins also bind and activate both neuropeptide FF receptors (NPFFR1 and NPFFR2) [11]. As NPFF receptors are coupled with $G\alpha_{i/o}$, their activation inhibits cAMP production. The Gβγ heterodimer released from $G_{i/o}$ proteins was found to inhibit voltage-gated Ca^{2+} channels. Moreover, it is capable of potentiating G_q signaling via physical interaction with PLC [3].

Kisspeptin is expressed in several regions of the rat central nervous system, including hypothalamic nuclei [e.g., arcuate nucleus, anteroventral paraventricular nucleus (AVPV)], thalamic nuclei, the amygdala, hippocampus, lateral septum, the bed nucleus of stria terminalis, striatum, nucleus accumbens (NAc), periaqueductal grey, and locus coeruleus [12,13]. Likewise, Kiss1r has been localized in rats in the hypothalamus (e.g., paraventricular, arcuate and supraoptic nucleus), thalamus, hippocampus, amygdala, septum, striatum, raphe nuclei, and cortex [5,14].

The expression of NPFF1 receptor mRNA has been detected in the lateral septum, in thalamic and brainstem nuclei, as well as in the ventral tegmental area (VTA), NAc, the bed nucleus of the stria terminalis, the amygdala and hippocampus. NPFF2 receptor mRNA expression has been reported in thalamic nuclei, in the hypothalamus, hippocampus, VTA, the A5 noradrenergic cell group and also in the dorsal horn of the spinal cord [15,16].

Following the original discovery of its metastasis suppressor role in melanoma [1], the anti-metastatic activity of kisspeptin has been found in a variety of tumors, including bladder, ovary, colorectal, pancreas, pituitary, prostate and thyroid cancer [17].

The involvement of kisspeptin in reproduction has been a topic of extensive research since it was discovered in 2003 that kisspeptin is a potent stimulator of gonadotropin secretion [18]. The role of kisspeptin in the regulation of puberty is underlined by the finding that various loss-of-function mutations of *KISS1R* and *KISS1* are associated with isolated hypogonadotropic hypogonadism, whereas activating mutations result in central precocious puberty [19]. Hypothalamic *Kiss1* neuron populations are responsible for the regulation of the estrous cycle by mediating positive and negative feedback of gonadal steroids on gonadotropin secretion [20]. The sexually dimorphic *Kiss1* neuron population of the AVPV is responsible for the positive feedback of estrogen, thus it contributes to the surge-like secretion of GnRH. However, pulsatile GnRH secretion is regulated by the KNDy neurons (coexpressing kisspeptin, neurokinin B, and dynorphin) of the arcuate nucleus that mediate the negative feedback of estrogen [21]. Compelling evidence has suggested that KNDy neurons in the arcuate nucleus function as a major integrator of various modifiers of the reproductive axis, including metabolic signals, olfactory clues, and circadian rhythm [22–25].

Similarly to other members of the RF-amide family [26], kisspeptin has also been implicated in the regulation of nociception [27]. In a recent study, Kp-13 lowered the nociceptive threshold in mice, decreased the analgesic effect of morphine, diminished morphine tolerance and caused mechanical hypersensitivity [28].

Based on the expression of *Kiss1* and *Kiss1r* in limbic brain structures [29,30], several studies have investigated the behavioral effects of kisspeptin.

An antidepressant-like effect of kisspeptin has been reported in rats [31], and intravenous kisspeptin has also decreased negative mood in human subjects [32].

Kisspeptin neurons in the rostral periventricular area of the 3rd ventricle (RP3V) seem to regulate sexual behavior in rodents, as they are activated by male urinary odors in female mice and facilitate copulatory behavior in a NO-dependent pathway [33,34].

An interplay between kisspeptin and the hypothalamic-pituitary-adrenal (HPA) axis was suggested in 2009, when Kinsey-Jones et al. discovered that stress-induced elevation of plasma corticosterone suppresses hypothalamic kisspeptin signaling in rodents [35]. Since that time, several studies have been conducted with controversial results.

In paraventricular nucleus-derived cell lines, Kp-10 increased the gene expression of arginine vasopressin (AVP) and oxytocin, while suppressing the expression of corticotropin releasing hormone (CRH). However, it failed to influence the activity of the HPA axis in vivo, as intraperitoneally (ip.) administered Kp-10 had no effect on plasma corticosterone and adrenocorticotropic hormone (ACTH) levels in rats [36]. Likewise, kisspeptin administration had no effect on anxiety in human subjects [32].

In 2013, our group reported an anxiogenic effect of intracerebroventricularly (icv.) administered Kp-13 in rats. Kp-13 not only induced a significant increase in plasma corticosterone level, but also decreased the number of entries into the open arms and the time spent in them in the elevated plus maze test. Moreover, it has stimulated spontaneous locomotion and it also had a hyperthermic effect lasting for several hours after treatment [37].

An anxiogenic property of kisspeptin signaling has also been proposed by the experiments of Delmas et al., in which *Kiss1r* KO mice have spent more time in the open arms in the elevated plus maze test, indicating a suppression of anxiety. The most pronounced anxiolytic effect was observed when kisspeptin signaling in GnRH neurons was selectively rescued in *Kiss1r* KO animals, suggesting a modulatory role of gonadal steroids. Interestingly, no significant effect of *Kiss1r* KO was detected on the behavioral parameters of the open field test [38].

In zebrafish, however, the central administration of kisspeptin has been associated with an anxiolytic tendency in the novel-tank diving test and a significantly reduced fear response to alarm substance [39].

In a recent study, a Cre-dependent, stimulatory DREADD (Designer Receptors Exclusively Activated by Designer Drugs) viral construct has been targeted to the *Kiss1* neurons of the posterodorsal medial amygdala (MePD) in mice. Upon selective activation of MePD *Kiss1* neurons by clozapine-N-oxide, a significant increase in open arm exploration has been observed in the elevated plus maze, suggesting an anxiolytic role of this neuron population [40].

There are several possible explanations for the ambiguous results reported in the literature. On one hand, the route of administration could be a determining factor. Peripheral administration of Kp has failed to influence the activity of the HPA axis in rats (0.13 µg/µL Kp-54 ip.) [36] and the activity of the limbic system in human subjects (1 nmol/kg/h Kp-54 iv. over 75 min) [32]. In contrast, central Kp-13 (1 or 2 µg icv.) had a pronounced anxiogenic effect in rats [37]. It is likely that the doses applied by Rao et al. [36] and Comninos et al. [32] were too low to exert an anxiogenic effect. In their investigation into the effect of peripheral or central Kp administration on the reproductive axis in rats, Thomson et al. have found that 1 nmol of icv. Kp-10 was sufficient to significantly raise plasma luteinizing hormone (LH) concentration, but a 100-fold dose was required for the same effect in case of ip. treatment [41]. Likewise, the selective activation of MePD *Kiss1* neurons [40] points to the function of a distinct neuron population, whereas central kisspeptin treatment [37] reflects a general central effect by activating neurons bearing Kiss1r throughout the brain.

On the other hand, the differences could also be attributed to the variety of species involved in these experiments. The kisspeptin system of zebrafish is strikingly different from the mammalian one, both in terms of anatomy and function [39,42], thus the results of studies on zebrafish should be interpreted with caution.

Some studies have also reported that kisspeptin might play a role in the regulation of locomotor activity. Icv. Kp-13 has induced an increase in not only spontaneous, but also in exploratory locomotion in male Sprague-Dawley rats [37]. In line with these results, Tolson et al. have found that *Kiss1r* KO female mice exhibit decreased locomotor activity and energy expenditure, leading to obesity [43].

It has been discovered that kisspeptin attenuates morphine effect [28], and is expressed in the NAc [44], pointing to its possible involvement in the regulation of mesocorticolimbic dopaminergic activity. Interestingly, the centers of reward and addiction have also been implicated in the regulation of locomotion. First, quinpirole (a D2 receptor agonist) injected into the NAc has suppressed exploratory locomotion in rats [45], whereas bicuculline (a $GABA_A$ receptor antagonist) administration into the nucleus induced hyperactivity with prolonged exploratory behavior in rats [46]. Second, the selective activation of dopaminergic neurons in the VTA by DREADD has induced a pronounced and sustained hyperactivity in rats, which effect could be reproduced by activating selectively activating the dopaminergic pathway between the VTA and NAc [47]. Thus, it is possible that kisspeptin might influence locomotion by modulating the activity of the VTA or NAc.

Nowadays kisspeptin analogs and antagonists are attracting considerable attention due to their potential therapeutic use in various gynecological conditions, including infertility, polycystic ovary syndrome and precocious puberty [48]. The shortest natural bioactive form of kisspeptin is the 10 amino acid long Kp-10, which has higher affinity to Kiss1r than Kp-54 [49]. According to molecular docking studies, ASN4, SER5, GLY7, ARG9 and PHE10 of Kp-10 are involved in the formation of hydrogen bonds between the peptide and Kiss1r [50]. Consequently, shorter kisspeptin fragments containing these amino acids might be able to bind and possibly activate the receptor.

The aim of the current study was to investigate whether the 8 amino acid long fragment of kisspeptin is capable of influencing the behavior of rats similarly to kisspeptin. Following icv. treatment with Kp-8, elevated plus maze (EPM), computerized open field (OF), and marble burying (MB) tests were performed. Serum corticosterone and luteinizing hormone concentrations were measured to assess the activation of the HPA axis and Kiss1 receptors, respectively. Moreover, dopamine release from the VTA and NAc and GABA release from the NAc were measured using ex vivo superfusion to further characterize the mechanism of action.

2. Materials and Methods

2.1. Animals and Housing Conditions

Adult male Wistar rats (Domaszék, Csongrád, Hungary) weighing 150–250 g were used for the experiments at the age of 6–8 weeks. The animals were housed under controlled conditions at constant room temperature, with a 12–12-h light dark cycle (lights on from 6:00 a.m.). The rats were allowed free access to commercial food and tap water.

The animals were kept and handled during the experiments in accordance with the instructions of the University of Szeged Ethical Committee for the Protection of Animals in Research, which approved these experiments. Permission for the experiments (number: X./1207/2018, date: 6 July 2018.) has been granted by the Government Office of Csongrád County Directorate of Food Chain Safety and Animal Health. Each animal was used for only one experimental procedure.

2.2. Intracerebroventricular Cannulation

A stainless steel Luer cannula (10 mm long) was implanted in the right lateral cerebral ventricle for icv. administration. The cannula was inserted under sodium pentobarbital (Euthasol, Phylaxia-Sanofi, 35 mg/kg, ip.) anaesthesia, according to the following stereotaxic coordinates: 0.2 mm posterior and 1.7 mm lateral to the bregma, and 3.7 mm deep from the dural surface [37]. Subsequently, it was secured to the skull with dental cement and acrylate. The experiments started after a recovery period of 1 week. All experiments were carried out between 8:00 a.m. and 10:00 a.m.

2.3. Peptide Synthesis

Kisspeptin-8 (WNSFGLRF-NH2) was synthesized on a Rink Amide MBHA resin (Bachem, Bubendorf, Switzerland, subst.: 0.52 mmol/g) using N^α-9-Fluorenylmethoxycarbonyl (Fmoc) protected amino acids (IRIS Biotech GmbH, Marktredwitz, Germany) by manual solid phase peptide synthesis by the Department of Medical Chemistry (University of Szeged). The resin was swollen in dichloromethane (DCM). The Fmoc group was removed by treating the peptide-resin with 20% piperidine/N,N-dimethylformamide (DMF) solution twice (5 + 15 min). Solvents were purchased from VWR (Radnor, PA, USA).

The amino acids were activated with N,N'-dicyclohexylcarbodiimide and 1-hydroxybenzotriazole in 50% DCM/DMF. The peptide-resin was incubated with this mixture for 3 h. The resin was washed with DMF (3×) and DCM (3×) after the deprotection and coupling steps.

The assembled peptides were cleaved from the resin by treating it with the following cleavage cocktail for 3 h: 90% trifluoroacetic acid (TFA) (Pierce, Rockford, IL, USA), 5% water, 2% dithiotreitol, 2% triisopropylsilane.

The peptides were precipitated with diethyl ether, dissolved in a mixture of acetonitrile (ACN) and water and lyophilized. The crude peptides were analyzed by HPLC (Hewlett-Packard Agilent 1100 system, column: Luna, c18 (2), 250 × 4.6 mm, 5 µm, 100 Å, Phenomenex, Aschaffenburg, Germany) and ESI-MS. The peptides were purified on a preparative HPLC column (Phenomenex Luna, c18 (2), 250 × 21.2 mm, 10 µm, 100 Å) using a Shimadzu 20-LC system. The fractions were analyzed on the above mentioned analytical HPLC system and measured by electrospray ionization mass spectrometry (ESI-MS) (see Appendix A Figures A1 and A2 for the results). The pure fractions were pooled and freeze-dried.

2.4. Treatment

The rats were treated icv. in a volume of 2 µL over 30 s using a Hamilton microsyringe (Merck KGaA, Darmstadt, Germany). The doses applied were 0.1 or 1 µg of Kp-8 dissolved in 0.9% saline. Control animals were injected with 2 µL of 0.9% saline alone. The animals were treated 30 min prior to the behavioral tests. Collection of trunk blood for LH ELISA, corticosterone ELISA and serum corticosterone measurement were carried out 15 min and 30 min after icv. treatment, respectively.

2.5. Behavioral Tests

2.5.1. Elevated Plus Maze Test

The EPM apparatus is a plus-shaped platform 50 cm above the ground. The maze consists of four arms (50 cm × 10 cm each): two opposing open arms and two closed arms enclosed by a 10 cm high wall. The test is based on two conflicting motivations of rodents: to avoid open, brightly lit spaces and to explore novel environment. The avoidance of open arms reflects anxiety-like behavior [51]. 30 min after icv. treatment the rats were placed in the maze facing one of the open arms, then their behavior was recorded by a camera suspended above the maze for 5 min. The time spent in each arm, as well as the number of entries per arm were registered by an observer blind to the experimental groups. The percentage of entries into the open arms and the percentage of time spent in the open arms were also calculated. The experiments were conducted between 8 a.m. and 10 a.m. and the apparatus was cleaned with 96% ethyl-alcohol after each session.

2.5.2. Computerized Open Field Test

The novelty-induced locomotor activity of rats was assessed using the Conducta 1.0 System (Experimetria Ltd., Budapest, Hungary). The system consists of black plastic OF arenas (inside dimensions: 48 × 48 cm, height: 40 cm) with 5 horizontal rows of infrared diodes on the walls to register both horizontal and vertical locomotion. The center of each box is illuminated by a LED lightbulb (230 lumen) from above the box. The central zone of the arena is defined as a 24 × 24 cm area in the center of the box. 30 min after icv. treatment the rats were placed in the center of the box and their behavior was recorded by the Conducta computer program for 60 min. Six behavioral parameters were measured during the experiment: total time and total distance of ambulation, immobility time, number of rearings (vertical locomotion), time spent in the central zone (central area of 24 × 24 cm), and distance travelled in the central zone. The OF experiments were conducted between 8 a.m. and 10 a.m. and the apparatus was cleaned with 96% ethyl-alcohol after each session.

2.5.3. Marble Burying Test

MB is a regularly used paradigm for the assessment of anxiety-like and compulsive-like behavior [52]. Our protocol was based on the method described by Schneider and Popik [53]. The animals were removed from their plexiglass home cages (420 × 275 × 180 mm) and temporarily moved into another cage before the experiment. Meanwhile the home cage was prepared for the experiment by increasing the depth of bedding material to 5 cm. Following icv. treatment one animal was placed back into the home cage for 30 min in order to acclimatize to the thick bedding. Then 9 glass marbles of 2.5 cm diameter were arranged in 3 rows along the shorter wall of the cage. The experiment was conducted for 10 min and recorded by a video camera above the cage. After the session, the animal was removed from the cage and the number of buried marbles (>50% marble covered by bedding material) was counted. The marbles were cleaned with 96% ethyl-alcohol after each session. After the experiment, the video recording was evaluated. The count and duration of two types of goal-oriented interactions with marbles (burying of marbles and moving marbles without burying them) were assessed.

2.6. Serum Corticosterone, Luteinizing Hormone and Total Protein Concentration Measurement

For the measurement of serum corticosterone and protein concentration, the animals were decapitated 30 min after icv. treatment. For the assessment of serum LH, decapitation was performed 15 min after icv. treatment. Trunk blood was collected into test tubes and left at room temperature for 30 min to clot, then it was centrifuged for 10 min at 3500 rpm. The samples were stored at −80 °C until the assays were performed. Serum corticosterone concentration was measured using a competitive corticosterone ELISA kit (Cayman Chemical, Ann Arbor, MI, USA), according to the manufacturer's instruction. Serum LH concentration was determined using a sandwich LH ELISA kit (Wuhan Xinquidi Biological Technology Co., Wuhan, China), according to the manufacturer's instructions. The Pierce Coomassie (Bradford) Protein Assay Kit (Thermo Fisher Scientific, Waltham, MA, USA) was used, according to the manufacturer's instructions for the measurement of total serum protein concentration. The absorbance was measured at 595 nm with a NanoDrop One^C microvolume spectrophotometer (Thermo Fisher Scientific, Waltham, MA, USA).

2.7. Ex Vivo Superfusion

Before the ex vivo superfusion, the animals did not undergo icv. cannulation. The rats were rapidly decapitated, and their brains were removed from the skull. Dissection was performed with the help of a brain matrix, a tissue puncher and razor blades, on a filter paper moistened with phosphate-buffered saline, on top of a Petri dish filled with ice. The NAc was removed from both sides, following the method of isolation described by Heffner [54]. The VTA was isolated as described by Salvatore et al. [55]. The tissue was cut to 300 μm slices and incubated for 30 min in 5 mL of Krebs solution (Reanal, Hungary) bubbled with carbogen gas (5% CO_2 and 95% O_2). Then 5 μL of [3H]GABA (PerkinElmer Inc., Waltham, MA, USA) was added to the NAc and 5 μL of [3H]Dopamine (PerkinElmer Inc., Waltham, MA, USA) was added to the VTA or the NAc. Afterwards the slices were transferred evenly into the four cylindrical chambers of the superfusion system (Experimetria Ltd., Budapest, Hungary), and superfusion with carbogen-bubbled Krebs solution was started at body temperature (37 °C). A constant flow rate of 227, 7 μL/min was maintained with a peristaltic pump (Minipuls 2, Gilson, Middleton, WI, USA). After 30 min of superfusion, the collection of superfusates into Eppendorf tubes was started with a multichannel fraction collector (FC 203B, Gilson, Middleton, WI, USA). Fractions were collected every two minutes for 32 min. At 6 min, 1 μg of Kp-8 dissolved in 1 mL of Krebs solution was added directly into the chambers. From the 12th minute of fraction collection, electrical stimulation of square-wave impulses was delivered for two minutes (ST-

02 electrical stimulator, Experimetria Ltd., Budapest, Hungary). Then, the tissue from each chamber was transferred into a beaker containing 600 µL of Krebs solution for ultrasonic homogenization (Branson Sonifier 250, Emerson Electric Co., St. Louis, MO, USA).

Afterwards 3 mL of Ultima Gold scintillation cocktail (Perkin-Elmer Inc., Waltham, MA, USA) was pipetted into 4 rows of 17 scintillation vials. Subsequently, 200 µL of the 16 fractions collected and of the suspension of the tissue from the corresponding chamber were added into each row of vials. The samples were homogenized mechanically for 30 min.

The radioactivity of samples was detected with a liquid scintillation spectrometer (Tri-carb 2100 TR, Hewlett-Packard Inc., Palo Alto, CA, USA). Fractional dopamine or GABA release (FR) was calculated from the counts per minute (CPM), according to the equation below, in which i stands for the number of fraction and $n = 16$. CPM_{17} refers to the CPM of the homogenized tissue sample corresponding to the fraction:

$$FR_i = 100 \cdot \frac{CPM_i}{4 \cdot CPM_{17} + \sum_{i+1}^{n} CPM_i}$$

2.8. Statistical Analysis

Data are presented as mean + SEM. Statistical analysis and graph editing were performed using the GraphPad Prism 8 software. One-way ANOVA with Holm-Sidak's post-hoc test was applied for the analysis of EPM results. One-way ANOVA with Dunnett's post-hoc test was used for the analysis of cumulative OF results, as well as for the evaluation of serum corticosterone, LH and total protein measurements. Two-way RM ANOVA with Holm–Sidak's post-hoc test was performed for the evaluation of 5-min intervals in the OF test as well as for the interpretation of dopamine and GABA release from the NAc. Mixed-effects analysis with Holm–Sidak's multiple comparison test was performed for the evaluation of fractional dopamine release from the VTA. Kruskal–Wallis test with Dunn's post-hoc test was performed for the analysis of MB results. Curve fitting for ELISA tests was performed according to the manufacturers' instructions.

3. Results
3.1. Behavioral Tests
3.1.1. Elevated Plus Maze

The 0.1 µg dose of Kp-8 significantly reduced the percentage of entries into the open arms of the plus maze (Figure 1a, $F_{(2, 20)} = 9.196$, $p = 0.0007$), as well as the percentage of time spent in the open arms of the maze (Figure 1b, $F_{(2, 20)} = 4.431$, $p = 0.0202$). A decrease in the total number of entries into the arms was induced by both 0.1 µg and 1 µg of Kp-8 (Figure 1c, $F_{(2, 20)} = 5.927$, $p = 0.0153$). There was no significant difference among the groups in the total time spent in the arms (Figure 1d, $F_{(2, 20)} = 1.932$, $p = 0.1710$).

3.1.2. Computerized Open Field Test

The cumulative results obtained after 60 min of data collection did not show any significant change in behavior (see Appendix B Figure A3).

However, significant differences were found following the analysis of each 5-min interval. As seen in Figure 2a, the two-factor RM-ANOVA on the distance travelled in the arena revealed a significant main effect for the time factor ($F_{(5.389, 183.2)} = 113.8$, $p < 0.0001$). Following a peak in the first five minutes the ambulation distance was steeply decreasing until a lower level of basal locomotor activity was reached around 30 min. The distance travelled at 50–55 and 55–60 min was lower in the 1 µg Kp-8 group than in the control group ($p = 0.0334$ and $p = 0.0410$, respectively).

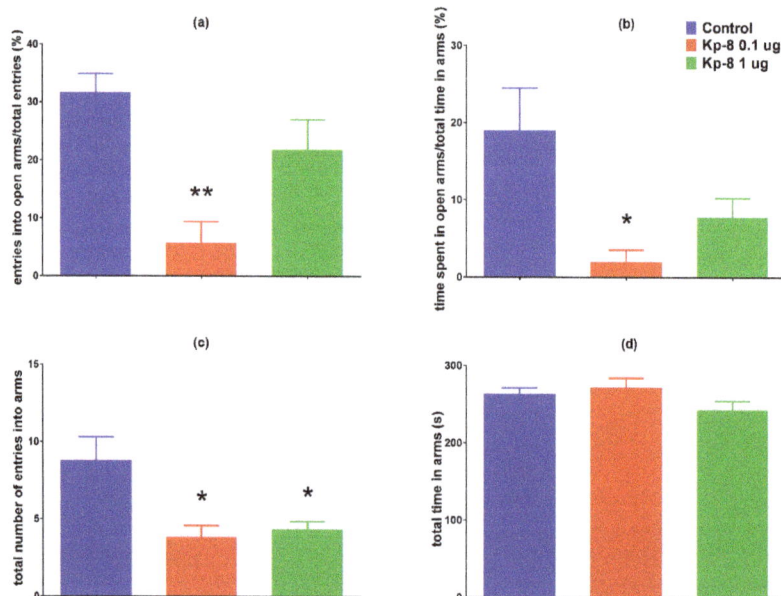

Figure 1. Elevated plus maze results: (**a**) percentage of entries into open arms, (**b**) percentage of time spent in the open arms, (**c**) total number of entries into arms, (**d**) total time spent in the arms of the maze, $n = 7$–9, * $p < 0.05$ vs. control, ** $p < 0.01$ vs. control.

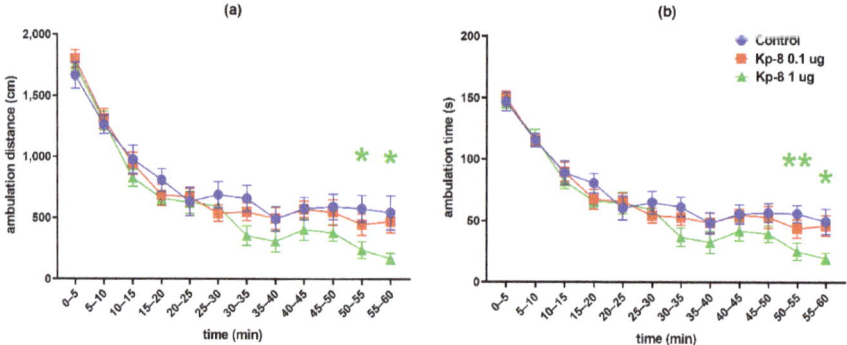

Figure 2. Open field test results in 5-min intervals: (**a**) total distance travelled in the arena, (**b**) total ambulation time. The color of * refers to the treatment group which significantly differs from the control group. $n = 12$–13, * $p < 0.05$ vs. control, ** $p < 0.01$ vs. control.

Regarding total ambulation time, there was a significant main effect for the time factor ($F (6.138, 208.7) = 98.03$, $p < 0.0001$) with a similar pattern of steep then mild decrease (Figure 2b). The 1 µg Kp-8 group spent less time with ambulation than the control group at 50–55 min ($p = 0.0090$) and 55–60 min ($p = 0.0326$), as well.

The two-way ANOVA on immobility yielded a significant main effect for the time factor ($F (5.396, 183.5) = 34.51$, $p < 0.0001$) and interaction ($F (22, 374) = 2.249$, $p = 0.0012$). The time spent immobile was increasing during the experiment, showing a tendency reciprocal to that of ambulation time and distance (Figure 3a). Compared to control, the 1 µg dose of Kp-8 significantly increased immobility at 50–55 and 55–60 min ($p = 0.0202$ and $p = 0.0186$, respectively).

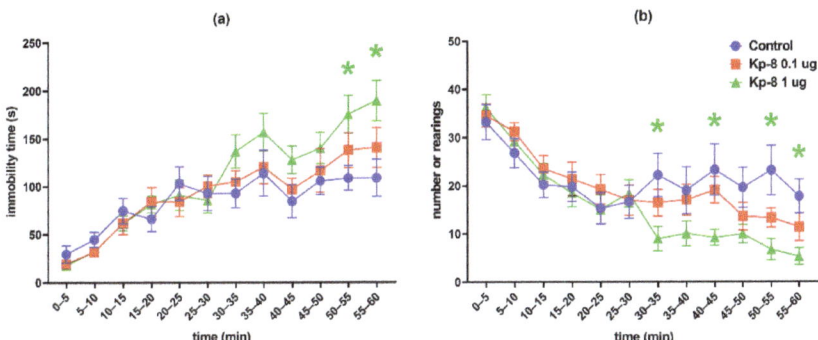

Figure 3. Open field test results in 5-min intervals: (**a**) total time spent immobile, (**b**) total number of rearings. The color of * refers to the treatment group which significantly differs from the control group. n = 12–13, * $p < 0.05$ vs. control.

Considering the number of rearing sessions, a significant main effect for the time factor was detected (F (6.756, 229.7) = 7.52, $p < 0.0001$), along with a statistically significant interaction between time and treatment (F (22, 374) = 3.095, $p < 0.0001$). As seen in Figure 3b, a pronounced difference started to appear among treatment groups from 30 min. There was a significant decrease in the number of rearings in the 1 µg Kp-8 group at 30–35 min ($p = 0.0369$), 40–45 min ($p = 0.0445$), 50–55 min ($p = 0.0182$) and 55–60 min ($p = 0.0108$).

Having calculated the average velocity for each timeframe, a significant main effect for the time factor (F (4.044, 129.4) = 12.17, $p < 0.0001$) and interaction (F (22, 352) = 1.940, $p = 0.0073$) could be seen, as shown in Figure 4c. There was no significant difference between treatment groups until 55 min, when the speed of the 1 µg Kp-8 group dropped ($p = 0.0479$).

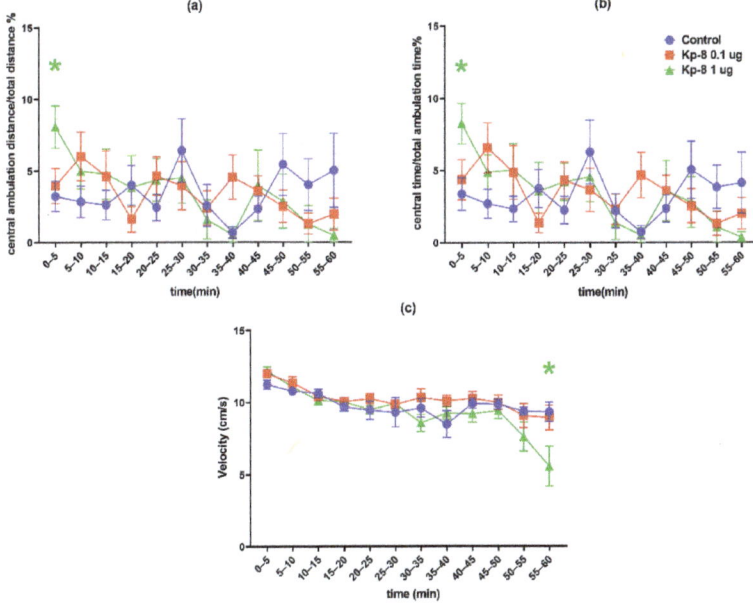

Figure 4. Open field test results in 5-min intervals: (**a**) percentage of distance travelled in the central zone of the arena, (**b**) percentage of time spent in the central zone of the arena, (**c**) average velocity of ambulation. The color of * refers to the treatment group which significantly differs from the control group. n = 12–13, * $p < 0.05$ vs. control.

Figure 4a shows the percentage of central ambulation distance, calculated by dividing the distance travelled in the central zone of the arena by the total ambulation distance, multiplied by 100. Time factor (F (6.920, 235.3) = 2.207, p = 0.0351) and interaction between time and treatment (F (22, 374) = 1.767, p = 0.0185) both significantly accounted for the variation, but there was no difference among the groups, except in the first 5 min, when the central ambulation distance of the 1 µg Kp-8 group was higher than that of control (p = 0.0429).

The percentage of central ambulation time was calculated by multiplying the ratio of central time and total ambulation time by 100, as shown in Figure 4b. There was a significant main effect for the time factor (F (6.981, 237.3) = 2931, p = 0.0059), as well as for the interaction (F (22, 374) = 1.945, p = 0.0070). In the first 5 min, the central ambulation time of the 1 µg Kp-8 group significantly exceeded the central time of the control group (p = 0.0409), otherwise there was no difference among the groups.

3.1.3. Marble Burying Test

There was no significant difference in the number of buried marbles among the groups (Figure 5a). Two types of goal-oriented interactions with the marbles were distinguished: marble burying and marble moving.

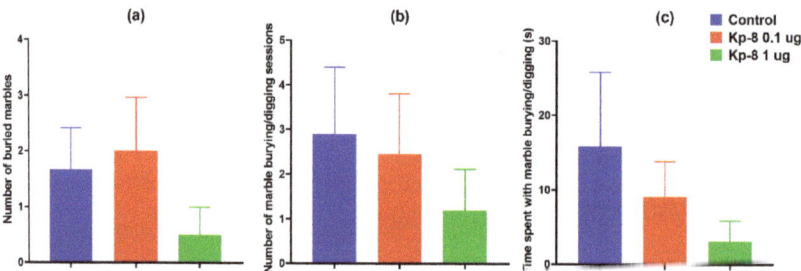

Figure 5. Results of marble burying test: (a) number of buried marbles (at least 50% covered with bedding material), (b) number of marble burying sessions, (c) duration of marble burying activity, n = 9–10.

Marble burying is an interaction involving digging around the marbles, resulting in marbles covered with bedding material. As seen in Figure 5b,c, neither the number of marble burying sessions, nor the duration of marble burying activity changed significantly with treatment, although a tendency of reduced burying activity was observable.

Marble moving is an interaction that involves rolling, moving the marbles with the forelegs, without successfully covering it with bedding material. Similarly to marble burying, there was no significant difference in the number and duration of marble moving among the groups (Figure 6a,b), although a tendency of suppressed marble moving could be seen in the groups treated with Kp-8.

However, taken the two types of interactions together, the 1 µg Kp-8 group interacted with the marbles fewer times than the control group (Figure 6c, p = 0.0499) and they also spent less time with goal-oriented interactions with the marbles (Figure 6d, p = 0.0274).

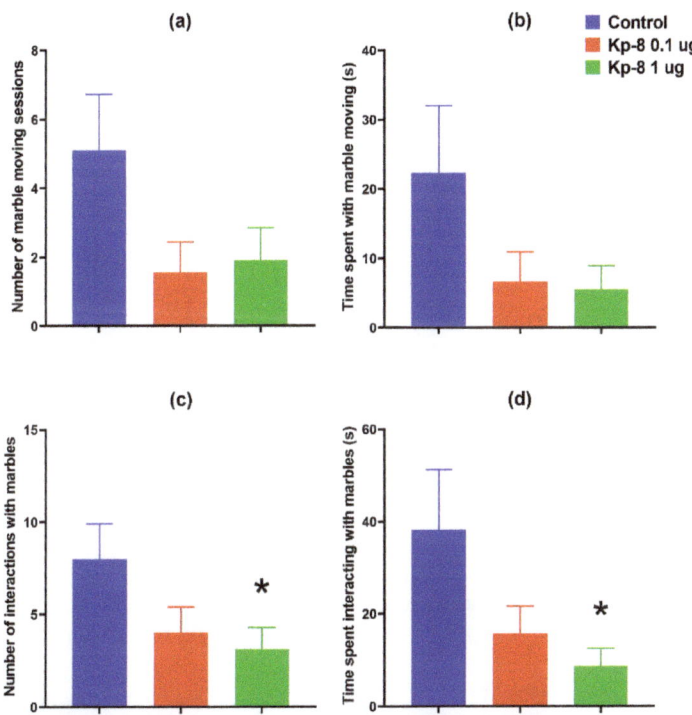

Figure 6. Results of marble burying test: (**a**) number of marble moving sessions, (**b**) duration of marble moving activity, (**c**) total number of interactions with marbles, (**d**) total duration of interactions with marbles, * $p < 0.05$ vs. control. $n = 9–10$.

3.2. Serum Corticosterone, LH and Total Protein

The results of serum corticosterone and LH measurement can be seen in Figure 7. One-way ANOVA showed a significant effect of Kp-8 treatment both on corticosterone ($F_{(2, 10)} = 12.02$, $p = 0.0022$) and LH concentration ($F_{(2, 15)} = 41.31$, $p < 0.0001$). A robust increase in serum corticosterone concentration was detected 30 min after icv. treatment with 1 µg of Kp-8 ($p = 0.001$ vs. control). The 0.1 µg dose had a tendency to elevate corticosterone concentration, but the change was not significant ($p = 0.306$ vs. control). The 1 µg dose of Kp-8 also raised serum LH concentration 15 min after icv. treatment ($p = 0.0001$ vs. control), but the 0.1 µg dose had no effect on LH ($p = 0.961$ vs. control). There was no difference in serum protein concentration among the groups ($F_{(2, 17)} = 2.365$, $p = 0.124$, $n = 5–8$): The mean serum protein concentrations with SD were 45.74 ± 4.898, 40.44 ± 3.115 and 45.13 ± 7.045 g/L in the control, 0.1 µg and 1 µg groups, respectively.

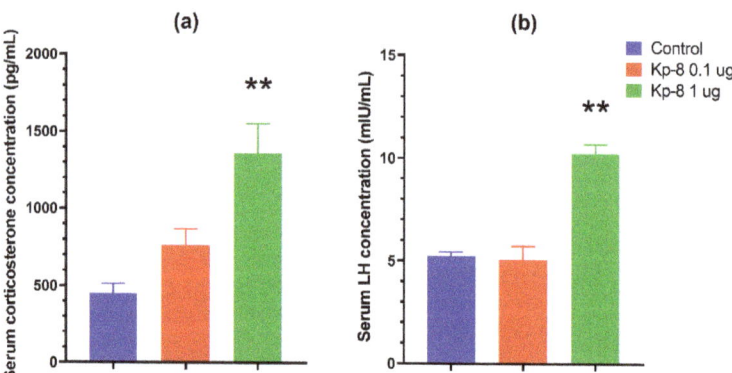

Figure 7. ELISA results: (**a**) serum corticosterone concentration (pg/mL), n = 4–5, ** $p < 0.01$ vs. control, (**b**) serum LH concentration (mIU/mL), n = 4–9, ** $p < 0.01$ vs. control.

3.3. Ex Vivo Superfusion

Figure 8 shows fractional dopamine release from the VTA. A p value was not calculated for the time factor (F (15.00, 104.0) = 16.41). There was no significant main effect neither for the treatment factor (F (1, 7) = 0.0008258, p = 0.9779), nor for the interaction between treatment and time (F (15, 104) = 0.5151, p = 0.9273). There was no significant difference between the groups at any other time point.

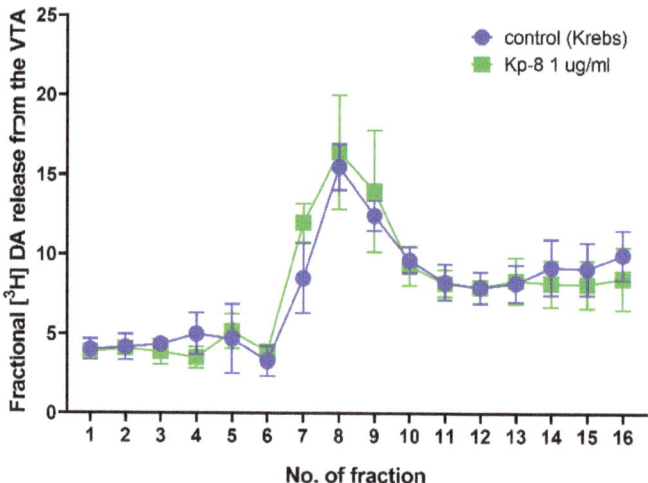

Figure 8. Fractional dopamine release from the ventral tegmental area. n = 4–5.

Likewise, Kp-8 did not influence fractional dopamine release from the NAc (Figure 9). However, there was a significant main effect for the time factor (F (3.134, 40.75) = 22.48, $p < 0.0001$). No significant main effect was found for the treatment factor (F (1, 13) = 0.0007717, p = 0.9783), and for the interaction between treatment and time (F (15, 195) = 0.4387, p = 0.9658). No significant difference could be detected at any specific time point between the groups.

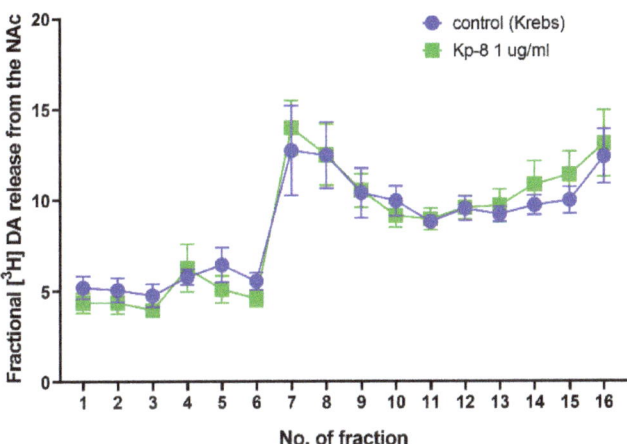

Figure 9. Fractional dopamine release from the nucleus accumbens. $n = 7–8$.

As shown in Figure 10, Kp-8 increased fractional GABA release from the NAc. There was a significant main effect for the time (F (2.227, 17.82) = 60.49, $p < 0.0001$) and interaction (F (15, 120) = 7.395, $p < 0.0001$) factors. In the seventh fraction, following electrical stimulation, fractional GABA release was significantly higher from the Kp-8 treated brain slices than from the control tissue ($p = 0.0039$).

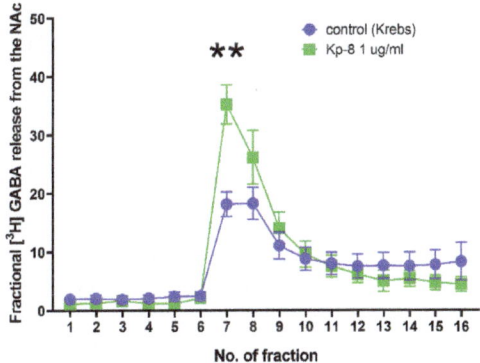

Figure 10. Fractional GABA release from the nucleus accumbens. ** $p < 0.01$ vs. control, $n = 5$.

4. Discussion

Short kisspeptin analogs are promising candidates in the treatment of infertility and other gynecological conditions [48]. Kisspeptins exert their effect on the reproductive axis via Kiss1r [4], but they also bind to and activate NPFF1 and NPFF2 receptors with lower affinity [11]. In our study, we investigated the behavioral and biological effects of icv. Kp-8 in male rats via performing a battery of behavioral tests (EPM, OF, MB), determining serum corticosterone and LH levels, as well as measuring dopamine release from the VTA and NAc, and GABA release from the NAc.

The 0.1 µg dose of Kp-8 (but not the 1 µg dose) decreased the percentage of open arm entries and open arm time in the EPM, which is characteristic of anxiety-like behavior [51]. It is in accordance with our previous experiments in which a preference for closed arms has been observed following icv. treatment with Kp-13 [37]. Still, it must be noted that only a higher dose of Kp-13 has exerted an anxiogenic action, whereas in the case of Kp-8 an approximately 10-times lower dose was effective. The dose–response curve of Kp-8 shows a bell-shape (or inverted U-shape), that has been reported in several studies involving neuropeptides [56–58]. This phenomenon, when a lower dose is stimulatory, whereas a higher dose is inhibitory or ineffective, is called hormesis [59]. A review by Calabrese has reported a wide range of explanations for hormetic responses, including receptorial and intracellular mechanisms. For example, the same substance might have a stimulatory effect in a low dose, but an inhibitory effect in a high dose either via the same receptor (often mediated by a so-called 'molecular switch'), or via different receptors to which it has higher and lower affinity, respectively [60]. Based on a review on RF-amides and their receptors, kisspeptins in general can bind to their cognant receptor, Kiss1r, and to NPFF receptors with different affinity [3], the latter of which depends on the length of the peptide: the full length Kp (in rats Kp-52) has a lower affinity to NPFF receptors, whereas the shorter endogenous derivatives' binding affinity to NPFF receptors is higher. Furthermore, Rouméas et al. have performed systemic N-terminus deletions and benzoylations of Kp-10, which has revealed a progressive loss of affinity of the shorter fragments to Kiss1r and a conserved high affinity to NPFF receptors. In contrast, these shorter benzoylated fragments could still act as full agonists on Kiss1r, whereas on NPFF receptors a partial agonistic action has been observed [61]. How the benzoylation affects the affinity profile of these Kp-10 fragments is not known, yet it is possible that the unmodified Kp-8 also has an altered binding profile. In point of fact, agonists of NPFF1 and NPFF2 receptors have been implicated in anxiety [62,63]. Indeed, both Kiss1r and NPFF receptors could mediate the anxiety-like action of Kp-8, and we cannot rule out the possible activation of other receptors, as well.

Kp-8 also induced an elevation in serum corticosterone concentration: the 0.1 µg dose showed a tendency to increase it, whereas the 1 µg dose was significant. Corticosterone elevation is indicative of the activation of the HPA axis, the parvocellular neurons in the hypothalamic paraventricular nucleus (PVN) might have released CRH and AVP, followed by the secretion of ACTH from the pituitary, which consequently triggered the secretion of glucocorticoids from the adrenal cortex. In a study by Rao et al., Kp induced an increase in AVP mRNA expression in PVN derived cell lines [36], and thus it is possible that Kp-8 activated the axis by increasing AVP release. Moreover, the activity of the HPA axis is modulated by limbic brain regions, including the amygdala [64]—an expression site of both Kp and Kiss1r [65]—which stimulates the HPA axis and regulates the behavioral response to stress [64,66]. The increase in glucocorticoid signaling in itself is also associated with anxiety-like behavior [67]. This result ties well with our previous study in which icv. Kp-13 has also caused an elevation in corticosterone concentration in a higher dose [37].

However, in the first 5 min of computerized open field test, the animals treated with 1 µg of Kp-8 spent more time in the central zone of the arena, which is considered a sign of anxiolysis [68]. As there was no difference in central locomotor activity at any other time point, this result should be interpreted with caution. At the beginning of the OF, the animals are placed in the center of the arena, so it is possible that the increase in central time reflects an initial latency in approaching the periphery rather than a real anxiolytic effect.

In addition, it is not uncommon to have discrepancies between the EPM and OF results. For example, chlordiazepoxide has reduced anxiety-like behavior in the EPM, but has had no significant effect in the OF in Lewis rats [69]. Although the principles of OF and EPM are similar, the two tests seem to load on different factors of anxiety [70]. Moreover, the approach of open arms in the EPM and central locomotion in the OF seem to be independently inherited in rats [71].

Altogether Kp-8 seemed to increase anxiety-like behavior and activate the HPA axis. These results are in accordance with the anxiogenic effect of icv. Kp-13 in rats [37] and the anxiolysis observed in *Kiss1r* KO mice [38]. However, Kp has not influenced anxiety in rats in the study by Rao et al. [36], which might be attributed to the peripheral route of administration and the relatively low dose of Kp used in the experiment. Likewise, intravenous Kp has had no effect on anxiety in human subjects [32]. Apart from the route of administration, another important factor to consider is the species: the Kp system of zebrafish greatly differs from that of mammals, which might explain the anxiolytic property of kisspeptin observed in the study of Ogawa et al. [39]. Moreover, when compared to a systemic treatment, the regional modulation of neuronal activity can have strikingly different consequences. For example, the selective activation of kisspeptin neurons in the medial posterodorsal amygdala has decreased anxiety [40].

The number of total arm entries in the EPM reflects the general locomotor activity of the animals [72]. Both the 0.1 and 1 μg doses of Kp-8 reduced the number of arm entries, suggesting that Kp-8 might cause hypolocomotion.

The 60-min OF also yielded some remarkable results. When placed in a novel environment, all groups exhibited a pronounced exploratory activity with intense ambulation and a high number of rearings. Following a gradual decline until approximately 30 min, activity returned to a basal level. From that point, differences have started to appear among the groups, as there was a decrease in ambulation and rearing activity, as well as an increase in immobility in the group treated with 1 μg of Kp-8. These results point to a decrease in spontaneous locomotion.

Kp-8 has also significantly reduced the number and time of goal-oriented interaction with marbles in the MB. Although MB has long been considered a test for anxiety-like behavior, now several authors have expressed doubts about it [73]. According to Thomas, the number of buried marbles does not correlate with other anxiety-like traits, namely central time in the open field test and light-dark transitions in the light-dark box test [74]. The utility of the test as a screening tool for anxiety has also been questioned based on the findings that most anxiolytics and antidepressant drugs reduce marble burying behavior secondary to drug-induced hypolocomotion [73]. It has been suggested that digging and burying are species-specific, innate behavioral patterns that are likely triggered by an exploratory drive [75] or by the bedding itself [76]. Nowadays marble burying is regarded as a sign of repetitive, compulsive-like behavior, which is highly dependent on general locomotor activity [52]. Consequently, the reduction in goal-oriented interactions with the marbles is most likely a sign of suppressed locomotion in our study.

These findings contrast with the results reported by our group on the effects of icv. Kp-13, as it has increased exploratory and spontaneous locomotion in rats [37]. In a study by Tolson et al., *Kiss1r* KO female mice have exhibited a decrease in spontaneous locomotion and energy expenditure, but the mutation has had no such effect in male animals [43], pointing to a possibly gender-dependent effect.

Icv. Kp-8 has stimulated LH release in our study, which is a sign of reproductive axis activation, secondary to Kiss1R binding and activation in the hypothalamus. Kiss1R is expressed on hypothalamic GnRH neurons [4], and upon its activation repetitive LH pulses are generated [77]. In our study, the 1 μg dose of Kp-8 caused a significant increase in LH concentration. This is in accordance with literature data as icv. injection of a similar dose of Kp-10 has exerted an LH surge [41]. It must be noted though, that 0.1 μg of Kp-8 did not affect LH release. This is not surprising since Thomson et al. have obtained a similar result when Kp-10 was administered icv in a similarly low dose [41]. Furthermore, in a study by Pheng et al., icv. administered Kp-10 at a similarly low dose was unable to stimulate LH release in male rats, only the full length Kp-52 did. The authors have postulated that slower degradation of Kp-52 might explain their results, but it is also possible that the different binding profiles of Kp-52 and Kp-10 are in the background [78]. This also might explain our result, since Kp-8 similarly to Kp-10 might bind with higher affinity to the NPFF receptors, more specifically to NPFF1 receptor. One of the ligands of NPFF1 receptor is the RF-amide-related peptide 3 (RFRP-3), which has an inhibitory effect on the reproductive axis in adult male rats [79,80]. Thus, it is possible that at a lower dose, the two opposing actions of Kp-8 result in no change in LH concentration. Nevertheless, further studies are required to determine the affinity of Kp-8 to its receptors and the degree of calcium mobilization upon receptor activation. As the hypolocomotor effect of Kp-8 seems to be in contrast with previous studies on kisspeptin and locomotion [37,43], it is likely that this effect is mediated by other mechanisms.

One possible explanation is the activation of NPFF receptors. Kp-8 has activated human NPFF2 receptors in *Xenopus* oocytes [81], and its N-terminally benzoylated form has shown to fully preserve the affinity of Kp-10 to NPFF1 and NPFF2 receptors [61], which are universally activated by all members of the RF-amide family [3].

It is noteworthy that several members of the RF-amide family have been reported to modulate locomotor activity, pointing to the possible role of NPFF receptors in the regulation of locomotion. Similarly to Kp-8, icv. treatment with RF-amide related peptide 1 (RFRP-1) has reduced total locomotor activity and has also induced anxiety-like behavior and HPA axis activation [63]. Likewise, intra-VTA injection of NPFF has reduced spontaneous locomotion in rats [82]. Interestingly, icv. NPFF has inhibited morphine-induced hyperlocomotion, but has failed to affect the locomotor activity of naïve rats [83]. Although icv. neuropeptide AF (NPAF) has also had an anxiogenic effect, contrary to RFRP-1 and NPFF, it has stimulated spontaneous and exploratory locomotion [56].

Another possible reason for the development of hypolocomotion is the modulation of the mesocorticolimbic dopaminergic system. Based on the expression of kisspeptin in the NAc, as well as the expression of NPFF1 and NPFF2 receptors in the NAc and VTA [16,44], it was reasonable to investigate whether Kp-8 has a direct effect on the VTA-NAc circuitry. The dopaminergic pathway connecting the VTA and NAc has long been implicated in the regulation of locomotion. As a matter of fact, VTA dopaminergic neurons are responsible for the locomotor-enhancing effect of cocaine [84]. Our hypothesis was that Kp-8 might suppress locomotion by directly modulating the activity of VTA dopaminergic neurons. However, in our ex vivo superfusion study, Kp-8 has not affected dopamine release from slices obtained from the VTA and NAc.

As the interaction between Kp and GABA is known from the literature [85,86], it also seemed possible that Kp-8 might directly affect GABA release in NAc. GABAergic neurons in the NAc have been shown to inhibit dopaminergic projections from the VTA [87]. In fact, GABAergic activity can also be connected with the suppression of locomotion, as locomotor activity has increased when $GABA_A$ receptor antagonists were injected into the NAc core [16]. In our study, Kp-8 significantly increased GABA release from NAc slices. This result suggests that Kp-8 might directly modulate the activity of GABAergic neurons in NAc, which could contribute to the suppression of locomotor activity. It must be mentioned, however, that ex vivo superfusion measures only the direct effect of Kp-8 on live tissue slices obtained from the NAc, but the complex assessment of the whole VTA-NAc circuitry is beyond the scope of this method. Consequently, further studies (e.g., in vivo microdialysis) are required to confirm these findings on the circuit level.

When considering the receptors involved, it is possible that Kp-8 alters GABA release via NPFF1 or NPFF2 receptors, which are abundantly expressed in the VTA and the NAc, and likely involved in the modulation of both dopaminergic and GABAergic neuronal activity [16]. The role of NPFF receptors is further supported by the results of Cador et al., who have reported a decrease in novelty-induced locomotion upon intra-VTA NPFF treatment. Kiss1r expression, however, has only been detected in the NAc of humans, but not in rodents [88], so it is unlikely that Kp-8 could modulate NAc activity via Kiss1r.

Furthermore, the contribution of altered metabolism and thermoregulation should not be ruled out in the background of altered locomotor activity. Kisspeptin's stimulatory effect on locomotion seemed to be coupled with metabolic effects in the literature. Icv. Kp-13 has induced hyperthermia [37], and *Kiss1r* KO has resulted in obesity, increased adiposity and impaired glucose tolerance in female mice [43]. Kp could also be involved in hypothalamic appetite regulation by exciting proopiomelanocortin (POMC) neurons and inhibiting neuropeptide Y/Agouti-related peptide (NPY/AgRP) neurons, resulting in an anorexigenic effect [89]. Although only a few studies have addressed the metabolic effects of other RF-amides, they have usually revealed significant results. Icv. NPFF has reduced food intake in food-deprived rats [90] and also had a hypothermic effect in mice [91]. Moreover, the stimulation of central NPFF1 and NPFF2 receptors have evoked hypothermia and hyperthermia, respectively [92].

Alternatively, Kp-8 might modulate the activity of other, locomotion-related systems differently than the naturally occurring kisspeptins, resulting in an opposing effect of locomotion. For example, central Kp-10 treatment has stimulated vasopressin release in rats [93], and vasopressin has induced hyperlocomotion by acting on V1a receptors on hypothalamic orexin/hypocretin neurons in mice [94]. Furthermore, kisspeptin has been shown to induce BDNF expression in the hippocampus [95] and the lack of active BDNF in tissue plasminogen activator deficient mice has been associated with a decrease in nocturnal wheel running activity [96]. It is a question of future research to investigate whether Kp-8 could modulate vasopressin release and BDNF secretion in a similar or different fashion as other kisspeptins.

Author Contributions: Conceptualization, G.S., G.T., and K.C.; data curation, K.E.I. and K.C.; formal analysis, Z.B. (Zsolt Bagosi); funding acquisition, G.S.; investigation, K.E.I., É.B., and Z.B. (Zsolt Bozsó); methodology, É.B., Z.B. (Zsolt Bagosi), and Z.B. (Zsolt Bozsó); project administration, K.E.I.; resources, G.T.; supervision, G.S. and K.C.; visualization, K.E.I.; writing—original draft, K.E.I.; writing—review & editing, K.C. All authors have read and agreed to the published version of the manuscript.

Funding: This research was funded by the Hungarian Government and the European Union through the EFOP-3.6.2-16-2017-00006 grant.

Institutional Review Board Statement: The study was conducted according to the guidelines of the Declaration of Helsinki and approved by the University of Szeged Ethical Committee for the Protection of Animals in Research. Permission for the experiments (number: X./1207/2018, date: 6 July 2018.) has been granted by the Government Office of Csongrád County Directorate of Food Chain Safety and Animal Health.

Data Availability Statement: Data is contained within the article.

Acknowledgments: We thank Ágnes Pál, Gusztáv Kiss and Veronika Romhányi for the excellent technical support during the experiments.

Conflicts of Interest: The authors declare no conflict of interest.

Appendix A

Following solid-phase peptide synthesis, Kp-8 was analyzed using HPLC and ESI-MS, the results of which are shown in Figures A1 and A2, respectively.

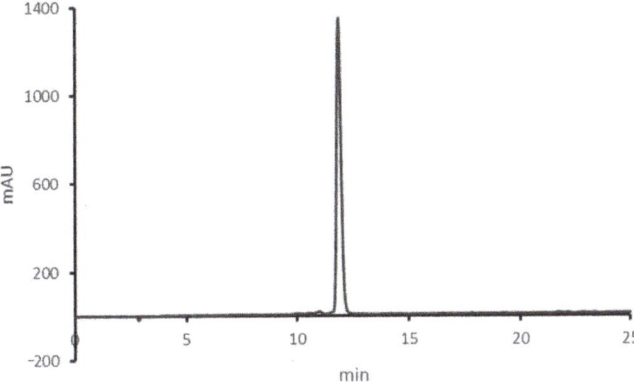

Figure A1. HPLC trace of Kisspeptin-8. Column: Phenomenex Luna C18, 5 µ, 100 Å, 4.6 mm × 250 mm, flow rate: 1 mL/min, wavelength: 220 nm, A eluent: 0.1% TFA in water, B eluent: 0.1% TFA/80% ACN/water, gradient: 30–55% eluent B in eluent A over 25 min.

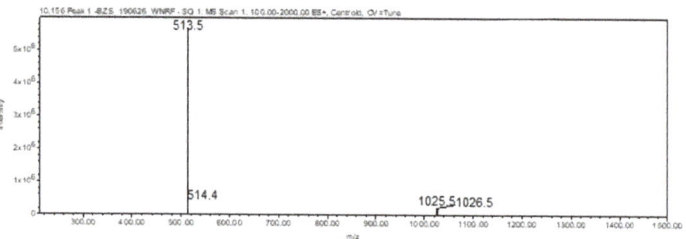

Figure A2. The ESI-MS trace of Kp-8 peptide.

Appendix B

During the computerized open field test, data were collected for 60 min, in 5-min timeframes. The cumulative results obtained after 60 min of data collection can be seen in Figure A3. There was no significant difference in any of the parameters measured: total distance of ambulation (Figure A3a, $F(2, 34) = 1.691$, $p = 0.1994$), total time of ambulation (Figure A3b, $F(2, 34) = 1.728$, $p = 0.1928$), time spent immobile (Figure A3c, $F(2, 34) = 1.274$, $p = 0.2927$), number of rearings (Figure A3d, $F(2, 34) = 1.522$, $p = 0.2328$), percentage of central ambulation distance (Figure A3e, $F(2, 34) = 0.6885$, $p = 0.5092$), and percentage of central ambulation time (Figure A3f, $F(2, 34) = 0.7265$, $p = 0.4910$).

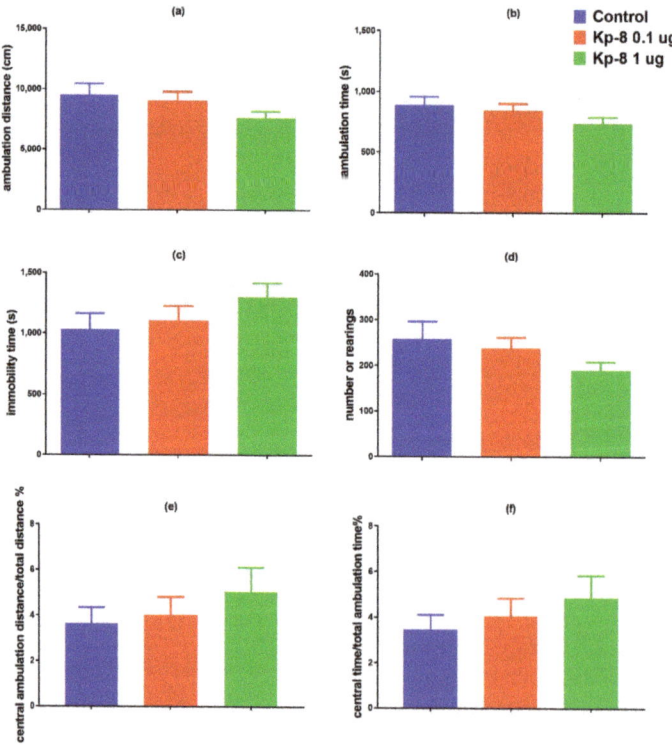

Figure A3. Cumulative data of 60-min open field test: (**a**) total distance of ambulation, (**b**) total time of ambulation, (**c**) total time spent immobile, (**d**) number of rearings, (**e**) percentage of distance travelled in the central zone, (**f**) percentage of time spent in the central zone, $n = 12$–13.

References

1. Lee, J.; Miele, M.E.; Hicks, D.J.; Karen, K.; Trent, J.; Weissman, B.; Welch, D.R. KiSS-1, a Novel Human Malignant Melanoma Metastasis-Suppressor Gene. *J. Natl. Cancer Inst.* **1996**, *88*, 1731–1737. [CrossRef] [PubMed]
2. Kotani, M.; Detheux, M.; Vandenbogaerde, A.; Communi, D.; Vanderwinden, J.M.; Le Poul, E.; Brézillon, S.; Tyldesley, R.; Suarez-Huerta, N.; Vandeput, F.; et al. The Metastasis Suppressor Gene KiSS-1 Encodes Kisspeptins, the Natural Ligands of the Orphan G Protein-coupled Receptor GPR54. *J. Biol. Chem.* **2001**, *276*, 34631–34636. [CrossRef] [PubMed]
3. Quillet, R.; Ayachi, S.; Bihel, F.; Elhabazi, K.; Ilien, B.; Simonin, F. RF-amide neuropeptides and their receptors in Mammals: Pharmacological properties, drug development and main physiological functions. *Pharmacol. Ther.* **2016**, *160*, 84–132. [CrossRef] [PubMed]
4. Franssen, D.; Tena-Sempere, M. The kisspeptin receptor: A key G-protein-coupled receptor in the control of the reproductive axis. *Best Pract. Res. Clin. Endocrinol. Metab.* **2018**, *32*, 107–123. [CrossRef]
5. Lee, D.K.; Nguyen, T.; O'Neill, G.P.; Cheng, R.; Liu, Y.; Howard, A.D.; Coulombe, N.; Tan, C.P.; Tang-Nguyen, A.-T.; George, S.R.; et al. Discovery of a receptor related to the galanin receptors. *FEBS Lett.* **1999**, *446*, 103–107. [CrossRef]
6. Ohtaki, T.; Shintani, Y.; Honda, S.I.; Matsumoto, H.; Hori, A.; Kanehashi, K.; Terao, Y.; Kumano, S.; Takatsu, Y.; Masuda, Y.; et al. Metastasis suppressor gene KiSS-1 encodes peptide ligand of a G-protein-coupled receptor. *Nature* **2001**, *411*, 613–617. [CrossRef]
7. Cargnello, M.; Roux, P.P. Activation and Function of the MAPKs and Their Substrates, the MAPK-Activated Protein Kinases. *Microbiol. Mol. Biol. Rev.* **2011**, *75*, 50–83. [CrossRef]
8. Peng, J.; Tang, M.; Zhang, B.P.; Zhang, P.; Zhong, T.; Zong, T.; Yang, B.; Kuang, H. Bin Kisspeptin stimulates progesterone secretion via the Erk1/2 mitogen-activated protein kinase signaling pathway in rat luteal cells. *Fertil. Steril.* **2013**, *99*, 1436–1443.e1. [CrossRef]
9. Taylor, J.; Pampillo, M.; Bhattacharya, M.; Babwah, A.V. Kisspeptin/KISS1R signaling potentiates extravillous trophoblast adhesion to type-I collagen in a PKC- and ERK1/2-dependent manner. *Mol. Reprod. Dev.* **2014**, *81*, 42–54. [CrossRef]
10. Bowe, J.E.; Chander, A.; Liu, B.; Persaud, S.J.; Jones, P.M. The permissive effects of glucose on receptor-operated potentiation of insulin secretion from mouse islets: A role for ERK1/2 activation and cytoskeletal remodelling. *Diabetologia* **2013**, *56*, 783–791. [CrossRef]
11. Oishi, S.; Misu, R.; Tomita, K.; Setsuda, S.; Masuda, R.; Ohno, H.; Ieda, N.; Tsukamura, H.; Inoue, N.; Hirasawa, A.; et al. Activation of Neuropeptide FF Receptors by Kisspeptin Receptor Ligands. *ACS Med. Chem. Lett.* **2010**, *2*, 53–57. [CrossRef] [PubMed]
12. Brailoiu, G.C.; Dun, S.L.; Ohsawa, M.; Yin, D.; Yang, J.; Jaw, K.C.; Brailoiu, E.; Dun, N.J. KiSS-1 expression and metastin-like immunoreactivity in the rat brain. *J. Comp. Neurol.* **2005**, *481*, 314–329. [CrossRef] [PubMed]
13. Overgaard, A.; Tena-Sempere, M.; Franceschini, I.; Desroziers, E.; Simonneaux, V.; Mikkelsen, J.D. Comparative analysis of kisspeptin-immunoreactivity reveals genuine differences in the hypothalamic Kiss1 systems between rats and mice. *Peptides* **2013**, *45*, 85–90. [CrossRef] [PubMed]
14. Higo, S.; Honda, S.; Iijima, N.; Ozawa, H. Mapping of Kisspeptin Receptor mRNA in the Whole Rat Brain and its Co-Localisation with Oxytocin in the Paraventricular Nucleus. *J. Neuroendocrinol.* **2016**, *28*, 1–8. [CrossRef]
15. Bonini, J.A.; Jones, K.A.; Adham, N.; Forray, C.; Artymyshyn, R.; Durkin, M.M.; Smith, K.E.; Tamm, J.A.; Boteju, L.W.; Lakhlani, P.P.; et al. Identification and characterization of two G protein-coupled receptors for neuropeptide FF. *J. Biol. Chem.* **2000**, *275*, 39324–39331. [CrossRef]
16. Wu, C.H.; Tao, P.L.; Huang, E.Y.K. Distribution of neuropeptide FF (NPFF) receptors in correlation with morphine-induced reward in the rat brain. *Peptides* **2010**, *31*, 1374–1382. [CrossRef]
17. Guzman, S.; Brackstone, M.; Radovick, S.; Babwah, A.V.; Bhattacharya, M.M. KISS1/KISS1R in Cancer: Friend or Foe? *Front. Endocrinol.* **2018**, *9*, 1–9. [CrossRef]
18. Seminara, S.B.; Messager, S.; Dixon, J.; Slaugenhaupt, S.A.; O'Rahilly, S.; Carlton, M.B.L.; Bo-Abbas, Y.; Schwinof, K.M.; Chatzidaki, E.E.; Gusella, J.F.; et al. The GPR54 Gene as a Regulator of Puberty. *N. Engl. J. Med.* **2003**, *349*, 1614–1627. [CrossRef]
19. Trevisan, C.M.; Montagna, E.; De Oliveira, R.; Christofolini, D.M.; Barbosa, C.P.; Crandall, K.A.; Bianco, B. Kisspeptin/GPR54 System: What Do We Know about Its Role in Human Reproduction? *Cell. Physiol. Biochem.* **2018**, *870*, 1259–1276. [CrossRef]
20. Putteeraj, M.; Soga, T.; Ubuka, T.; Parhar, I.S. A "timed" kiss is essential for reproduction: Lessons from mammalian studies. *Front. Endocrinol.* **2016**, *7*, 1–10. [CrossRef]
21. Pinilla, L.; Aguilar, E.; Dieguez, C.; Millar, R.P.; Tena-Sempere, M. Kisspeptins and Reproduction: Physiological Roles and Regulatory Mechanisms. *Physiol. Rev.* **2012**, *92*, 1235–1316. [CrossRef] [PubMed]
22. Manfredi-Lozano, M.; Roa, J.; Tena-Sempere, M. Connecting metabolism and gonadal function: Novel central neuropeptide pathways involved in the metabolic control of puberty and fertility. *Front. Neuroendocrinol.* **2018**, *48*, 37–49. [CrossRef] [PubMed]
23. Watanabe, Y.; Ikegami, K.; Ishigaki, R.; Ieda, N.; Uenoyama, Y.; Maeda, K.I.; Tsukamura, H.; Inoue, N. Enhancement of the luteinising hormone surge by male olfactory signals is associated with anteroventral periventricular Kiss1 cell activation in female rats. *J. Neuroendocrinol.* **2017**, *29*, 1–9. [CrossRef] [PubMed]
24. Yeo, S.H.; Colledge, W.H. The role of Kiss1 neurons as integrators of endocrine, metabolic, and environmental factors in the hypothalamic-pituitary-gonadal axis. *Front. Endocrinol.* **2018**, *9*, 188. [CrossRef] [PubMed]
25. Padilla, S.L.; Perez, J.G.; Ben-hamo, M.; Bussi, I.L.; Palmiter, R.D.; Iglesia, H.O. De Kisspeptin Neurons in the Arcuate Nucleus of the Hypothalamus Orchestrate Circadian Rhythms and Metabolism. *Curr. Biol.* **2019**, *29*, 592–604.e4. [CrossRef]

26. Ayachi, S.; Simonin, F. Involvement of Mammalian RF-Amide Peptides and Their Receptors in the Modulation of Nociception in Rodents. *Front. Endocrinol.* **2014**, *5*, 158. [CrossRef]
27. Elhabazi, K.; Humbert, J.P.; Bertin, I.; Schmitt, M.; Bihel, F.; Bourguignon, J.J.; Bucher, B.; Becker, J.A.J.; Sorg, T.; Meziane, H.; et al. Endogenous mammalian RF-amide peptides, including PrRP, kisspeptin and 26RFa, modulate nociception and morphine analgesia via NPFF receptors. *Neuropharmacology* **2013**, *75*, 164–171. [CrossRef]
28. Csabafi, K.; Bagosi, Z.; Dobó, É.; Szakács, J.; Telegdy, G.; Szabó, G. Kisspeptin modulates pain sensitivity of CFLP mice. *Peptides* **2018**, *105*, 21–27. [CrossRef]
29. Clarkson, J.; d'Anglemont de Tassigny, X.; Colledge, W.H.; Caraty, A.; Herbison, A.E. Distribution of kisspeptin neurones in the adult female mouse brain. *J. Neuroendocrinol.* **2009**, *21*, 673–682. [CrossRef]
30. Herbison, A.E.; De Tassigny, X.D.A.; Doran, J.; Colledge, W.H. Distribution and postnatal development of Gpr54 gene expression in mouse brain and gonadotropin-releasing hormone neurons. *Endocrinology* **2010**, *151*, 312–321. [CrossRef]
31. Tanaka, M.; Csabafi, K.; Telegdy, G. Neurotransmissions of antidepressant-like effects of kisspeptin-13. *Regul. Pept.* **2013**, *180*, 1–4. [CrossRef] [PubMed]
32. Comninos, A.N.; Wall, M.B.; Demetriou, L.; Thomas, S.A.; Wilson, S.R.; Jayasena, C.N.; Bloom, S.R.; Bassett, P.; Hönigsperger, C.; Mehta, A.; et al. Kisspeptin modulates sexual and emotional brain processing in humans. *J. Clin. Investig.* **2017**, *127*, 709–719. [CrossRef] [PubMed]
33. Bakker, J.; Pierman, S.; González-Martínez, D. Effects of aromatase mutation (ArKO) on the sexual differentiation of kisspeptin neuronal numbers and their activation by same versus opposite sex urinary pheromones. *Horm. Behav.* **2010**, *57*, 390–395. [CrossRef] [PubMed]
34. Hellier, V.; Brock, O.; Candlish, M.; Desroziers, E.; Aoki, M.; Mayer, C.; Piet, R.; Herbison, A.; Colledge, W.H.; Prévot, V.; et al. Female sexual behavior in mice is controlled by kisspeptin neurons. *Nat. Commun.* **2018**, *9*, 1–2. [CrossRef]
35. Kinsey-Jones, J.S.; Li, X.F.; Knox, A.M.I.; Wilkinson, E.S.; Zhu, X.L.; Chaudhary, A.A.; Milligan, S.R.; Lightman, S.L.; O'Byrne, K.T. Down-regulation of hypothalamic kisspeptin and its receptor, Kiss1r, mRNA expression is associated with stress-induced suppression of luteinising hormone secretion in the female rat. *J. Neuroendocrinol.* **2009**, *21*, 20–29. [CrossRef]
36. Rao, Y.S.; Mott, N.N.; Pak, T.R. Effects of kisspeptin on parameters of the HPA axis. *Endocrine* **2011**, *39*, 220–228. [CrossRef]
37. Csabafi, K.; Jászberényi, M.; Bagosi, Z.; Lipták, N.; Telegdy, G. Effects of kisspeptin-13 on the hypothalamic-pituitary-adrenal axis, thermoregulation, anxiety and locomotor activity in rats. *Behav. Brain Res.* **2013**, *241*, 56–61. [CrossRef]
38. Delmas, S.; Porteous, R.; Bergin, D.H.; Herbison, A.E. Altered aspects of anxiety-related behavior in kisspeptin receptor-deleted male mice. *Sci. Rep.* **2018**, *8*, 2–8. [CrossRef]
39. Ogawa, S.; Parhar, I.S. Biological significance of kisspeptin-Kiss 1 receptor signaling in the habenula of teleost species. *Front. Endocrinol.* **2018**, *9*, 1–8. [CrossRef]
40. Adekunbi, D.A.; Li, X.F.; Lass, G.; Shetty, K.; Adegoke, O.A.; Yeo, S.H.; Colledge, W.H.; Lightman, S.L.; O'Byrne, K.T. Kisspeptin neurones in the posterodorsal medial amygdala modulate sexual partner preference and anxiety in male mice. *J. Neuroendocrinol.* **2018**, *30*, 1–9. [CrossRef]
41. Thomson, E.L.; Patterson, M.; Murphy, K.G.; Smith, K.L.; Dhillo, W.S.; Todd, J.F.; Ghatei, M.A.; Bloom, S.R. Central and peripheral administration of kisspeptin-10 stimulates the hypothalamic-pituitary-gonadal axis. *J. Neuroendocrinol.* **2004**, *16*, 850–858. [CrossRef] [PubMed]
42. Ogawa, S.; Sivalingam, M.; Anthonysamy, R.; Parhar, I.S. Distribution of Kiss2 receptor in the brain and its localization in neuroendocrine cells in the zebrafish. *Cell Tissue Res.* **2020**, *379*, 349–372. [CrossRef] [PubMed]
43. Tolson, K.P.; Garcia, C.; Yen, S.; Simonds, S.; Stefanidis, A.; Lawrence, A.; Smith, J.T.; Kauffman, A.S. Impaired kisspeptin signaling decreases metabolism and promotes glucose intolerance and obesity. *J. Clin. Investig.* **2014**, *124*, 3075–3079. [CrossRef] [PubMed]
44. Desroziers, E.; Mikkelsen, J.; Simonneaux, V.; Keller, M.; Tillet, Y.; Caraty, A.; Franceschini, I. Mapping of kisspeptin fibres in the brain of the pro-oestrous rat. *J. Neuroendocrinol.* **2010**, *22*, 1101–1112. [CrossRef] [PubMed]
45. Mogenson, G.J.; Wu, M. Effects of administration of dopamine D2 agonist quinpirole on exploratory locomotion. *Brain Res.* **1991**, *551*, 216–220. [CrossRef]
46. Yael, D.; Tahary, O.; Gurovich, B.; Belelovsky, K.; Bar-Gad, I. Disinhibition of the nucleus accumbens leads to macro-scale hyperactivity consisting of micro-scale behavioral segments encoded by striatal activity. *J. Neurosci.* **2019**, *39*, 5897–5909. [CrossRef] [PubMed]
47. Boekhoudt, L.; Omrani, A.; Luijendijk, M.C.M.; Wolterink-Donselaar, I.G.; Wijbrans, E.C.; van der Plasse, G.; Adan, R.A.H. Chemogenetic activation of dopamine neurons in the ventral tegmental area, but not substantia nigra, induces hyperactivity in rats. *Eur. Neuropsychopharmacol.* **2016**, *26*, 1784–1793. [CrossRef]
48. Szeliga, A.; Podfigurna, A.; Bala, G.; Meczekalski, B. Kisspeptin and neurokinin B analogs use in gynecological endocrinology: Where do we stand? *J. Endocrinol. Investig.* **2020**, *43*, 555–561. [CrossRef]
49. Asami, T.; Nishizawa, N.; Ishibashi, Y.; Nishibori, K.; Nakayama, M.; Horikoshi, Y.; Matsumoto, S.I.; Yamaguchi, M.; Matsumoto, H.; Tarui, N.; et al. Serum stability of selected decapeptide agonists of KISS1R using pseudopeptides. *Bioorg. Med. Chem. Lett.* **2012**, *22*, 6391–6396. [CrossRef]
50. Rather, M.A.; Basha, S.H.; Bhat, I.A.; Sharma, N.; Nandanpawar, P.; Badhe, M.; Gireesh-Babu, P.; Chaudhari, A.; Sundaray, J.K.; Sharma, R. Characterization, molecular docking, dynamics simulation and metadynamics of kisspeptin receptor with kisspeptin. *Int. J. Biol. Macromol.* **2017**, *101*, 241–253. [CrossRef]

51. Walf, A.A.; Frye, C.A. The use of the elevated plus maze as an assay of anxiety-related behavior in rodents. *Nat. Protoc.* **2007**, *2*, 322–328. [CrossRef] [PubMed]
52. de Brouwer, G.; Wolmarans, D.W. Back to basics: A methodological perspective on marble-burying behavior as a screening test for psychiatric illness. *Behav. Process.* **2018**, *157*, 590–600. [CrossRef] [PubMed]
53. Schneider, T.; Popik, P. Attenuation of estrous cycle-dependent marble burying in female rats by acute treatment with progesterone and antidepressants. *Psychoneuroendocrinology* **2007**, *32*, 651–659. [CrossRef] [PubMed]
54. Heffner, T.G.; Hartman, J.A.; Seiden, L.S. A rapid method for the regional dissection of the rat brain. *Pharmacol. Biochem. Behav.* **1980**, *13*, 453–456. [CrossRef]
55. Salvatore, M.F.; Pruett, B.S.; Dempsey, C.; Fields, V. Comprehensive profiling of dopamine regulation in substantia nigra and ventral tegmental area. *J. Vis. Exp.* **2012**, 1–7. [CrossRef] [PubMed]
56. Jászberényi, M.; Bagosi, Z.; Thurzó, B.; Földesi, I.; Szabó, G.; Telegdy, G. Endocrine, behavioral and autonomic effects of neuropeptide AF. *Horm. Behav.* **2009**, *56*, 24–34. [CrossRef]
57. Kushikata, T.; Yoshida, H.; Kudo, M.; Salvadori, S.; Calo, G.; Hirota, K. The effects of neuropeptide S on general anesthesia in rats. *Anesth. Analg.* **2011**, *112*, 845–849. [CrossRef]
58. Gyires, K.; Zádori, Z.S. Brain neuropeptides in gastric mucosal protection. *Curr. Opin. Pharmacol.* **2014**, *19*, 24–30. [CrossRef]
59. Kastin, A.J.; Pan, W. Peptides and hormesis. *Crit. Rev. Toxicol.* **2008**, *38*, 629–631. [CrossRef]
60. Calabrese, E.J. Hormetic mechanisms. *Crit. Rev. Toxicol.* **2013**, *43*, 580–606. [CrossRef]
61. Rouméas, L.; Humbert, J.P.; Schneider, S.; Doebelin, C.; Bertin, I.; Schmitt, M.; Bourguignon, J.J.; Simonin, F.; Bihel, F. Effects of systematic N-terminus deletions and benzoylations of endogenous RF-amide peptides on NPFF1R, NPFF2R, GPR10, GPR54 and GPR103. *Peptides* **2015**, *71*, 156–161. [CrossRef] [PubMed]
62. Palotai, M.; Telegdy, G.; Tanaka, M.; Bagosi, Z.; Jászberényi, M. Neuropeptide AF induces anxiety-like and antidepressant-like behavior in mice. *Behav. Brain Res.* **2014**, *274*, 264–269. [CrossRef] [PubMed]
63. Kaewwongse, M.; Takayanagi, Y.; Onaka, T. Effects of RFamide-Related Peptide (RFRP)-1 and RFRP-3 on oxytocin release and anxiety-related behaviour in rats. *J. Neuroendocrinol.* **2011**, *23*, 20–27. [CrossRef]
64. Aguilera, G. The Hypothalamic–Pituitary–Adrenal Axis and Neuroendocrine Responses to Stress. In *Handbook of Neuroendocrinology*; Elsevier: London, UK, 2012; pp. 175–196.
65. Mills, E.G.A.; O'Byrne, K.T.; Comninos, A.N. The Roles of the Amygdala Kisspeptin System. *Semin. Reprod. Med.* **2019**, *37*, 64–70. [CrossRef] [PubMed]
66. Herman, J.P.; McKlveen, J.M.; Ghosal, S.; Kopp, B.; Wulsin, A.; Makinson, R.; Scheimann, J.; Myers, B. Regulation of the Hypothalamic-Pituitary-Adrenocortical Stress Response. In *Comprehensive Physiology*; John Wiley & Sons, Inc.: Hoboken, NJ, USA, 2016; Volume 6, pp. 603–621.
67. Packard, A.E.B.; Egan, A.E.; Ulrich-Lai, Y.M. HPA axis interactions with behavioral systems. *Compr. Physiol.* **2016**, *6*, 1897–1934. [CrossRef]
68. Seibenhener, M.L.; Wooten, M.C. Use of the Open Field Maze to measure locomotor and anxiety-like behavior in mice. *J. Vis. Exp.* **2015**, e52434. [CrossRef]
69. Vendruscolo, L.F.; Takahashi, R.N.; Brüske, G.R.; Ramos, A. Evaluation of the anxiolytic-like effect of NKP608, a NK1-receptor antagonist, in two rat strains that differ in anxiety-related behaviors. *Psychopharmacology* **2003**, *170*, 287–293. [CrossRef]
70. Ramos, A. Animal models of anxiety: Do I need multiple tests? *Trends Pharmacol. Sci.* **2008**, *29*, 493–498. [CrossRef]
71. Ramos, A.; Mellerin, Y.; Mormède, P.; Chaouloff, F. A genetic and multifactorial analysis of anxiety-related behaviours in Lewis and SHR intercrosses. *Behav. Brain Res.* **1998**, *96*, 195–205. [CrossRef]
72. File, S.E.; Lippa, A.S.; Beer, B.; Lippa, M.T. Animal Tests of Anxiety. In *Current Protocols in Pharmacology*; John Wiley & Sons, Inc.: Hoboken, NJ, USA, 2005; Volume 31, pp. 241–251.
73. Dixit, P.V.; Sahu, R.; Mishra, D.K. Marble-burying behavior test as a murine model of compulsive-like behavior. *J. Pharmacol. Toxicol. Methods* **2020**, *102*, 106676. [CrossRef]
74. Thomas, A.; Burant, A.; Bui, N.; Graham, D.; Yuva-Paylor, L.A.; Paylor, R. Marble burying reflects a repetitive and perseverative behavior more than novelty-induced anxiety. *Psychopharmacology* **2009**, *204*, 361–373. [CrossRef] [PubMed]
75. Londei, T.; Valentini, A.M.V.; Leone, V.G. Investigative burying by laboratory mice may involve non-functional, compulsive, behaviour. *Behav. Brain Res.* **1998**, *94*, 249–254. [CrossRef]
76. Gyertyán, I. Analysis of the marble burying response: Marbles serve to measure digging rather than evoke burying. *Behav. Pharmacol.* **1995**, *6*, 24–31.
77. Han, S.Y.; McLennan, T.; Czieselsky, K.; Herbison, A.E. Selective optogenetic activation of arcuate kisspeptin neurons generates pulsatile luteinizing hormone secretion. *Proc. Natl. Acad. Sci. USA* **2015**, *112*, 13109–13114. [CrossRef]
78. Pheng, V.; Uenoyama, Y.; Homma, T.; Inamoto, Y.; Takase, K.; Yoshizawa-Kumagaye, K.; Isaka, S.; Watanabe, T.X.; Ohkura, S.; Tomikawa, J.; et al. Potencies of centrally-or peripherally-injected full-length kisspeptin or its C-terminal decapeptide on LH release in intact male rats. *J. Reprod. Dev.* **2009**, *55*, 378–382. [CrossRef]
79. Pineda, R.; Garcia-Galiano, D.; Sanchez-Garrido, M.A.; Romero, M.; Ruiz-Pino, F.; Aguilar, E.; Dijcks, F.A.; Blomenröhr, M.; Pinilla, L.; Van Noort, P.I.; et al. Characterization of the inhibitory roles of RFRP3, the mammalian ortholog of GnIH, in the control of gonadotropin secretion in the rat: In vivo and in vitro studies. *Am. J. Physiol. Endocrinol. Metab.* **2010**, *299*, 9–12. [CrossRef]

80. Hu, K.L.; Chang, H.M.; Li, R.; Yu, Y.; Qiao, J. Regulation of LH secretion by RFRP-3—From the hypothalamus to the pituitary. *Front. Neuroendocrinol.* **2019**, *52*, 12–21. [CrossRef]
81. Lyubimov, Y.; Engstrom, M.; Wurster, S.; Savola, J.M.; Korpi, E.R.; Panula, P. Human kisspeptins activate neuropeptide FF2 receptor. *Neuroscience* **2010**, *170*, 117–122. [CrossRef]
82. Cador, M.; Marco, N.; Stinus, L.; Simonnet, G. Interaction between neuropeptide FF and opioids in the ventral tegmental area in the behavioral response to novelty. *Neuroscience* **2002**, *110*, 309–318. [CrossRef]
83. Kotlinska, J.; Pachuta, A.; Dylag, T.; Silberring, J. The role of neuropeptide FF (NPFF) in the expression of sensitization to hyperlocomotor effect of morphine and ethanol. *Neuropeptides* **2007**, *41*, 51–58. [CrossRef]
84. Runegaard, A.H.; Sørensen, A.T.; Fitzpatrick, C.M.; Jørgensen, S.H.; Petersen, A.V.; Hansen, N.W.; Weikop, P.; Andreasen, J.T.; Mikkelsen, J.D.; Perrier, J.F.; et al. Locomotor- and reward-enhancing effects of cocaine are differentially regulated by chemogenetic stimulation of Gi-signaling in dopaminergic neurons. *eNeuro* **2018**, *5*, e0345-17.2018. [CrossRef] [PubMed]
85. Pielecka-Fortuna, J.; Moenter, S.M. Kisspeptin increases γ-aminobutyric acidergic and glutamatergic transmission directly to gonadotropin-releasing hormone neurons in an estradiol-dependent manner. *Endocrinology* **2010**, *151*, 291–300. [CrossRef] [PubMed]
86. Di Giorgio, N.P.; Bizzozzero-Hiriart, M.; Libertun, C.; Lux-Lantos, V. Unraveling the connection between GABA and kisspeptin in the control of reproduction. *Reproduction* **2019**, *157*, R225–R233. [CrossRef] [PubMed]
87. Yang, H.; de Jong, J.W.; Tak, Y.; Peck, J.; Bateup, H.S.; Lammel, S. Nucleus Accumbens Subnuclei Regulate Motivated Behavior via Direct Inhibition and Disinhibition of VTA Dopamine Subpopulations. *Neuron* **2018**, *97*, 434–449.e4. [CrossRef] [PubMed]
88. Gottsch, M.L.; Cunningham, M.J.; Smith, J.T.; Popa, S.M.; Acohido, B.V.; Crowley, W.F.; Seminara, S.; Clifton, D.K.; Steiner, R.A. A role for kisspeptins in the regulation of gonadotropin secretion in the mouse. *Endocrinology* **2004**, *145*, 4073–4077. [CrossRef]
89. Rønnekleiv, O.K.; Qiu, J.; Kelly, M.J. Arcuate Kisspeptin Neurons Coordinate Reproductive Activities with Metabolism. *Semin. Reprod. Med.* **2019**, *37*, 131–140. [CrossRef] [PubMed]
90. Murase, T.; Arima, H.; Kondo, K.; Oiso, Y. Neuropeptide FF reduces food intake in rats. *Peptides* **1996**, *17*, 353–354. [CrossRef]
91. Desprat, C.; Zajac, J.M. Hypothermic effects of neuropeptide FF analogues in mice. *Pharmacol. Biochem. Behav.* **1997**, *58*, 559–563. [CrossRef]
92. Moulédous, L.; Barthas, F.; Zajac, J.M. Opposite control of body temperature by NPFF1 and NPFF2 receptors in mice. *Neuropeptides* **2010**, *44*, 453–456. [CrossRef]
93. Ten, S.C.; Gu, S.Y.; Niu, Y.F.; An, X.F.; Yan, M.; He, M. Central administration of kisspeptin-10 inhibits water and sodium excretion of anesthetized male rats and the involvement of arginine vasopressin. *Endocr. Res.* **2010**, *35*, 128–136. [CrossRef]
94. Tsunematsu, T.; Fu, L.-Y.; Yamanaka, A.; Ichiki, K.; Tanoue, A.; Sakurai, T.; van den Pol, A.N. Vasopressin Increases Locomotion through a V1a Receptor in Orexin/Hypocretin Neurons: Implications for Water Homeostasis. *J. Neurosci.* **2008**, *28*, 228–238. [CrossRef] [PubMed]
95. Arai, A.C.; Orwig, N. Factors that regulate KiSS1 gene expression in the hippocampus. *Brain Res.* **2008**, *1243*, 10–18. [CrossRef] [PubMed]
96. Krizo, J.A.; Moreland, L.E.; Rastogi, A.; Mou, X.; Prosser, R.A.; Mintz, E.M. Regulation of Locomotor activity in fed, fasted, and food-restricted mice lacking tissue-type plasminogen activator. *BMC Physiol.* **2018**, *18*, 2. [CrossRef] [PubMed]

MDPI
St. Alban-Anlage 66
4052 Basel
Switzerland
Tel. +41 61 683 77 34
Fax +41 61 302 89 18
www.mdpi.com

Biomedicines Editorial Office
E-mail: biomedicines@mdpi.com
www.mdpi.com/journal/biomedicines

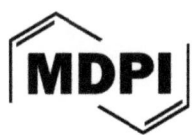

www.ingramcontent.com/pod-product-compliance
Lightning Source LLC
LaVergne TN
LVHW070500100526
838202LV00014B/1757